Palgrave Studies in International Relations

Series Editors
Knud Erik Jørgensen, Aarhus University, Aarhus, Denmark
J. Marshall Beier, Political Science, McMaster University, Milton, ON, Canada
Katrina Lee-Koo, Monash University, Melbourne, Australia

Palgrave Studies in International Relations provides scholars with the best theoretically-informed scholarship on the global issues of our time. The series includes cutting-edge monographs and edited collections which bridge schools of thought and cross the boundaries of conventional fields of study.

Knud Erik Jørgensen is Professor of International Relations at Aarhus University, Denmark, and at Yaşar University, Izmir, Turkey.

Daniel Serwer

Strengthening International Regimes

The Case of Radiation Protection

palgrave
macmillan

Daniel Serwer
School of Advanced International Studies
Johns Hopkins University
Washington, DC, USA

ISSN 2946-2673 ISSN 2946-2681 (electronic)
Palgrave Studies in International Relations
ISBN 978-3-031-53723-3 ISBN 978-3-031-53724-0 (eBook)
https://doi.org/10.1007/978-3-031-53724-0

Cover illustration: Piotr Krześlak/Alamy Stock Photo

This Palgrave Macmillan imprint is published by the registered company Springer Nature Switzerland AG
The registered company address is: Gewerbestrasse 11, 6330 Cham, Switzerland

Paper in this product is recyclable.

For our delightful grandchildren:
Drew Lilian, Hannah Beatrice, Caleb Lehman, and Ethan Isaac

Foreword

I encountered the International Commission on Radiological Protection (ICRP) more than 15 years ago when I was a Ph.D. student. While researching the fallout controversy, I quickly realized the vital importance of ICRP recommendations in all aspects of radiation protection around the world. However, scholars have rarely discussed the history of this nongovernmental expert body that has existed since 1928. My interest in the ICRP ceased to be merely academic in 2011, when a major earthquake and tsunami struck Japan, destroying the Fukushima Daiichi nuclear power plant. Seeing how frequently ICRP recommendations informed controversial decisions ranging from evacuation to compensation, my scholarly pursuit morphed into a personal quest to understand the enormously influential yet enigmatic organization.

It was at this pivotal moment that I discovered Dr. Daniel Serwer's 1976 dissertation on the formative years of radiation protection leading to the creation of ICRP and its partner institutions. It was like no other that I had ever read on the subject. Based on a judicious use of multilingual materials, the thesis offered a transatlantic perspective on the genesis of radiation protection prior to the atomic age. Moreover, it opened the black box of science for radiation protection, revealing its dynamic interactions with society at large. Written nearly half a century ago, Dr. Serwer's dissertation stands the test of time to date and is widely recognized as one of the foundational texts on the history of radiation protection. Deeply impressed by its unique and compelling insights, I sought his further work. To my chagrin, however, I could not find any related publications. I was mystified: where had he gone?

Little did I know that, after completing his Ph.D., Dr. Serwer ventured into the world of diplomacy. Throughout his distinguished career on the world stage, he emerged as a leading expert in conflict resolution and peacebuilding. His mediation efforts as special envoy to Bosnia and Herzegovina helped end the Bosnian War, and his leadership at the U.S. Institute of Peace shaped conflict prevention strategies in volatile regions from the Balkans to the Middle East. After many years of public service, he joined the Johns Hopkins School of Advanced International Studies, where he directed its highly successful Conflict Management Program.

I was surprised again when Dr. Serwer contacted me a few years ago with the exciting news about his return to the study of radiation protection. He envisioned much more than to bring his seminal dissertation up to date. His firsthand knowledge of international affairs, combined with his enduring concerns for peace and democracy, led him to revisit the subject with a fresh eye, as an unparalleled opportunity to study in granular detail the development of international norms over a century. The result is this truly multidisciplinary study reflective of Dr. Serwer's unique blend of scientific and diplomatic expertise. Theoretically rich and deeply researched, the book advances our understanding of epistemic communities as more diverse and dynamic than previous scholarship has suggested. Through his meticulous analysis of the interplay between science and society, Dr. Serwer also shows us the utmost importance of inclusive dialogue and mutual accommodation between stakeholders in a conflict for building robust norms. This masterful book stands as a landmark contribution to our understanding of how international norms emerge and evolve, offering invaluable lessons for the challenges of today and tomorrow in an ever-more complex world.

Washington, DC, USA Toshihiro Higuchi

Preface

This study bookends my professional life. I originally wrote on the history of radiation protection up to 1934 as a thesis with Thomas Kuhn at Princeton University's History of Science Program, for my doctorate in history in 1977. I was already then dividing my time between academic pursuits and international affairs, as I had spent most of the years 1970–1975 working at the United Nations, first on preparations for the 1972 Stockholm Conference on the Human Environment and later, courtesy of a Rockefeller Foundation fellowship, for the United Nations Environment Programme, to which the Conference had given birth.

I then worked on environmental issues associated with energy production and use at Brookhaven National Laboratory and joined the U.S. Foreign Service in 1977, focused initially on science and technology issues at the embassies in Rome and Brasilia and on energy issues at the State Department. I later served as Deputy Chief of Mission and Chargé d'affaires ad interim at the U.S. Embassy in Rome and as Special Envoy for the Bosnian Federation during and after the Bosnian war.

In 1998, I moved to the U.S. Institute of Peace to handle conflicts in the Balkans and the Middle East, and in 2010 to the Johns Hopkins School of Advanced International Studies to teach conflict management and do research, producing two books on war and peace issues. I am now Senior Fellow at SAIS's Foreign Policy Institute, which has provided me the opportunity to complete the history of radiation protection up to the present, as a study of how some international norms develop from interactions between science and society.

I spent much of my time at the United Nations, in the Foreign Service, and at USIP trying to build, rebuild, extend, or sometimes undermine, regimes. I often observed that societal interaction with regimes is more important than legalities in determining their strength, which results from public preference, professional expertise, and social interaction rather than enforcement. I returned to radiation protection in order to understand how the regime that regulates it became strong and resilient, despite many controversies and lack of legal force. Its norms have permitted society to garner the benefits of radiation while controlling the risks. That, I hoped, might suggest ways to govern other knowledge-based enterprises.

Our contemporary rules-based regime is now at risk, at home and abroad. We made the mistake of thinking it was self-sustaining. We imagined it would attract and tame our own worst instincts as well as gain the respect of others. That has proved illusory. We need to do more to make norms habitual and universal. We also need to recognize the limits and uncertainties of knowledge. In a regime that lasts, norms cannot remain static while knowledge progresses. We need regimes that can adapt as well as guide. Properly understood, perfection is a process, not an outcome.

Washington, DC, USA — Daniel Serwer

Acknowledgments

So much time has passed since I initiated the research for this book that many of those who deserve thanks are gone. I remember them fondly. Princeton Professor Thomas Kuhn, my thesis supervisor, and Francesco Sella, who makes a cameo appearance in this book as Secretary to the UN Scientific Committee on the Effects of Atomic Radiation, merit credit for, respectively, permitting and suggesting that I deal with radiation protection. David Sowby, then Secretary of the International Commission on Radiation Protection, and Leonard Hamilton, Scientist at Brookhaven National Laboratory, encouraged the enterprise. They also make cameo appearances in this volume, as does Alexander Hollaender, who spent his career mainly at Oak Ridge National Laboratory and with whom I visited Moscow in 1974 to discuss the International Register of Potentially Toxic Chemicals.

In recent years, colleagues at the Johns Hopkins School of Advanced International Studies have been generous, kind, and helpful. Deans Vali Nasr, Eliot Cohen, Kent Calder, and James Steinberg provided intellectual freedom, a stimulating environment, and much-appreciated research funds (thanks for that also to Associate Dean Mark Bailey). The Foreign Policy Institute under Cinnamon Dornsife offered a haven and stimulating colleagues. The indefatigable library staff, especially Stephen Sears, hunted innumerable resources. Professors I. William Zartman, Terry Hopmann, Sinisa Vukovic, and Dan Markey offered encouragement and many helpful suggestions, including that I read up on "epistemic communities."

The current Scientific Secretary of the ICRP, Christopher Clement, and its Historian, Georgetown Professor Toshihiro Higuchi, kindly granted me interviews and provided access to the ICRP archives. Professor Higuchi read and commented on a draft of this book, helping me to explicate its implications and deepening its connections to relevant scholarly literature. Roy Gutman, a Pulitzer Prize journalist and fellow Haverford College alumnus, deserves special credit for ploughing through material that is nothing like the issues he usually writes about and helping me to make it more comprehensible and incisive. Geoffrey Kabat, my classmate at Haverford who enjoyed a career in epidemiology, has read and commented on issues of particular interest to those who worry about toxic chemicals. My older brother, Philip Serwer, a professor of biochemistry in the Health Sciences Center of the University of Texas at San Antonio, tried to keep me both scientifically accurate and comprehensible, as did my Haverford roommate Thomas Howe, M.D.

My sons, Jared and Adam, have kindly tolerated my passion for this work, which is dedicated to their fabulous children. As always, my wife of 55 years, Jacquelyn Days Serwer, has provided the essential encouragement, time, and goodwill I needed to sustain a major writing project.

I received time, library, and financial support from the Johns Hopkins School of Advanced International Studies. I have no competing financial or nonfinancial interests, only a great deal of enthusiasm for what the International Commission on Radiological Protection has accomplished and for the model it offers for controlling other knowledge-rich enterprises that pose risks while also offering benefits.

About This Book

Strengthening International Regimes: The Case of Radiation Protection Will

- Analyze the evolution of the regulatory regime that sets international radiation protection norms and assess the factors that have driven its decisions,
- Examine why states have respected this regulatory regime as authoritative despite its lack of formal legal authority,
- Elucidate how the international radiation protection regime has maintained its global international legitimacy and credibility,
- Suggest lessons that should be applied to other technologies with both risks and benefits.

Because international regulatory regimes are inherently fragile, it is important to understand in detail how a strong one was constructed, sustained for the better part of a century, and still operates effectively, despite dramatic challenges and a lack of legal authority.

Contents

About the Author

Daniel Serwer is Professor at the Johns Hopkins School of Advanced International Studies and Senior Fellow at its Foreign Policy Institute. He was previously Vice President at the U.S. Institute of Peace and taught at Georgetown and George Washington Universities. From 1977 to 98 he served in the U.S. Foreign Service, first as a Science Counselor in Rome and Brasilia and eventually as a Minister Counselor and Chargé d'affaires in Rome and war-time Special Envoy for the Bosnian Federation. He worked on environmental issues at the United Nations from 1970 to 74.

Serwer edited with David Smock *Facilitating Dialogue: USIP's Work in Conflict Zones* (2012) and has written two other books, *Righting the Balance: How You Can Help Protect America* (2013) and *From War to Peace in the Balkans, the Middle East, and Ukraine* (2019). He is married to Jacquelyn Days Serwer, formerly chief curator of the Corcoran and Smithsonian American Art Museums as well as the National Museum of African American History and Culture. Elder son Jared is Associate Principal Architect at Perkins and Will and married to Korynn Schooley, Vice President of Achieve Atlanta. Younger son Adam is a writer for the Atlantic and author of *The Cruelty Is the Point* and married to Lt. Col. Alicia Williams, a surgeon with the U.S. Army.

CHAPTER 1

Introduction

The U.S.-centered, post-World War II, rules-based world order is at risk. It consists of various international "regimes" defined as "sets of implicit or explicit principles, norms, rules, and decision-making procedures around which actor expectations converge in a given issue-area."[1] Such regimes are inherently regulatory. They aim at affecting behavior. China is posing a global economic, technological, and military challenge to the current world order. Russia, Iran, and North Korea are posing regional military challenges. Europe, once content with American hegemony, is talking about "sovereignty" and trying to pursue its own technological and economic path, even as it remains in an aging Atlantic Alliance that would likely be fraying but for Russia's invasion of Ukraine. Geopolitical and geoeconomic rivalries appear stronger than regimes based on norms, defined as measures "of appropriate behavior for actors with a given identity."[2] Some norms are self-enforcing: "everyone wants to play their part given the expectation that others will play theirs."[3] But in today's world

[1] Krasner SD. International Regimes. Ithaca, NY: Cornell University Press; 1983:2.

[2] Finnemore M, Sikkink K. International Norm Dynamics and Political Change. International Organization. 1998;52(4):887–917.

[3] Young HP. Genetic and Cultural Evolution of Cooperation. Cambridge: Peter Hammerstein; 2003. The Power of Norms:389–99.

D. Serwer, *Strengthening International Regimes*,
Palgrave Studies in International Relations,
https://doi.org/10.1007/978-3-031-53724-0_1

it sometimes appears that no one agrees on the appropriate behavior of anyone, or is willing to play their part or trusts that others will.

There is also a challenge ***within*** the United States, which has been a mainstay of the post-World War II regime. Most Americans do not know what the "rules-based world order" consists of, what role the United States plays in it, and even less how it might benefit them. Many question how this order was created, who runs it, and what difference it makes. The potency of these domestic doubts was apparent throughout the Trump Administration, which withdrew from international engagements in the rules-based order, including membership in the World Health Organization, the Paris Climate Change accord, pending trade agreements in both the Pacific and the Atlantic, the Iran nuclear deal, and arms control agreements with Russia. Doubts about the virtues of the rules-based order persist for some Americans, even if the Biden Administration has sought to reverse many of these decisions. The next election could renew the American withdrawal from the rules-based world order.

At the same time, trust in the statements of scientists—one potential basis for universal norms that support world order—has declined in the United States, even while rising in other countries.[4] Political polarization surrounding climate change as well as the COVID-19 pandemic upended some Americans' confidence in scientists and physicians and fostered widespread doubts about climate change as well as anti-vaccination and anti-masking campaigns. Experts, initially uncertain about how to respond to the epidemic, changed their views as it spread. Unproven remedies gained currency. Angry populist rhetoric was common. Unedited social media undermined traditional news sources and enabled the rapid spread of unreliable information. Respect for expertise and professionalism reached a nadir. The efficacy of masks, the wisdom of school closings, and the origins of the virus are still hotly debated. Climate change has generated similar phenomena: denial, distrust, and disrespect for expertise.

[4] Kennedy B, Tyson A, Funk C. Americans' Trust in Scientists, Other Groups Declines [Internet]. Pew Research Center Science & Society. 2022. Available from: https://www.pewresearch.org/science/2022/02/15/americans-trust-in-scientists-other-groups-declines/, accessed October 31, 2023; Wellcome Global Monitor 2020: Covid-19 [Internet]. Wellcome. Available from: https://wellcome.org/reports/wellcome-global-monitor-covid-19/2020, accessed October 31, 2023.

Questions about the rules-based world order are often answered with generalities concerning relatively weak, although treaty-based, international regimes such as the Law of the Sea or the UN Charter's prohibition on the threat or use of force. Likewise, doubts about scientific validity often lack rigorous answers. This book, by contrast, analyzes the history of a particularly strong, knowledge-based but value-laden regime that sets norms in a controversial area of human endeavor on a global basis. Since 1928, a nongovernmental committee of self-appointed physicists, biologists, physicians, engineers, and other professionals with no formal legal authority has produced universally respected (even if not always followed) recommendations to protect people from "ionizing" radiation (the kind produced by X-rays, radium, and other radioactive elements but not by cell phones). The norms recommended by the International Commission on Radiological Protection (ICRP) are the basis of laws, industry standards, and regulations worldwide. Despite frequent controversy and revisions, occasional tightening, and significant costs to those obligated to meet them, these international norms have continued to command respect in medicine, electricity generation, storage of radioactive waste, and fabrication of nuclear weapons as well as in industries that handle radioactive materials and in scientific research. Even the current wave of populist doubts about scientific expertise in the United States seems not to have undermined the dominance of the longstanding international regime for radiation protection, which has already survived the inter-war period, World War II, and two versions of the post-World War II liberal order.[5] Though nothing is guaranteed, it looks set to survive longer, despite the return of multilateral geopolitics and geoeconomics. Perhaps this almost century-long experience based on non-state actors can elucidate, better than weak state-based regimes, what makes an international regime strong.

The radiation protection regime today provides global governance in the sense of Chhotray and Stoker: "rules of collective decision-making…where there are a plurality of actors or organisations and where

[5] Ikenberry GJ. Liberal Internationalism 3.0: America and the Dilemmas of Liberal World Order. Perspectives on Politics. 2009 Feb 12;7(1):71–87. The radiation protection regime is in practice hegemonic, in the sense that it is in practice universal, though I have preferred to use the term "dominant" to avoid the negative connotations of "hegemonic," see Koskenniemi M. Hegemonic Regimes. In: Young MA, editor. Regime Interaction in International Law. Cambridge: Cambridge University Press; 2012:305–24.

no formal control system can dictate the terms of the relationship between these actors and organisations."[6] The actors on radiation protection have included people who regard themselves as laboratory scientists and clinical physicians, specialists and generalists, professionals, and the lay public, in addition to governments, nongovernmental organizations, courts, corporations, and international organizations. Different people and institutions come to the issues ionizing radiation has posed with diverse perspectives and different knowledge. No one knows all that is required to reach rational conclusions. They have nevertheless managed to create a regime with universal legitimacy but no legal authority.

Assumptions and Perspectives

The process of decision-making in such a pluralistic world is an inherently conflictual practice that requires a good deal of social interaction as well as eventual compromise. States would eventually play roles in radiation protection, but the core of the norm-setting process even today lies outside governments. The material thus dictates what people who study international affairs label a "constructivist" approach in which identity and social relations produce shared meanings and values. We will have opportunities to delve deeply into the governance of radiation protection during almost 100 years and to trace the process by which it has produced changing outcomes, starting in particular countries and evolving eventually to span the globe. Some of the countries most active in this process—the United States, Germany, Britain, and France—were also among the most powerful in the world. The technology in question—beginning with X-rays and radium—was discovered and applied first there. But beyond that, little in this history will reflect state-centered realism. The Soviet Union, a great power after World War II, contributed little even though it used ionizing radiation extensively. Key contributions to

[6] Chhotary V, Stokes G. Governance Theory and Practice: A Cross-Disciplinary Approach. Basingstoke, Hampshire: Palgrave MacMillan; 2009;3. Others have noted that radiation protection is a subject of global governance, but with little understanding of its pre-Cold War history and the importance of the ICRP's norms, see Rentetzi, M. The Politics of Radiation Protection. N.T.M.; 2022;30:125–35. https://doi.org/10.1007/s00048-022-00332-z

radiation protection norms came during the Cold War from an Argentine and two Swedes, whose countries were marginal to the great power politics of the period.

Any study of this sort requires perspectives on modern science and its interactions with medicine, technology, and society. Medicine and technology are today often assumed to be endeavors rooted in a common body of scientific knowledge. By contrast, I view science and medicine as socially distinct institutions, the former housed mainly in laboratories and the latter mainly in clinics. While both are professions in the sense that they require specialized training, they draw on distinct bodies of knowledge, often apply different techniques, and utilize different criteria in coming to conclusions. Technology likewise has its own institutions and decision criteria: manufacturers, military institutions, and commercial enterprises have been involved from the beginning in the history of radiation protection and adoption of its norms. The scientific, medical, and technological communities are best distinguished not by the stated intentions of individuals, but rather by occupational roles, institutional affiliations, funding sources, and the means they use to convey information.

Different "methods of knowing" are dominant, though not exclusive, in these different communities. In the history of radiation protection, they correspond to those John Pickstone describes, though I was unaware of his work when writing this book. He uses the terms "natural history," "analysis," "experimentalism," and "technoscience."[7] What I label clinical case studies, reductionism, experiments, and applied science fit roughly into these categories, respectively. Radiation protection has employed all these ways of knowing. It originated in case studies in the clinic, has undergone several reductionist analyses as well as biological, physical, and epidemiological experiments, and has emerged today as an applied science. This trajectory has required that people who use these different methods communicate with each other and reach an agreement on their implications for formulating norms. That is a difficult and contentious

[7] Pickstone JV. Ways of Knowing: A New History of Science, Technology, and Medicine. Chicago: University of Chicago Press; 2000. I am indebted to Toshihiro Higuchi's reading of the draft manuscript for making this connection. Like Pickford, Thomas Kuhn influenced my thinking on the distinction between clinical case studies and the more mathematical tradition associated with the other methods.

process among people with distinct professional identities and criteria for reaching conclusions.

Within science and medicine there are distinct subdisciplines. In the case of ionizing radiation, the relevant science involves both biologists who study the effects of radiation as well as physicists who study how it is generated, its interactions with matter, and how to measure it. The relevant medicine and biology likewise involve different subdisciplines: radiologists, oncologists, geneticists, and epidemiologists, for example. The history of radiation protection entails a dizzying "interdisciplinary" array of interactions among these scholarly groups. Managing these interactions and reaching conclusions on norms to protect human health prompted the professionals involved to form what is known today as an interdisciplinary "epistemic community" of global experts, defined as a network of professionals with policy-relevant expertise in a particular area.[8] Not all expert groups constitute epistemic communities, which by definition share normative and causal beliefs, notions of validity, and a common policy enterprise.[9] Epistemic communities are not merely professional societies but policy-focused norm entrepreneurs.

The epistemic community associated with radiation protection was international from early on, initially involving professionals mainly from Europe and North America. It was from both the national and international levels of this international epistemic community that norms for measuring ionizing radiation as well as protecting people and eventually

[8] Or, if you prefer more rigor: "a network of professionals with recognized expertise and competence in a particular domain and an authoritative claim to policy-relevant knowledge within that domain or issue-area," Haas PM. Introduction: Epistemic Communities and International Policy Coordination. International Organization [Internet]. 1992;46(1):1–35. Available from: https://www.jstor.org/stable/2706951, accessed October 31, 2023. For a masterful update on epistemic community research in the subsequent 20 years, see Cross MKD. Rethinking Epistemic Communities Twenty Years Later. Review of International Studies [Internet]. 2012 Apr 11;39(1):137–60. Available from: https://www.cambridge.org/core/journals/review-of-international-studies/article/abs/rethinking-epistemic-communities-twenty-years-later/C7057E942EAFAED773470752746F8454, accessed November 1, 2023.

[9] Haas, Ibid. Secrecy and hierarchy militate against formation of epistemic communities, according to Cross MKD. The Limits of Epistemic Communities: EU Security Agencies. Politics and Governance. 2015 Mar 31;3(1):90–100. https://www.cogitatiopress.com/politicsandgovernance/article/view/78, accessed December 13, 2023. Neither of those factors was strong in the radiation protection community, except during World War II when it did not function as before or after.

the environment from its harmful biological effects emerged. Emanuel Adler and Peter M. Haas, writing in 1992, came to robust conclusions about epistemic communities[10]:

1. They can shape the preferences of nation states.
2. They can offer policy innovations and compromises otherwise hard to come by.
3. They can shape policy outcomes and persistence as well as norms and their diffusion.
4. They can order issues that might otherwise contribute to international anarchy.

This study of radiation protection will validate these conclusions but also go further. Much scholarly work on epistemic communities has focused on their relations with states while neglecting the technical details of their work and viewing them as coherent and harmonious. By contrast, the case of radiation protection will allow us to view the internal dynamics of an epistemic community of global experts, including its discussions of the scientific basis for tightening norms, as well as the expert community's interactions with the general public. This is possible due to the availability of large quantities of correspondence and other documentation. Social pressure, professional resistance to encroachment, institutional pluralism, and epistemic diversity will be central to the narrative.[11] That will enable the reader to see a much clearer picture of the motives, objectives, and modalities of norm formulation than is usually available. Specialists who pushed for norm tightening from within the community as well as competition from other professional organizations and public pressure have been driving forces. The history of radiation protection can also suggest ways that epistemic communities of international experts might contribute to resolving other issues, including some that are knowledge-rich but not technological in content.

With the notions of "scientific" medicine and "scientific" technology often comes the assumption that medical and technological decisions can

[10] Haas PM, Adler E. Knowledge, Power, and International Policy Coordination. International Organization, [Internet]. 1992;46(1):367–90. Available from: https://www.jstor.org/stable/2706960, accessed November 1, 2023.

[11] I am indebted to Toshihiro Higuchi's comments on a draft of this book for this formulation of its contributions.

be made on a "scientific" basis. But medical and technological decisions with social impacts, like those in this book, are often made under uncertain conditions, entailing controversial value judgments about risks and benefits. Many factors from beyond the science involved can therefore enter into consideration. Science, medicine, and technology as institutions are not insulated from the rest of society. Professional institutions and their members interact with social pressures, transmitted through personal contacts, lawsuits, protests, insurance companies, professional societies, government decisions, political pressures, legislation, the news media, and other mechanisms.[12] These pressures can affect not only the status and prerogatives of a profession or an epistemic community, but also its intellectual development, its self-protective mechanisms, its cohesion, its international connectedness, and its value judgments.

The public often looks to science, medicine, and technology for certainty and consequent authority. But these enterprises aim at discovery and improvement, which necessarily entails change and uncertainty. In any still-developing field in the twentieth and twenty-first centuries, the science, medicine, and technology of one decade may change profoundly from the previous one. Professionals may want the public to understand their enterprises and treat them with respect and even awe, but the public is often ill-equipped to comprehend the intricacies of professional enterprises, the uncertainties that lie within the range of their knowledge, and their changing understanding of the natural world. The result is often dread more than respect. Fear is a powerful motivation for public reaction, especially when it comes to "nuclear" questions.[13] Those most directly engaged with technology will often deny the validity and impact of public concern, preferring to portray themselves as relying on their specialized knowledge. But when professionals perceive a serious threat to their enterprise from a public that fears it, their epistemic communities may react by

[12] Other case studies that take a similar approach to the interactions between science, medicine, and society include Whorton JC. Before Silent Spring. Princeton, NJ: Princeton University; 1974; French RD. Antivivisection and Medical Science in Victorian Society. Princeton, NJ: Princeton University; 1975.

[13] For a survey of those fears, see Weart SR. The Rise of Nuclear Fear. Harvard University Press; 2012.

setting norms to protect both the enterprise and the public. Even without legal force, norms, when adopted widely, can solve daunting problems.[14]

The Science, Medicine, and Technology of Ionizing Radiation Evolved Rapidly

This study concerns the interactions among science, medicine, and technology within the social context of the United States, Europe (mainly Britain, France, Germany, Sweden, Switzerland, Austria, and the Soviet Union), and Japan through the two World Wars and one global Cold War of the twentieth century, up to the present. Only occasionally does the rest of the world appear on the screen. The professionals, publics, and governments of other countries were more norm-takers than norm-makers. The particular branches of science and medicine in question were both initially termed "radiology," which meant the study of the rays Röntgen discovered in 1895 and the radium the Curies discovered less than three years later. Together X-rays and radium opened a new chapter in the human relationship with nature. Products of science discovered in university laboratories, X-rays and radium were readily applied, especially in medicine. Despite their common denominator, however, the science and medicine of radiology were distinct from the start and for more than two decades thereafter. Comprised of physicists and chemists, the scientific radiological community came to include biologists as well. Their main institutional setting was the laboratory, usually associated with a university. Medical radiology began with applications of X-rays and radium for diagnostic and therapeutic purposes. The primary institutional setting for medical radiology was the clinic, sometimes private and sometimes attached to a hospital, university, or health spa.

The technology in question initially serviced mainly medical radiology, which required X-ray tubes, radium applicators, measuring instruments, protection devices, and a variety of auxiliary equipment. Scientists and

[14] At the individual level, see Nyborg K, Anderies JM, Dannenberg A, Lindahl T, Schill C, Schluter M, et al. Social Norms as Solutions. Science. 2016 Oct 6;354(6308):42–3, in economic life, see Young, note 3, and among states, see Thomas DC. The Helsinki Effect: International Norms, Human Rights, and the Demise of Communism. Princeton, NJ; Oxford: Princeton University Press; 2001. Even America's current polarized politics have not destroyed the popular consensus on human rights norms, Shattuck JHF, Raman S, Risse M. Holding Together: The Hijacking of Rights in America and How to Reclaim Them for Everyone. New York: The New Press; 2022.

physicians contributed to this clinical technology, but so did a diverse group of skilled craftspeople. Before the discovery of X-rays at the end of 1895, these artisans had been glassblowers, instrument makers, electricians, and mechanics. From 1896 onward, some became X-ray equipment manufacturers. Radium required laborious chemical techniques to separate it from the "pitchblende" ore in which it was found. Mining it and other minerals would pose risks that were not immediately recognized. Despite many claims to its "scientific" status, only during World War I did X-ray and radium technology begin to rely heavily on the science of radiology and on academically trained professionals from beyond medicine.

Once separated, radium could be readily used to make luminescent paint. This application proved important after World War I when nighttime flying became crucial to military aviation. The women who painted luminescent aircraft dials would pay a heavy price. So too did the miners who brought uranium out of the ground. During World War II, it was plutonium, created by bombardment of uranium with neutrons, that became a valuable military asset, along with uranium 239, a relatively rare isotope that had to be "enriched" from "natural" uranium (mainly uranium 238). Little known in nature, plutonium posed a greater health risk.

The scientific and medical personnel concerned with radiation protection during the World War II Manhattan Project acquired the appellation "health physics," which was possibly intended to hide its focus on radiation and radioactivity.[15] The corresponding military usage for radiation protection was "rad safe." Physicists and physicians worked closely together to protect the tens of thousands of workers potentially exposed to radiation throughout the Manhattan Project: from the demonstration of a chain reaction in Chicago in 1942 through the Trinity test of the first atomic bomb in 1945 to the nearly disastrous second test at Bikini Atoll in 1946. The collaboration between laboratory scientists and clinical physicians continued after the war when the fallout from atmospheric nuclear tests became a major international concern, leading to the Partial Test Ban Treaty in 1963 among the United States, the Soviet Union, and the United Kingdom.

[15] Hacker BC. The Dragon's Tail: Radiation Safety in the Manhattan Project, 1942–1946. Berkeley: University Of California Press; 1987.

Nuclear-generated electricity grew rapidly in the 1960s and 1970s. Government regulation became unavoidable but continued to rely on norms set by a nongovernmental, interdisciplinary, epistemic community. The United States today generates close to 20% of its electricity from 92 power plants that rely on controlled nuclear fission to generate the heat required to evaporate water and drive steam turbines to generate electricity. France relies on nuclear power for about 70% of its electricity requirements. Thirty countries use nuclear power and many more have reactors for research and production of radiopharmaceuticals. All still rely on the ICRP recommendations to limit the risks of ionizing radiation, despite the changed science, medicine, and technology involved.

The Health Effects Raised Public Concern

Early marveling at X-ray images and health claims for radium soon gave way to concern. In the early months of 1896, it became widely known that exposure to the X-ray tube caused human hair to fall out (epilation), reddened and inflamed skin (erythema), and could also cause more severe skin irritations (dermatitis). Both those responsible for applying radiation in the clinic and their patients suffered injuries. Today's controversies about the risks of nuclear reactors had their analogs more than 120 years ago, when newspaper editorials focused on the risks of exposure to X-rays and radium in medical use. Even today, medical irradiation on average contributes far more than routine reactor discharges and nuclear waste to the dose of ionizing radiation the average person receives from man-made sources.[16]

In 1902 and 1903, several less obvious effects were reported. X-rays and radium caused sterility in both males and females, changes in the blood and blood-forming organs, and cancer. In the two or three years before World War I, the effects on blood and blood-forming were found to lead to leukemia and to a sharp decline in red blood cells that was then termed "pernicious anemia" (not to be confused however with the autoimmune disease that term designates today). General recognition of these sometimes fatal consequences did not come until around 1920. Most of these biological effects were the results of exposure to X-rays

[16] World Health Organization. Ionizing Radiation and Health Effects [Internet]. www.who.int. 2023. Available from: https://www.who.int/news-room/fact-sheets/detail/ionizing-radiation-and-health-effects, accessed October 31, 2023.

and radium in medical use and among people working to improve the technology. They were discovered mainly in clinics, not laboratories.

In the 1920s, the health effects of radioactive materials in industry began to arouse concern. By 1930, public health officials had concluded that radium and mesothorium (a mixture of radium and actinium that results from the decay of thorium) caused inflammation of bone (osteitis) and bone sarcoma among radium dial painters. Lawsuits over the deaths of radium dial painters reached U.S. courts in the mid-1920s and stirred public concern for more than a decade thereafter. Radon, a gas produced by the radioactive decay of radium, was strongly suspected of causing lung cancer in arsenic and uranium miners exposed in the course of their work, though that aroused little public concern. A monument to X-ray and radium victims of all countries carried 169 names when it was dedicated in Hamburg in 1931. That number increased to over 400 after World War II. Many others remain anonymous.

Public controversy erupted again after the bombing of Hiroshima and Nagasaki in 1945 and in the 1950s over atmospheric testing of nuclear weapons and effects of radioactive fallout, including radiostrontium and radioiodine. Effects on children and genetic effects, for which it was believed there was no threshold, were particularly concerning until the 1963 Partial Test Ban Treaty. Thereafter, public concern focused on the risk of cancer from relatively low levels of radioactive effluent from nuclear power plants and the possibility of major nuclear reactor accidents. The accidents included damaged and lost nuclear weapons (aka Broken Arrows) as well as the three major ones at power stations in the United States (Three Mile Island, 1979), Soviet Union (Chernobyl, 1986), and Japan (Fukushima Daiichi, 2011).

Public Concern Generated Pressure for Protection

The discovery of the harmful effects of ionizing radiation generated a series of North American and European national and international institutions concerned with radiation protection during the first four decades of the twentieth century. Radiation protection recommendations first began appearing in the medical radiological literature around 1902. Before World War I, X-ray protection and X-ray measurement had become continuing concerns of the German Röntgen Society, which played a leadership role in this area as it did in medical radiology as a whole.

The Germans issued their first formal set of professional radiation protection guidelines in 1913, a precedent that the British Röntgen Society followed in 1915. Their purpose was to protect medical radiology from lawsuits and government regulation as well as patients and practitioners from biological effects.

After World War I, concern with radium as well as X-ray protection grew rapidly. While public criticism and lawsuits drove medical practitioners to adopt professional standards, uncertainty about how to measure doses raised questions that medical doctors were ill-prepared to answer. In 1925, the first International Congress of Radiology, a conference of mainly medical radiologists, created an International Commission on X-ray Units (ICRU) focused on how to measure radiation. In 1928, the second such Congress convened an International Commission on X-ray and Radium Protection. Physicists and physicians thereafter pursued an international consensus first on dose measurements and then on radiation protection measures. The two distinct "measures" remained linked thereafter.

By 1934, the Protection Commission had explicitly adopted a numerical "tolerance dose" as the basis for its X-ray protection recommendations, defined initially as the dose a person in normal health can tolerate. In most countries, the institutions concerned with radiation protection before World War II were still professional, not governmental. The scientific and medical radiological communities, not administrative or legal institutions, promulgated radiation protection recommendations, which I refer to as "norms" (reserving the term "standards" for legally enforceable obligations imposed by governments or formal international agreements). These professional institutions were reacting to threats from the broader society, conveyed primarily through courts, news media, and insurance companies. At critical junctures, professional perceptions of public reaction, combined with data on risks and pressure from professional specialists or encroachment from other institutions, would provide compelling motives for setting or tightening radiation protection norms.

After World War II, the Americans revived their own professional institution concerned with radiation measurement and protection (then the nongovernmental National Committee on Radiological Protection, now the Congressionally chartered National Council on Radiation Protection and Measurements, or NCRP in both cases) and also prompted the revival of the two pre-war international commissions (now the International

Commission on Radiological Units, or ICRU, and the ICRP). West Europeans and Canadians joined the international revivals. The United States was hegemonic in the immediate post-war period, in radiation protection as in many other things. In 1946, it created the civilian Atomic Energy Commission, heir to the military's Manhattan Project, with a mandate for both regulating atomic energy and promoting it. The AEC passed the responsibility for radiation protection to the Federal Radiation Council in 1959, which in turn passed it to the Environmental Protection Agency in 1970. Throughout Western Europe, as well as in Japan and the Soviet Union, governments had created comparable regulatory institutions. The United Nations created an intergovernmental Scientific Committee on the Effects of Atomic Radiation (UNSCEAR) in 1955 and the International Atomic Energy Agency (IAEA) in 1957. These governmental and intergovernmental institutions generally chose to use the ICRP recommendations as the basis for regulating radiation exposure.

Today, government authorities make the decisions on radiation standards that can be enforced legally. But more often than not, these decisions are the culmination of a process that has reached far beyond the officials formally responsible. That wider process relies on professional mechanisms and public pressures strikingly similar to those that existed before government institutions became involved. Governmental involvement has not removed decisions on complex medical and technical issues associated with radiation from the tug-and-pull of interactions among professionals, the public, and those who use ionizing radiation. The epistemic community associated with radiation protection is still essential in protecting not only the public but also the enterprises using radiation.

History of Science and International Relations Intersect

While often contested, sometimes breached, and focused as well as tightened over nearly a century, the ICRP's norms have stood the test of time and geography. They constitute a single, strong, science-based but value-laden regulatory regime accepted worldwide. This puts the ICRP at the intersection of important issues for two widely separate academic disciplines. One is the history of science, for which the impacts of science on society—and of society on science—have long been an important scholarly focus. The second is the field of international relations, which in recent decades has treated the formation, diffusion, and performance of international normative regimes as important subjects of study. These include non-binding, "soft" law, a category into which the ICRP's norms fit at the softest side of the spectrum, as they lack any legal authority. Using Edith Brown Weiss's categories, compliance is mainly the result of consensus on the underlying norms, though reputation and continuing relationships among epistemic community participants also contribute.[17]

This book aims to use radiation protection to probe key issues in both disciplines: how do science and medicine impact society? How does society impact science and medicine? When science and medicine create societal risks, how can an international normative regime be created to minimize them? What makes such a regime strong or weak? How do such regimes evolve, and why in some fields but not in others? Why did a global normative regime emerge for radiation but not for most chemicals or pharmaceuticals? Why do states accept norms that they do not themselves set? How and why does a regime gain universal international acceptance? How does a regime with no enforcement powers prevail in practice? What other technologies might benefit from the kind of norms that govern exposure to ionizing radiation? The final chapter will discuss the possibility of air pollution and toxic chemicals, ozone-depleting and climate change gases, and other hi-tech hazards, including nonionizing radiation, pharmaceuticals and medical devices, artificial intelligence, genome editing, and arms control. Might it even be possible to establish norms for non-technological risks like interstate war, currency manipulation, and trade?

The history of science regards science not only as the intellectual activity of lone researchers in isolated laboratories, but also as a social enterprise. Scientific ideas are developed, elaborated, and propagated within professional organizations and specific economic, political, social, and cultural contexts. This "external" perspective (in contrast to the "internal" one focused primarily on the evolution of scientific ideas) opens the history of science to the study of factors from outside science that may influence the scientific enterprise. Those factors can include not only ideas, but also finance, powerful elites, available technology, and historical events like war, revolution, recession, migration, empire-building, and

[17] Weiss EB. Conclusions: Understanding Compliance with Soft Law. In: Commitment and Compliance: The Role of Non-Binding Norms in the International Legal System. Oxford University Press; 2000.

other societal upheavals.[18] Tracing such influences from outside science on its intellectual and professional evolution is difficult. Scientific ideas have a life of their own, often one self-consciously well-insulated from societal events. A scientist's intellectual circle may be limited to a single person, or just a few.[19] Or cultural developments in the broader society may affect how scientists approach and solve problems, even if the mechanisms are obscure.[20] Radiation, unlike many scientific discoveries, had a quick and easily visible impact on society. The social reaction was likewise quick and visible. This strong, two-way interaction makes the study of the mechanisms of mutual influence far easier than in many other instances.

Radiation protection is also a good case for the study of international norms. The ICRP's history is now long, close to 100 years, far longer than many other contemporary international institutions. The radiation protection regime is also more widely accepted than many other normative regimes. There are sometimes multiple regimes covering different parts of the world, for example for the control of private security forces.[21] Some regimes are universal but with so many exceptions and so much surrounding "gray area" it is doubtful they still regulate behavior, like the prohibition on the use of military force.[22] A longstanding, universal regime in a controversial area of human endeavor is a relative rarity.

International relations scholars have investigated the existence and persistence of international regimes from contrasting perspectives for

[18] For example, Smith C. Wise MN. Energy and Empire: A Biographical Study of Lord Kelvin. Cambridge: Cambridge University Press; 1989.

[19] For example, Serwer D. Unmechanischer Zwang: Pauli, Heisenberg, and the Rejection of the Mechanical Atom, 1923–1925. Historical Studies in the Physical Sciences. 1977 Jan 1;8:189–256. https://doi.org/10.2307/27757371, accessed November 1, 2023.

[20] For example, Forman P. Weimar Culture, Causality, and Quantum Theory, 1918–1927: Adaptation by German Physicists and Mathematicians to a Hostile Intellectual Environment. Historical Studies in the Physical Sciences. 1971 Jan 1;3:1–115. https://doi.org/10.2307/27757315, accessed November 1, 2023.

[21] Boggero M. The Governance of Private Security. Springer; 2018. https://doi.org/10.1007/978-3-319-69593-8, accessed November 1, 2023.

[22] Kress C. On the Principle of Non-Use of Force in Current International Law [Internet]. Just Security. 2019. Available from: https://www.justsecurity.org/66372/on-the-principle-of-non-use-of-force-in-current-international-law/, accessed November 1, 2023.

decades.[23] Both realists and neoliberals see their origins in state power, but neither of those conceptual frameworks can account for the universal adoption of the ICRP's radiation protection standards. In the chaotic world of realism, a hegemon might impose standards on a lesser power, but there would be little reason for two powerful states to adopt a common set of norms, hence the struggle over 5G (fifth generation) telecommunication norms between China and the United States.[24] In the more cooperative neoliberal view, international norms are the product of state decisions to level the playing field based on mutual interests, thus allowing equitable competition. But states did not create the international regime for radiation protection, which does not regulate an international network. They adopted an already existing nongovernmental regime for reasons that included equitable competition but were not limited to it. The radiation protection regime is thus unlike the international regimes Zacher and Sutton analyze governing global networks like shipping, air transport, telecommunications, and postal services.[25]

The radiation norms are based on a self-selected and self-perpetuating epistemic community of physicists, physicians, engineers, biologists, and others whose recommendations states have chosen to use as the basis for regulating risk. Such "cognitivist" enterprises have generated a good deal of conceptual interest but detailed and careful analysis of the norm-creation process and what makes the norms they create resilient has been lacking.[26] How such communities form and evolve over decades, how they formulate and update norms, how the norms diffuse, and

[23] Hasenclever A, Mayer P, Rittberger V. Theories of International Regimes. Cambridge; New York: Cambridge University Press; 1997. For a comprehensive treatment of the intersection of international relations with science and technology, see Bueger C. From Expert Communities to Epistemic Arrangements: Situating Expertise in International Relations. In: Mayer M, Carpes M, Knoblich R, editor. The Global Politics of Science and Technology—Vol 1 Concepts from International Relations and Other Disciplines. Springer; 2014.

[24] Brake D, Bruer A. Mapping the International 5G Standards Landscape and How It Impacts U.S. Strategy and Policy [Internet]. https://www.itif.org/. 2021. Available from: https://itif.org/publications/2021/11/08/mapping-international-5g-standards-landscape-and-how-it-impacts-us-strategy.

[25] Zacher MW, Sutton BA. Governing Global Networks: International Regimes for Transportation and Communications. Cambridge: Cambridge University Press; 1995:i–vi. (Cambridge Studies in International Relations).

[26] Cross, note 8.

why states choose to adopt these norms are key questions to those who think international regimes are rooted at least partially in social relations rather than only in state power and national interests. Those matter for many purposes, but they are not the origin of the regime that governs protection from ionizing radiation. Social relations within an epistemic community, and its interactions with specialists, other professional institutions, and the broader public, are at the origins of the strong international regime for radiation protection.

These origins make the dissemination of international radiation protection norms a variant, albeit not a wildly divergent one, of the usual dissemination model, which posits a "life cycle" of norm emergence, norm cascade, and norm internalization.[27] In the case of radiation protection, the motives of those who originated the norms, the "norm entrepreneurs," are not the usual altruistic, empathetic, or ideational ones cited by Martha Finnemore but rather the preservation of professional economic activity. The "norm cascade" occurred mainly among professionals protecting the applications of radiation rather than among states. "Internalization" in state practice, "implementation," and "localization" are consequences of that professional norm cascade, not of legal obligation.[28] This makes the case of radiation protection distinct from that of many other environmental regimes, which are by contrast rooted in intergovernmental agreements. It has been demonstrated for such intergovernmental environmental regimes that non-state actors, including but not limited to scientific groups, contribute significantly to regime legitimacy by reducing uncertainties, improving compliance, and managing environmental problems, without diminishing the role of states.[29] In radiation protection, an epistemic community of global experts has contributed in addition to recommended norms that are the keystone of the regime states have adopted.

Even if it sometimes exhibits behavior that might be described colloquially as "clubby," the ICRP is not a "club" in the academic sense.[30]

[27] Finnemore, note 2.

[28] Betts A, Orchard P. Implementation and World Politics. OUP Oxford; 2014. On localization, see Schnyder M. Global Norms in Local Contexts. Springer; 2023, https://link.springer.com/book/10.1007/978-3-031-41108-3, accessed November 23, 2023.

[29] Breitmeier H. The Legitimacy of International Regimes. Routledge; 2016.

[30] Prakash A, Potoski M. The International Organization for Standardization as a Global Governor: A Club Theory Perspective. In: Avant DA, Finnemore M, Sell SK, editor.

Unlike the International Organization for Standardization, likewise a nongovernmental norm-setter, the Commission has no formal membership standards offering branding or other privileges to members beyond that of helping to set norms intended for universal adoption. The public goods the Commission produces are neither “excludable” nor “rival.” Anyone can take advantage of the norms without denying advantage to others. They entail large positive externalities. They allow even non-participating states to adopt norms without paying the associated production costs. They also ensure that beneficial radiation-producing activities are widely accepted within and between states, so long as the norms are observed. But membership in the Commission and its Subcommittees confers reputational advantages primarily to individuals, not to governments, firms, or associations. Observation of the norms the Commission sets is not a formal requirement for membership, though it is far more often than not the case. Unlike a club, the ICRP does little to monitor compliance, relying instead on its reputation, epistemic strength, and its own mostly professional version of the norm cascade.

Thus, if we ask with respect to radiation protection “who governs with what authority?” the answer lies in a nongovernmental organization with no formal delegation of authority. Professional specialists (including successively physicists, geneticists, and national radiation protection specialists) acting within the ICRP have played a particularly strong role throughout its almost 100-year history. Using the categorization of Avant, Finnemore, and Sell, the ICRP’s authority is rooted in professional expertise and the capacity of specialists to deal with complex issues, supplemented after World War II by implicit state delegation, as evidenced in government financing for the Commission.[31] Only occasionally will we see people in national authority positions, mainly in the United States, perceive reasons to deviate or contest the international norms. Neither utilitarianism nor the “logic of appropriateness” suggests that they do so most of the time.[32] Habit, duty, professional integrity,

Who Governs the Globe. Cambridge: Cambridge University Press; 2010:72–101. The ICRP resembles the International Electrotechnical Commission more than the International Organization for Standardization, though the ICRP in principle eschews “national” delegations, see Büthe T. The Power of Norms; The Norms of Power: Who Governs International Electrical and Electronic Technology. Ibid.:292–332.

[31] Ibid.:9–14.

[32] These factors are discussed in note 2.

economic efficiency, and personal safety often all point in the same direction. Conformity to the internationally agreed norms is then the rational outcome. They emerged from a more cooperative and less adversarial process than is usual in negotiating treaties or other "hard" law formalities and will thus confirm, as Abbott and Snidal suggest, that "soft legalization…is easier to achieve, provides strategies for dealing with uncertainty, infringes less on sovereignty, and facilitates compromise among differentiated actors."[33] These are great advantages in dealing with knowledge-rich issues, especially those in which the knowledge involved can be expected to change.

Internationalism as an ideology played little apparent role in the development of radiation protection norms, even if it motivated some individuals.[34] The proponents of radiation protection have held widely diverse views on the international issues of their times—from British chauvinist to German Fascist after World War I as well as Communist fellow traveler to Cold Warrior after World War II. But in their work on radiation protection, they regarded "politics" as anathema and governments as suspect. They believed that an elite group of professional experts would do a better job of setting norms than politicians or bureaucrats. They might occasionally appeal to the universal character of science in after-dinner speeches, and they were certainly convinced that valid scientific results were independent of geography, but their motives for international cooperation were more pragmatic than idealistic. Participating in international norm-setting gave the scientists and physicians involved purchase on national norms, and participating in national norm-setting gave them influence on international decisions.

The epistemic community of radiation protection experts aimed to dominate the pertinent norm-setting process globally and ensure that no competitive regime would arise. That concern made the proponents sensitive to competition from other professional organizations and to public

[33] Abbott KW, Snidal D. Hard and Soft Law in International Governance. International Organization. 2000;54(3):421–56.

[34] The ideologies available in the century under discussion have been many and varied, see Somsen GJ. A History of Universalism: Conceptions of the Internationally of Science from the Enlightenment to the Cold War. Minerva [Internet]. 2008;46(3):361–79. Available from: https://www.jstor.org/stable/41821469, accessed December 1, 2023; and Sluga G. Internationalism in the Age of Nationalism. Philadelphia: University of Pennsylvania Press; 2013. Project Muse, https://www.muse.jhu.edu/book/22233, accessed December 1, 2023.

pressure. Encroachment threatened dominance. The community has been willing to expand participation beyond its origins in Western Europe and North America but only slowly to individuals the existing participants deem technically qualified. The proponents of radiation protection initially conducted their proceedings behind closed doors and eschewed any explicit consideration of values, which necessarily entails the possibility of regional or national variations. But they eventually came to accept, acknowledge, and analyze inputs from stakeholders outside their professional circles, the ethical implications of their decisions, and the legitimacy of national adaptations of their recommended norms.

Sources

Many episodes in the history of radiation protection have been subjected to close examination, based on extensive primary source materials. The radium dial painters, who suffered terribly from ingesting an element that acts chemically like calcium and therefore deposits in bones, are the subject of a detailed case study of occupational health as well as a more recent and even more disturbing best-seller.[35] Nobel Prize winner Hermann Muller, who demonstrated that X-rays cause genetic mutation and played an important role in making that discovery relevant to radiation protection norms, is the subject of an excellent biography based on his archives.[36] *The Dragon's Tail* chronicles the role of radiation protection during the Manhattan Project.[37] If ever there was a moment when departure from the still relatively new international regime was possible and even justified, that might have been it. The urgent and top-secret Manhattan Project adopted, but did not always observe, international norms established before the war, though no one working on it had been involved in their development.

After War World II, the U.S. military tried to hide the worst radiation-induced impacts of the bombings of Hiroshima and Nagasaki, exposed

[35] Clark C. Radium Girls: Women and Industrial Health Reform, 1910–1935. Chapel Hill: University of North Carolina Press; 1997; and Moore K. The Radium Girls: The Dark Story of America's Shining Women. Turtleback Books; 2018.

[36] Carlson EA. Genes, Radiation, and Society: The Life and Work of H. J. Muller. Cornell University Press; 1981.

[37] Hacker, note 13.

U.S. soldiers, sailors, and private citizens, and downplayed the risks associated with fallout from atomic bomb tests. These issues have been well-documented.[38] The story of how radioactive fallout from atmospheric tests of atomic weapons generated momentum in favor of the Partial Test Ban Treaty has been admirably told.[39] Other fallout controversies have also been treated in depth.[40] The American military nuclear accidents of the post-war period, including at least six still missing atomic bombs, are no longer shrouded in secrecy, though the number of missing Soviet and Russian ones is still unknown.[41] The civilian nuclear accidents of the post-war period have all been documented.[42]

Up until World War II, this book relies mainly on primary sources, both in the scientific literature and in the few remaining unpublished documents held mainly by radiology-related institutions at the time the research was done in the mid-1970s. After World War II, the main primary sources come from three large collections: the ICRP archives, a voluminous collection with commentary by American physicist Lauriston Taylor,[43] and two of the four volumes by Swedish engineer Bo Lindell.[44] Taylor and Lindell both served on the ICRP Main Commission; Lindell

[38] Advisory Committee on Human Radiation Experiments, Final Report. October 1995. Superintendent of Documents, U.S. Government Printing Office.

[39] Higuchi T. Political Fallout. Stanford University Press; 2020.

[40] Hacker BC. Elements of Controversy: The Atomic Energy Commission and Radiation Safety in Nuclear Weapons Testing, 1947–1974. Berkeley: University Of California Press; 1994.

[41] The risks associated with nuclear weapons in peacetime, including the crash of a nuclear-armed US Air Force B-52 at Thule, Greenland in 1968, are discussed in Sagan S. Limits of Safety: The Limits of Safety: Organizations, Accidents, and Nuclear Weapons. Princeton University Press, 1995.

[42] Suciu P. The U.S. Military Is Missing Six Nuclear Weapons [Internet]. The National Interest. 2021. Available from: https://nationalinterest.org/blog/reboot/us-military-missing-six-nuclear-weapons-180032, accessed November 1, 2023; Union of Concerned Scientists. A Brief History of Nuclear Accidents Worldwide [Internet]. Union of Concerned Scientists. 2013. Available from: https://www.ucsusa.org/resources/brief-history-nuclear-accidents-worldwide, accessed November 1, 2023.

[43] Taylor L. Organization for Radiation Protection: The Operations of the ICRP and NCRP, 1928–1974. 1979. U.S. Department of Energy; DOE/TIC-10124, 1979. Taylor played a key role in both organizations as well as in the International Commission on Radiological Units for more than 45 years.

[44] Lindell B. The History of Radiation, Radioactivity, and Radiological Protection. Pandora's Box, Part I: The Time Before World War II. 1996. Atlantis. The Sword of

chaired it. The current ICRP Scientific Secretary, Christopher Clement, kindly approved access to the ICRP archives. Georgetown Professor Toshihiro Higuchi, the ICRP historian, generously provided guidance to the documents he has digitized. They are not yet ordered in a useful way, so consulting them requires scrolling through (many) tens of thousands of pages (blessedly online). Rolf Sievert, who preceded Lindell as the key Swede on the ICRP and served as its first chair, left voluminous papers that would have been valuable had they not been inexplicably destroyed at the Swedish National Archives.[45] I have not consulted the Taylor archives at Harvard, admirably exploited however in a Harvard doctoral dissertation, nor his interviews of early radiation workers at the American Institute of Physics.[46] Nor have I tried to decipher the Swedish material in the ICRP archives, which includes letters between Lindell and his mentor Sievert.

During and after World War II, high quality secondary sources are thankfully abundant. Barton C. Hacker and Samuel J. Walker have written indispensable volumes, the former with support from the U.S. Department of Energy and the latter the U.S. Nuclear Regulatory Commission.[47] James L. Nolan, Jr. has used his father's documents, dating from his medical service in the Manhattan Project, to document the moral

Damocles, Part II: the 1940s. 1999. Bo Lindell and Nordic Society for Radiation Protection. The Labours of Hercules, Part III (1950–1966). 2020. Bo Lindell and Nordic Society for Radiation Protection. The Toil of Sisyphus, Part IV (1967–1999+). 2020. Bo Lindell and Nordic Society for Radiation Protection. All available at https://nsfs.org/?page_id=1364, accessed November 1, 2023. Parts III and IV contain ample primary source material with commentary.

[45] Sisyphus, ibid.: 297.

[46] Lauriston Sale Taylor papers, 1904-1999 (inclusive), 1928-1989 (bulk). H MS c334. Harvard Medical Library, Francis A. Countway Library of Medicine, Boston, Mass. https://id.lib.harvard.edu/ead/med00144/catalog, accessed November 1, 2023. The Harvard archives has been deeply mined in Whittemore GF. The National Committee on Radiation Protection, 1928–1960: From Professional Guidelines to Government Regulation. Harvard University Ph.D. Dissertation, 1986.

[47] Hacker, note 15. Hacker BC. Elements of Controversy: The Atomic Energy Commission and Radiation Safety in Nuclear Weapons Testing, 1947–1974. Berkeley: University Of California Press; 1994. J. Samuel Walker. Permissible Dose. Berkeley: University of California Press; 2000.

dilemmas of that work.[48] I have had no reason to doubt their presentations of the historical facts, which are based on extensive primary source materials. But I offer my own interpretation of events when it comes to how radiation protection norms were set. Neither Hacker nor Walker shares my view of the importance of public pressure to the norm-tightening process. Nor do they emphasize the roles of specialists and fear of encroachment by other institutions that I emphasize here. The Final Report of the Advisory Committee on Human Radiation Experiments is likewise definitive on the facts. It would be pointless to try to reproduce its deep dive into primary sources.[49]

Methods and Objectives

This book will look to many at first sight like a single case study of a specific subject: international radiation protection norms. From that perspective, the "case" is a technology (ionizing radiation) that proved to have both serious risks and gigantic benefits. We can hope, and will show in the concluding chapter, that it illuminates how to handle other technologies with both risks and benefits. But looked at more closely, the history of the radiation protection regime appears to be a series of case studies, because the history provides changing circumstances, technologies, personalities, and institutions. In John Gerring's terms, the "units" are the radiation protection norms of a given time and place.[50] The places started with German and British professional institutions from 1900 to 1920, then moved in 1928 to the International Commission on X-ray and Radium Protection and its successor organization after World War II until the present. Each "unit" entailed a diachronic tightening of the norms, we will find in different degrees at different times to two main factors: scientific data and professional concern about limits or encroachment on professional prerogatives.

The potential limits or encroachment came from three sources: public concern, pressure from specialists near or within the profession, and the

[48] Nolan, JL Jr. Atomic Doctors: Conscience and Complicity at the Dawn of the Nuclear Age. Cambridge: Harvard University Press; 2020.

[49] Advisory Committee on Human Radiation Experiments, note 35.

[50] Gerring J. What Is a Case Study and What Is It Good for? The American Political Science Review [Internet]. 2004;98(2):341–54. Available from: https://www.jstor.org/stable/4145316, accessed November 1, 2023.

threat of encroachment by other professional organizations. We will trace in detail the causal process by which these four factors led to the occasional tightening of norms. None of these factors (including data, despite the claims of scientists involved) were sufficient on their own to cause the tightening of norms, but two or more together could do so. We will also find that the legitimacy of the international radiation protection regime has not depended on legal mandates, geographic diversity of the participants, or institutional authority (all of which were trailing indicators of legitimacy), but rather on epistemic dominance based on co-optation of norm-setting participants, supplemented in recent decades by openness to stakeholder input.

Throughout, I have tried to ask the same structured, focused questions and to provide nuanced answers reflecting the complexities of each phase of the narrative, in accordance with George and Bennett's methodology.[51] The basic questions include the following:

> What does it mean for medicine and technology to be "scientific"?
> Why do professionals set norms for themselves?
> How are decisions with social impacts made under conditions of scientific uncertainty?
> Why do professionals seek international cooperation on norms?
> Why and how do international institutions that set norms gain and sustain their legitimacy?
> What roles do various sorts of professionals and organizations play in controlling the risks arising from science, medicine, and technology?

The result is not a complete history of radiation dosimetry and protection, whether in individual countries or internationally. Both the national and international institutions involved developed elaborate substructures (committees, task forces, and more informal groups) to enable them not only to recommend basic radiation protection norms but also to

[51] George AL, Bennett A. Case Studies and Theory Development in the Social Sciences. Cambridge, Mass.; London: Mit; 2005:45–7.

translate them into practical procedures that could be applied in laboratories, clinics, industry, and emergencies. This effort raised a dizzying array of issues, both organizational and technical, most of which will have to await more comprehensive treatment. These include the implications of radiation exposure for supersonic transport, pregnant women, television watchers, wearers of luminous watches, shoe-fitting fluoroscopes, radiopharmaceuticals, patients undergoing diagnosis and therapy, homes built with radioactive material, handling and disposal of radioactive waste, accidental high-level exposure, as well as many other issues. They also include a host of technical concepts concerning relative biological effectiveness, critical organs, standard man, dose commitments, effective dose equivalent, dose rate effects, attenuation curves, annual limits on intake, maximum permissible concentrations in air, water, and food as well as other parameters that the ICRP had to develop in order for the basic radiation protection standards to be applied in real-world situations. A 1984 list of symbols used in ICRP publications ran to eleven pages.[52] A draft compilation of basic concepts ran to 35 pages.[53]

Nor does this volume cover the organization of the ICRP, its committees and task forces, its choice of specific members, its many meetings over almost a century, or most of the personal interactions among its members and with other institutions.[54] Sometimes cooperative and sometimes contentious work on the myriad of radiation protection issues is what made the scientists and physicians an epistemic community with a common but changing set of procedures for solving problems (what Thomas Kuhn called a "paradigm") that produced policy in the form of

[52] "Stockholm meeting 1984," ICRP Archives, Box W-18, Archive files 33, Secretariate-General Distr- Main Comm.pdf, 16–27.

[53] A Compilation of the Major Concepts and Quantities in Use by ICRP, March 1984, ICRP/84/MC-09, ICRP Archives, Archive Files, MC 1984-86 B.pdf, 37–72.

[54] Many of the organizational and policy issues omitted here are elucidated in Clarke RH, Valentin J. The History of ICRP and the Evolution of its Policies: Invited by the Commission in October 2008. Annals of the ICRP. 2009;39(1):75–110. Available from: https://doi.org/10.1016/j.icrp.2009.07.009, accessed November 1, 2023.

norms for radiation doses.[55] But only when personal and organizational issues impinge on the broader questions listed above do they enter this narrative. Likewise, I treat implementation at the national level mostly as a given and cite anecdotal evidence to that effect, until it is not. Then it is important to ask how implementation failure relates to the question of regime legitimacy. My attention to the contestation that sometimes contributed to norms and adjustments in them is not comprehensive. I treat it only where I can document a clear impact on the epistemic groups making the normative decisions, which happens far less frequently than the contestation.[56]

The focus here is on the evolution of the basic radiation protection norms and the international institutions that set them. A central element of the norms was originally termed the "tolerance dose" before World War II, but its intellectual descendants came to be known thereafter as "maximum permissible doses" or just "dose limits." Even among these, I have focused on the most basic norms for the protection of radiation workers and members of the general public. Looked at from the conflict management perspective, they function in the norm-setting process as "focal points" on which an epistemic group of global experts settles in particular circumstances, after discussion of various possible salient points.[57] After an initial three decades during which numerical limits were not set but medical practice unquestionably lowered exposures of both practitioners and patients, the dose limits were tightened (lowered) by about one order of magnitude between 1928 and 1990.[58] The actual doses to workers in the United States fell by far more. This is one expert illustration of the progression (Fig. 1.1):

[55] Kuhn T. The Structure of Scientific Revolutions. Chicago: University of Chicago Press; 1962.

[56] For examples of more comprehensive treatment, see Wiener A. Contestation and Constitution of Norms in Global International Relations. Cambridge: Cambridge University Press; 2018.

[57] Schuessler R, van der Rijt J-W. Focal Points in Negotiation. Palgrave MacMillan; 2019:45.

[58] Linet MS, Kim KP, Miller DL, Kleinerman RA, Simon S, de Gonzalez AB. Historical Review of Cancer Risks in Medical Radiation Workers. Radiation Research [Internet]. 2010 Dec 1;174(6):793–808. Available from: https://www.ncbi.nlm.nih.gov/pmc/articles/PMC4098897/, accessed November 1, 2023.

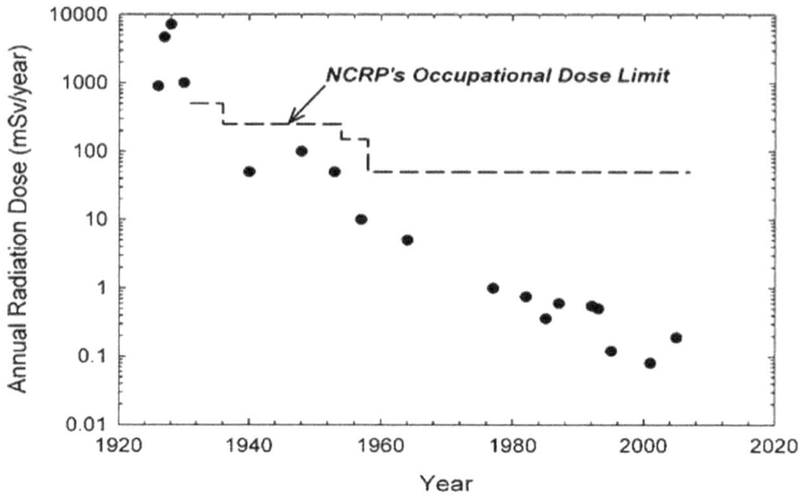

Fig. 1.1 Annual occupational radiation dose per year[59]

Other important norms—related to justifying the use of radiation and optimizing its risks and benefits—are also crucial to radiation protection and at least in part responsible for the drop in actual doses, but they were not formulated numerically and are therefore more difficult to trace through decades of adjustments.

The main changes in the international norms are documented in ICRP publications approved by the "Main Commission" that set forth its basic radiation protection rationale and norms. These include its recommendations adopted in 1928, 1934, 1950, 1953, 1956 (amendments), 1958 (now known as Publication 1), 1962 (Publication 6), 1965 (Publication 9), 1977 (Publication 26), 1990 (Publication 60), and 2007 (Publication

[59] Ibid., © 2023 Radiation Research Society, reproduced with permission.

103).[60] The post-World War II narrative presented here focuses mainly on the contributing factors to tightening decisions summarized in Table 1.1: New data or other scientific arguments, specialist pressure from within the radiation protection epistemic community, heightened public concern, and the threat or reality of institutional competition.

The ICRP is now planning for its next "Review and Revision of the System of Radiological Protection."[61] I detect no sign at present of the factors that have contributed to tightened permissible limits in the past, but they could of course emerge in what will likely be years before the next recommendations are adopted.

The basic radiation protection recommendations reflect only a fraction of the ICRP's work, which includes about 200 other publications, produced by committees and task forces with hundreds of members and now also subject to public input and comment. The ICRP also hosts dozens of meetings each year to disseminate its approach to radiation protection. But it remains a nongovernmental, self-selected body with no legal authority to enforce its recommendations, which are nevertheless used worldwide by governments and international organizations as the basis for standards incorporated in regulations and laws. There is still no formal governmental control over the ICRP, but its funding and the success of its recommendations depend on government agencies who also contribute personnel to ICRP activities.

Good or Bad?

Some readers will wonder if this history has provided the world with adequate protection from ionizing radiation. Should there have been more direct governmental control? Should the norms be tightened

[60] AICRP [Internet]. www.icrp.org. Available from: https://www.icrp.org/page.asp?id=5, accessed November 1, 2023.

[61] "ICRP Main Commission Meetings 15–17 September 2022 Rome, Italy & 5 November 2022 Vancouver, Canada," ICRP ref 4855-1037-4988 released January, 24, 2023, https://www.icrp.org/admin/Summary%20of%20Sept%20and%20Nov%202022%20Main%20Commission%20Meetings%20Rome%20and%20Vancouver.pdf, accessed November 1, 2023.

Table 1.1 Key decisions on tightening permissible limits and contributing factors

ICRP Recommendations	*New data or other scientific arguments*	*Specialist pressure*	*Heightened public concern*	*Institutional competition*	*Tightening of permissible limits?*
1950/1951[a]	Prewar Ra data and wartime experiments	Geneticists	Hiroshima/Nagasaki aftermath	No	Occupational: 0.2 r/day to 0.3 r/week
1953/1955[a]	Muller arguments	Geneticists	Testing/fallout	No	1/10 for general population
1956/1958[a]	Leukemia	Geneticists	Testing/fallout	NAS and UNSCEAR	Occupational: 0.3 r/week to 0.1 rem/week to the gonad plus generational limit
1958/1959[a] (Pub 1)	No	No	Testing/fallout	No	No
1962/1964[a] (Pub 6)	No	No	Testing/fallout	No	No
1965/1966[a] (Pub 9)	No	No	No	No	No
1977 (Pub 26)	Risk calculations	Gofman and Tamplin Beninson and Lindell	Nuclear power growth	NAS 1972	Public: language tightened towards 1 mSv/year
1990/1991[a] (Pub 60)	Risk calculations	Beninson and Lindell	TMI, Chernobyl, environmental activists	No	Occupational: 50 mSv to 20 mSv/year; public: 5 mSV to 1 mSv/year
2007 (Pub 103)	No	Roger Clarke	Attenuated	No	No

[a]The first date is the year in which the decision was made. The second is the date of publication

further? Should we have gotten to where we are now more quickly? These are legitimate questions, but definitive answers can only emerge in interactions between the relevant epistemic community and the public, then ultimately from government authorities. A historian can recount past decisions based on the often-uncertain information available and seek to explain why and how they were made. Take Lauriston Taylor as an example. His is perhaps the most frequent name cited in subsequent chapters. Readers will note that his preferences and expectations were repeatedly invalidated during (and after) his several decades-long tenure as a national and international leader on radiation protection issues. Others prevailed over his views that the public should not be protected more than radiation workers, that radiation protection norms should not be formalized in legislation, and that genetic effects should not be considered for the general public. But he changed his mind on these (and other) issues and also collected documents that enable us to understand the views he and others held and why. It would be a mistake to ask more than that in a retrospective analysis. He merits appreciation, not opprobrium, even if you disagree with his views (which I hope I would have done at the time).

I could have taken a different approach, faulting not only Taylor but many others for their failure to anticipate tightening of the radiation protection norms and the harm done in the meanwhile. I could have cherry-picked early warnings and blamed the X-ray equipment manufacturers, the Curies, physicians, bomb builders, and the nuclear industry for hesitation and delays. Certainly, each of these did at times resist radiation protection norms, which I have noted where it made a difference. Muckraking of this sort might have gained a wider audience, and it lends support to the early collection of epidemiological data, certainly a good idea.[62] But it would also have obscured the main point: an epistemic community of global experts took those concerns into account and enabled the use of radiation in many beneficial ways while preventing harm to many millions of people. Might it have been done faster and better? Surely the answer is yes, especially in the years before World War

[62] Lambert B. Radiation: Early Warnings; Late Effects. In: Harremoës P, editor. Late Lessons from Early Warnings: The Precautionary Principle 1896–2000 [Internet]. Environmental Issue Report No. 22. European Environmental Agency; 2001. Available from: https://www.eea.europa.eu/publications/environmental_issue_report_2001_22, accessed December 12, 2023.

I when there were no international norms. But it got done. I wish the same could be said for other risks of modern life, which are more often the subject of adversarial processes rather than cooperative regimes like the one for radiation protection. The radiation protection regime did not, however, get built only because of disinterested scientific inquiry or professional self-regulation, which many of the scientists and physicians involved might claim. Today's global regime for radiation protection owes its existence also to perceptions of public pressure, to specialist concern, and to fear of institutional competition.

While it has in recent decades followed the trend of opening up its norm-setting process to knowledgeable segments of the broader society, the ICRP and the epistemic community that surrounds it has remained remarkably resistant to isomorphic change, that is to the tendency of social institutions to grow to resemble each other. It is an early and remarkably resilient and effective example of what is now termed the "depoliticization" and "scientization" of global governance effected through an epistemic community that has sought to balance risks and benefits.[63] Governments and intergovernmental organizations have chosen to rely on the norms its experts recommend. This relative isolation from the give and take of politics has enabled the use of a particularly risky but highly beneficial technology.

Chapter Outline

We start in Chapter 2 where "radiology" began: with the discovery of X-rays in late 1895 and radium in 1898 in laboratories and their application in medical clinics. Medical radiology used these discoveries without substantial input from laboratory experiments or scientific theory. Medical professionals, though themselves subject to risk, did not immediately act to protect themselves and their patients from harmful biological effects. Lawsuits and insurance requirements, not self-regulation, elicited a professional response aimed at protecting the medical profession as well as patients. Practical rules of thumb and simple measurement devices rather than scientific precision were the rule. Radiation protection lagged.

[63] Stone D. Global Governance Depoliticized: Knowledge Networks, Scientization, and Anti-Policy. In: Paul Fawcett, and Others, editor. Anti-Politics, Depoliticization, and Governance. Oxford: Online edition, Oxford Academic; 2017. https://doi-org.proxy1.library.jhu.edu/10.1093/oso/9780198748977.003.0005, accessed November 12, 2023.

Professional attention to X-ray protection would rise rapidly in the decade before World War I under social pressure, but radium protection would continue to lag, as we shall see in Chapter 3. The inverse was true for radiological measurements. Measurement techniques in X-ray clinics were practical but rudimentary and unstandardized. Radium measurements using more precise laboratory techniques became internationally comparable, due largely to pressure from physicists and commercial requirements.

World War I would enlarge and enrich medical radiology, as described in Chapter 4. Scientific understanding of the physics of X-rays and radium as well as biological understanding of their effects on living beings advanced but still offered little benefit to their application in medicine. The War dramatically increased the number of X-ray practitioners as well as the number of physicists engaged in medical radiology, especially in Germany. That influx would have important post-war consequences.

German war-time scientific achievements were not readily accepted in Allied countries, especially France and Britain. A post-war Allied boycott of German science slowed recognition that the Germans were on a productive track, one that enabled X-ray therapy deep within the human body but required a reevaluation of methods of measuring radiation. Chapter 5 recounts how international standardization of X-ray dose measurements became a post-war professional necessity stemming from international scientific and medical competition. That necessity led to resuscitation of international cooperation with Germany.

Two different dimensions of competition eventually led to internationally accepted standards for measuring X-rays and radium as well as for protecting people from exposure to them. This is the focus of Chapter 6. The first dimension was post-war national competition, in particular between institutions in Allied countries and the German-language academic and medical world. The second was competition within individual countries between more educated and specialized professionals, especially physicists, and less educated and less specialized professionals. Professionalization favored science-based norms. Along with them came nongovernmental national and international institutions committed to their formulation, dissemination, and application. Before World War II, the International Commission on X-ray and Radium Protection played a central role.

During and immediately after World War II, the Manhattan Project applied the Commission's norms, at considerable cost and inconvenience.

In Chapter 7 we examine why a secret crash program to develop the most powerful weapons ever known paid attention to radiation standards that lacked legal force. Retention and recruitment of personnel and fear of labor unrest as well as lawsuits were major factors. Post-war, the Americans reactivated their own national institution for radiation protection and catalyzed the revival of international cooperation, including the ICRP. Public controversy re-emerged during post-war atmospheric atomic bomb testing. Genetic effects discovered before World War II in scientific laboratories far removed from medical radiology took on new significance with the post-World War II exposure of large populations to radioactive fallout. As public controversy raged, concerns expressed mainly by geneticists and the threat of encroachment by other institutions incentivized tightening of the ICRP norms.

Numerical radiation protection norms set in the 1950s lasted until the late 1980s, when under pressure from specialists within its own epistemic community and from the public the ICRP explicitly tightened its recommended permissible doses. As recounted in Chapter 8, the dozens of "Broken Arrow" incidents involving lost or damaged nuclear weapons were not a major factor. The nuclear incident at Three Mile Island in 1979 caused minimal health impacts, but in its aftermath public pressure, combined with data on how radiation was affecting survivors at Hiroshima and Nagasaki, incentivized the tightening of norms for the exposure of the general population. That had already been mostly accomplished under pressure from radiation protection specialists by the time of the Chernobyl incident in 1986, but the occupational norm was also lowered after that, in part due to public concerns.

Other technologies pose risks comparable if not greater than ionizing radiation. They are the focus of Chapter 9. Air pollution and toxic chemicals as well as pharmaceuticals and medical devices are possible analogues, but they are not the subjects of international regimes comparable to the one that exists for ionizing radiation. Even the existing regime for nonionizing radiation has not gained the same dominant position. Why not? By contrast, the world successfully resolved threats to the ozone layer, and the Intergovernmental Panel on Climate Change has begun to achieve a normative role analogous to that of the ICRP, likewise without legal authority. How did this happen? Other potentially beneficial technologies like genetic manipulation and artificial intelligence also pose serious risks and will need norms for their application. What should be learned from the case of ionizing radiation and applied to these other technologies? How can resilient norms be established? What is the proper role of scientists and other experts? To what degree should norms be national or global? How can reasonable balances be struck between benefits and risks?

What we will find contrasts sharply with present practice, which often deploys adversarial processes in setting norms and in many other aspects of contemporary national and international governance. There has long been doubt among psychologists that adversarial processes are a good way to integrate science and values.[64] They are inherently slow and procedurally complex, ill-adapted to knowledge-rich issues, and more suited to stop or prohibit rather than to protect and balance. An epistemic community working cooperatively can more readily mobilize knowledge, balance risks and benefits, reach consensus, and gain legitimacy. In the case of radiation protection, the key factors that led to norm tightening were new data on risks, specialist pressure from within the relevant professions, fear of encroachment by other institutions, and concern about public reaction and possible consequent restrictions. When these factors were present, the epistemic community felt compelled to react constructively and did so to protect people from harm as well as to preserve the benefits of technology. That is an approach we should consider more often.

[64] For example, Hammond KR, Adelman L. Science, Values, and Human Judgment. Science. 1976 Oct 22;194(4263):389–96.

CHAPTER 2

Science Discovers, Medicine Applies, Protection Lags, 1896–1902

Wilhelm Conrad Röntgen, a professor of physics at the University of Würzburg, had been experimenting with rays produced by a high-voltage electric discharge at the negative pole (or cathode) of a partially evacuated glass bulb or tube.[1] The precise nature of cathode rays, which today

[1] For the historian of science, the classic telling of this story is Röntgen WC, Sarton G. The Discovery of X-Rays. Isis. 1937 Mar;26(2):349–69. Most of the details there and elsewhere come from Glasser O. Wilhelm Conrad Röntgen and the Early History of Röntgen Rays. Springfield, Illinois: Charles C. Thomas; 1934, which for lack of other materials is usually treated as a primary source. A. Romer has briefly discussed the lack of reliable primary sources and the consequent limitations on writing the history of the discovery of X-rays in Romer A. Accident and Professor Röntgen. American Journal of Physics. 1959;27:275–7. A full, critical discussion of the sources with reprints of the original articles in English and German can be found in Klickstein HS. Wilhelm Conrad Röntgen "On a New Kind of Rays": A Bibliographical Study. Mallinckrodt Chemical Works; 1966. This excellent study is not readily available in even the best libraries. I am indebted to the Mallinckrodt Chemical Works for providing me with a copy. There are many variations on Sarton and Glasser, including Jauncey GEM. The Birth and Early Infancy of X-Rays. American Journal of Physics. 1945;13:362–79; Crane AW. The Research Trail of the X-Ray. In: Bruwer AJ, editor. Classic Descriptions in Diagnostic Röntgenology. Springfield, Illinois: Charles C. Thomas; 1964; and Underwood EA. W. C. Röntgen and the Early Development of Radiology. Proceedings of the Royal Society of Medicine. 1945;145(38):697–706. Nitske WR. The Life of Wilhelm Conrad Röntgen: Discoverer of the X-Ray. Tuscon: University of Arizona Press; 1971 is derivative of Glasser, despite some embellishments. Not all the embellishments are accurate.

D. Serwer, *Strengthening International Regimes*,
Palgrave Studies in International Relations,
https://doi.org/10.1007/978-3-031-53724-0_2

we regard as electrons, was then in dispute. The designation "ray" merely implied that whatever their nature, cathode rays propagated in straight lines, like rays of light. Philipp Lenard, a young physicist at Bonn, had found that he could make cathode rays pass through a thin metal foil inserted like a window into the glass wall of the discharge tube.[2] Alerted by Lenard's work to the possibility of rays outside the tube, Röntgen late in 1895 found much more penetrating rays than those Lenard had observed. These new rays originated wherever the cathode rays struck the wall of the discharge tube regardless of whether it was equipped with a foil window. Like cathode rays, Röntgen's new rays exposed photographic plates and could not be reflected or refracted by readily available mirrors or prisms, but unlike cathode rays they could not be deflected by a magnet and their absorption in matter did not appear to depend solely on density.

The apparatus required to produce X-rays was widely available in the 1890s, and the equipment Röntgen used differed in only small ways from that of his predecessors and successors. Central to the apparatus was the discharge tube, an evacuated glass bulb with metal electrodes sealed into its walls. Glass blowers had been making such tubes for physicists since the 1850s, mainly for electrical experiments. Röntgen purchased some of his tubes commercially, and both scientific and medical radiology soon depended heavily on commercial tube manufacturers. Röntgen permitted his cathode rays to strike the glass wall of the tube; shortly after his discovery, it became standard to allow them to strike a metal target (the anticathode) placed in the center of the tube, a procedure that produced a higher intensity of X-rays. To evacuate his tube, Röntgen used a common vacuum pump in which liquid mercury falling repeatedly into a tube with a closed-end created a vacuum. Röntgen kept the tube attached to the pump in order to maintain a sufficiently high vacuum, but this procedure soon became unnecessary. The vacuum could be made high enough, and the seals tight enough, to permit a manufacturer to evacuate the tube in advance. To excite his discharge tube, Röntgen used a Ruhmkorff coil, which was one of the standard electrical induction coils of the day and continued in use for more than a decade after 1896. This coil converted a low-voltage current of about 20 amperes to a much higher voltage current of several milliamperes. Röntgen might also have used, as some of his successors did, a generator of static electricity (known as an "influence

[2] Lenard P (Bonn, Physik. Inst. d. Univ.). Ueber Kathoden-strahlen Vom Atmosphärischen Druck Und Im Äussersten Vacuum. Ann Phys. 1894;51:225–67.

machine") to produce the high-voltage electric discharge. Induction coils were readily available from electrical equipment manufacturers.

Röntgen's discovery was rapidly disseminated and confirmed elsewhere, as the photographs he distributed aroused immediate attention and his laboratory equipment was widely available. Röntgen submitted a paper for publication describing his findings in late 1895.[3] On New Year's Day of 1896, he sent reprints of this "preliminary communication" to colleagues, enclosing photographs demonstrating the ability of X-rays to penetrate matter. The most spectacular showed the bones of a hand. Such photographs would soon become as well-known to the world of the 1890s as photographs of the earth taken from space were to the 1960s. One of the reprints and a set of photographs fell into the hands of a Viennese journalist who wrote an account of the discovery that spread rapidly from Vienna to London, New York, and Paris, and from there to the rest of the world. Before the end of the first week of 1896, the news of X-rays was known throughout Europe and the United States. The technology would spread rapidly and eventually trigger a popular backlash.[4]

Biological Effects and Medical Applications Do Not Require Scientific Explanation

Röntgen has been celebrated ever since his discovery for his contribution to medicine as well as to physics. Medical interest in X-rays lay initially in their diagnostic potential, discussed even in the first newspaper reports of the discovery. Within a few weeks, both physicians and nonphysicians reported numerous diagnostic successes. From swallowed pins and pennies, attention shifted quickly to embedded bullets, broken limbs, kidney stones, and soft tissues, some of which were readily made visible by the injection of opaque substances. Many examinations were undertaken to determine what a given pathological condition might look

[3] Röntgen WC. Eine neue Art von Strahlen (Vorläufige Mitteilung). Sitzungsber Phys Med Ges. 1895;Würzburg:132–41, am 28 Dezember wurde als Beitrag eingereicht. Translations can be found in numerous places, including the following: Glasser, note 1, 16–28; Klickstein, ibid.; and Feather N. X-Rays and the Electric Conductivity of Gases. Alembic Club Reprint No 22. Edinburgh: E. and S. Livingstone; 1958.

[4] The initial popular craze in the United States, followed by "commodification" and "backlash," is described in detail in Lavine M. The First Atomic Age. Palgrave MacMillan; 2013.

like in the sometimes-deceptive shadow images that X-rays projected onto a photographic plate (radiography) or onto a fluorescent screen (radioscopy). The demand for refinements in technique was met with a flood of inventions. Contrast media, devices for taking stereoscopic pictures, localization techniques for foreign bodies, regulators to control the vacuum in the X-ray tube, and improved X-ray plates and films were often invented independently in several different places. The reason for simultaneous discoveries was a common set of technological capabilities existing in many places in Europe. New techniques developed from scattered beginnings, small improvement by small improvement. With hundreds of people contributing, overall progress was rapid.[5]

It is often assumed that a technique based on scientific discovery necessarily relies on scientific knowledge and that such a technique thereby offers the certainty in its results that is associated with the underlying science. There are, of course, techniques that do rely heavily on science in both medicine and technology. This pattern is not, however, a necessary one, especially in the early days after a discovery. X-rays were unquestionably "scientific" in pedigree. They were discovered by an academic physicist working within a laboratory tradition of experimentation with cathode ray tubes. But academic science would not reach consensus on the nature of X-rays for more than a decade in the future. An explanation of how X-rays interact with matter came even later. Röntgen made medical radiology possible without contributing further to it. He and most of his colleagues in physical laboratories generally left medical applications to others. The relatively few technical innovations the physicists offered did not usually rely on the specialized knowledge of their discipline. For more than two decades, advances in diagnostic radiology were

[5] For accounts of early techniques, see: Bruwer AJ. Classic Descriptions in Diagnostic Röntgenology. Springfield, Illinois: Charles C. Thomas; 1964; Pizon P. La Radiologie En France, 1896–1904. Paris: l'Expansion Scientifique Française; 1970; Brecher R, Brecher E. The Rays: A History of Radiology in the United States and Canada. Baltimore: Williams and Wilkins; 1969; Schinz HR. Sechzig Jahre Medizinische Radiologie: Probleme und Empirie. Stuttgart: Georg Thieme; 1959; Møller PF. History and Development of Radiology in Denmark, 1896–1950. Copenhagen: Nyt Nordisk Verlag-Arnold Busek; 1968. These references are but the cream of a vast retrospective literature, some of which is listed in the "Annotated 'Radiohistoric' Bibliography" in Grigg ERN. The Trail of Invisible Light. Springfield, Illinois: C. C. Thomas; 1965:822–64.

more often the result of trial-and-error tinkering (bricolage) than applied science.[6]

Similarly, the discovery that exposure to an X-ray tube could cause "physiological" effects, as the effects we would now term "biological" were then called, was independent of both physical and biological science. In the first few months of 1896, several investigators, thinking that X-rays resembled ultraviolet light, had anticipated that they might affect bacteria. The experiments undertaken to test this expectation yielded negative results. X-rays did not appear to kill bacteria, as had been hoped, or even to limit their growth.[7] At about the same time that this disappointment was becoming apparent, the first reports of other, unanticipated, biological effects began to appear. A number of diagnostic practitioners reported that patients were suffering from loss of hair (epilation), reddening and inflammation of the skin (usually termed "erythema"), and a more severe dermatitis resembling a third degree burn.[8] Both practitioners and patients were surprised that the effects often appeared after a delay, sometimes of hours and sometimes of days or weeks, but the appearance of epilation, erythema, and dermatitis on parts of the body that had been close to the X-ray tube during irradiation made it clear that the tube was in some way responsible. Clinical accidents, not scientific knowledge or laboratory experiments, first revealed the biological effects of exposure to the X-ray tube.

Dermatologists, already emerging as a specialty group within medicine, seized this discovery as a promising tool and applied the X-ray tube to the treatment of a wide variety of skin diseases. Sometimes the X-ray tube

[6] For the meaning of bricolage and its relationship to science, see Lévi-Strauss C. The Savage Mind. Chicago: The University of Chicago Press; 1962:16–22. Tinkering and trial-and-error are close in meaning.

[7] Mink F. Zur Frage über die Einwirkung der Röntgensche Strahlen auf Bakterien und ihre ev. therapeutische Verwendbarkeit,. München Med Wschr. 1896 Feb 14;143:101–2 and March 3;202 and 3 March 1896;202; and Lyon TG (Senior Assistant Physician to the Victoria Park Chest Hospital). The Röntgen Rays as a Cure for Disease. Lancet. 74 (1 February 1896) 326 and (22 February 1896):513–4.

[8] The first report was probably Daniel J (Physical Laboratory at Vanderbilt University). The X-Rays. Science. 1896 Apr 10;562–3, signed 23 March 1896, but there was a flood of similar reports soon thereafter, see for example Marcuse. Dermatitis und Alopecie nach Durchleuchtungsversuchen mit Röntgenstrahlen. Deut Med Wschr. 1896 Jul 23;22:481–3. For other early reports, see Glasser O. First Observations on the Physiological Effects of Röntgen Rays on the Human Skin. American Journal of Physics. 1932;28:75–80.

worked, especially in conditions such as eczema, lupus vulgaris (tuberculosis of the skin), and hypertrichosis (excessive growth of hair).[9] The success in the treatment of lupus vulgaris, which was known to be caused by the tubercle bacillus, stood in direct contradiction to what little was known from experiments about the effect of X-rays on bacteria. The contradiction prompted further experimentation, but it did not slow the therapeutic use of the X-ray tube in cases of lupus vulgaris and other bacterial skin diseases.[10] By 1900, success with rodent ulcer (a tumor of epithelial cells) had been reported.[11] With the shift in medical and popular attention around the turn of the century from tuberculosis to cancer, X-rays took on greater promise in both the professional and the public mind. The possibility of a cancer cure, and later a cancer cause, was to remain a major factor in the growth of biological and medical work with X-rays, and later with radium.

Progress in X-ray therapy, as in diagnosis, was largely the result of small contributions, many of which were made independently in several places. Neither theory nor laboratory experiments played a major role. Trial and error, only occasionally guided by conceptions of the nature of X-rays and their interactions with biological material, was the basic technique. The standard that prevailed among practitioners was not intelligibility but effectiveness. It mattered little whether the biological effects of the X-ray tube could be understood. If the treatment worked, it could be used in the clinic, regardless of whether scientists understood the mechanism. There were no legal, cultural, or other constraints. The subject of treatment was the patient, and the results were reported as case histories.

[9] Freund L. Ein mit Röntgen-Strahlen behandelter Fall von Naevus pigmentosus piliferus. München Med Wschr. 1897 Mar 6;47:429–33, based on a lecture at the k. k. Gesellschaft der Aerzte in Wien on 15 January 1897, and Albers-Schönberg. Über die Behandlung des Lupus und des chronischen Ekzems mit Röntgenstrahlen. Fortschr Röntgenstr. 1898;2:20–9.

[10] Albers-Schönberg, ibid., and an editorial, The Action of X-Rays on Microorganisms. Arch Rönt Ray. 1898;3(3):1–2. provide extensive references. Claims of unequivocal success in killing bacteria and in inhibiting their growth also helped to promote further efforts, see for example Rieder H. Wirkung der Röntgenstrahlen auf Bakterien. Munchen Med Wschr. 1898;45:101–4.

[11] See Sjögren T, Sederholm E. (Stockholm) Beitrag zur therapeutischen Verwertung der therapeutischen Verwertung der Röntgenstrahlen. Fortschr Röntgenstr. 1900;4:145–70. where they claimed priority on the basis of a report to the Gesellschaft der schwedischen Ärzte on 19 December 1899.

A physician might append a few words at the end of an article speculating that the effects of X-rays on biological material were similar to their effects on the photographic plate, and therefore chemical or "actinic" in character. Or he might guess that the biological effects were essentially "trophoneurotic," affecting the electrical condition of the nervous system first and only secondarily causing damage to other tissues.[12] But these speculations remained at a general level, often testifying more to the assumption that biological facts could be explained in physical terms (a practice known as reductionism) than to any detailed scientific explanation or continuing interest in unraveling the mechanisms at work.

Science Offers Little

Why was scientific input into medical radiology so meager? Especially in Germany, where there was a long tradition of close connections between academic science and clinical medicine, practical applications of physical and chemical knowledge might be expected. The annual Conferences of German Scientists and Physicians had been meeting since 1822, and Röntgen's "preliminary communication" had been published in the Proceedings of the Physical-Medical Society of Würzburg, a society devoted to invigorating medicine with scientific methods.[13] The explanation for the paucity of applied science even in this science-based branch of medicine is two-fold. Neither biology nor physics had much to offer in these early years of the use of X-rays in medicine. Nor could medicine make ready use of the limited scientific knowledge available. X-rays had not only taken everyone by surprise, but their physical nature and biological effects would remain controversial for decades to come.

The physicist faced three interrelated problems: the nature of the X-rays; the processes generating them in a discharge tube; and the mechanism of the interaction of X-rays with matter. We today regard X-rays as electromagnetic waves of shorter wavelengths than visible light.

[12] For an example of the comparison with the photographic plate, seeGocht. (Assistenzarzt, aus der chirurgischen Abteilung des Neuen allgemeinen Krankenhaus in Hamburg) Therapeutische Verwendung der Röntgenstrahlen. Fortschr Röntgenstr. 1897;1:14–22. For an example of emphasis on trophoneurosis, see Albers-Schönberg, note 9.

[13] On the history of the Versammlungen der Gesellschaft Deutscher Naturforscher und Ärzte, see Thomas RH. Liberalism, Nationalism and the German Intellectuals. Cambridge: W. Heffer; 1951.

According to quantum theory, such electromagnetic waves have a dual nature and can also display particle characteristics. But that concept still lay in the future in the late nineteenth century. In 1897 and 1898 a theory emerged that achieved widespread acceptance among physicists by 1900. This theory treated X-rays as electromagnetic pulses generated by the deceleration of cathode rays, which were by then viewed as streams of negatively charged particles. If in passing through matter, X-rays interacted primarily with elastically bound electrons, such pulses might be very penetrating and also cause the already known emission of secondary X-rays. This "pulse" theory was challenged by those physicists who believed X-rays to be particles arising from the discharge of cathode rays when they struck a solid body. In 1907 the English physicist William Henry Bragg would precipitate a major controversy over the nature of X-rays (and the gamma rays of radium) with the claim that they were particles rather than pulses. The pulse theory, however, remained dominant until at least 1912.[14]

Productive though it was of physical experiment and discovery, the pulse theory had little to offer medical practitioners. Even if they understood the theory, those who were using X-rays for therapy and diagnosis had no means of linking their biological materials with the physicist's picture of matter. Not until well after 1900 did research on the biochemical effects of radiation prove fruitful. First the colloidal aggregate theory of proteins and later the chromosome theory of heredity would eventually provide a bridge between the physical process of ionization and the observed biological effects. In the years before 1900, however, the medical use of X-rays established itself without any firm link to scientific theory and experiment. Biology and physics took longer to make something useful of this discovery than did medicine, which put it to work in the clinic almost immediately. Clinical tinkering worked.

Similarly, radium had been put to use in medicine without relying on scientific knowledge soon after its discovery in 1898. Marie and Pierre Curie discovered this radioactive element in their laboratory while trying to find the reason for the surprisingly intense emission, discovered in 1896 by French physicist Henri Becquerel, of rays similar to X-rays from

[14] On the pulse theory, Wheaton BR. Impulse X-Rays and Radiant Intensity: The Double Edge of Analogy. Historical Studies in the Physical Sciences. 1981 Jan 1;11(2):367–90. Available from: https://doi.org/10.2307/27757484.

the uranium ore pitchblende.[15] Radium would initially attract far less public attention than X-rays, and physicists would continue to dispute whether the rays emitted by radium were identical to X-rays. But physicians were already referring by 1900 to the "radioactivity of the X-ray tube. The parallels were apparent. Both newly discovered phenomena affected photographic plates, caused fluorescence, and ionized air. It was a small step to imagine that radium, like the X-ray tube, might have biological effects. Once sufficient quantities of radium became available, it was another small step to the relevant clinical trials. A series of reports in 1900 and 1901 put the matter beyond doubt: radium, like the X-ray tube, could "burn."[16] Radium was then quickly applied in therapy, beginning as X-rays had with dermatological ailments.

Medical, biological, and popular interest in radium increased further with the discovery that a radioactive gas, known today as radon but then called "radium emanation," was present in the atmosphere, in soil, and in mineral springs.[17] In Continental Europe, mineral springs were frequently used in therapy, and it appeared reasonable to suggest that the curative effects of drinking and bathing in these waters might depend on the presence of radium emanation. The measurement of emanation in mineral waters soon became a minor outdoor sport, with wide surveys conducted in France, Germany, and Austria. Radium also quickly took on a metaphorical significance as the "secret of life," as Luis Campos has

[15] For the Becquerel papers in translation, see Romer A. The Discovery of Radioactivity and Transmutation. New York: Dover; 1964. For the Curie papers in translation and a narrative account of this work, see Romer A. Radiochemistry and the Discovery of Isotopes. New York: Dover; 1970:63–75 and the Historical Essay:3–8. See also Badash L. Chance Favors the Prepared Mind: Henri Becquerel and the Discovery of Radioactivity. Archives Internationales d'Histoire des Sciences. 1965;70:55–66.

[16] Becquerel H, Curie P. Actions Physiologiques Des Rayons Du Radium. Comptes rendus de l'Académie des Sciences (Paris). 1901;132:1289–91. is the standard reference, but largely because of the fame of the authors. They were aware of Giesel F. Ueber radioaktiven Stoffe. Ber Deut Chem Ges. 1900;33:3569–71, received 7 December 1900, and of a report by Walkhoff in *Photographische Rundschau* (October 1900).

[17] Elster J, Geitel H. (Wolfenbüttl) Über die Radioaktivität der im Erdboden enthaltenen Luft. Phys Zeit. 1902;3. received 3 September 1902. See also Gerlach W. Johann Philipp Ludwig Julius Elster. In: Dictionary of Scientific Biography. New York: Charles Scribner's Sons; 1971:354–7.

documented.[18] In the minds of some biologists, it would continue to play an almost metaphysical role for decades to come.

Radium, however, still posed fundamental problems for both physicists and chemists. The notion that its radioactivity arose from the transmutation of one element into another, a notion that we today regard as true, was put forward around the turn of the century, but the Curies continued to believe even then in the theory that had led them to use the term "radioactive."[19] This theory held that there were highly penetrating rays throughout space to which certain elements, the radioactive ones, were sensitive, and from which they could extract energy that was reemitted. Debate on this scientific problem, however, had no discernible bearing on the burgeoning interest in medical uses of radium and radium emanation, which developed apace on the basis of clinical trials. Tinkering worked again.

Medical Radiology Nevertheless Expands Rapidly

Despite their initial lack of grounding in contemporary science, X-ray diagnosis and X-ray and radium therapy were clinical successes and spread rapidly. Well before 1900, diagnostic X-rays were prerequisite to many surgical procedures.[20] By early 1901, one American hospital had made 8000 diagnostic X-ray exposures in 3000 cases.[21] By 1900 there were at least several hundred diagnostic X-ray installations in each of the most technologically adept of the countries of the time: Austria, France,

[18] Campos LA. Radium and the Secret of Life. Chicago: University Of Chicago Press; 2016.

[19] For the development of the idea of transmutation, see the original papers and narrative in Romer (1964), note 15:86–150. For Marie Curie's original presentation of this theory, see her first article on Becquerel rays, "Rays Emitted by the Compounds of Uranium and Thorium" (originally "Rayons émis par les composés de l'uranium et du thorium") Comptes rendus de l'Académie des Sciences (Paris). 1898 Apr 12;126:1101–3. as translated in Romer, ibid.:65–8, especially 67–8. For the Curies continuing defense, see for example their "On Radioactive Substances" (originally "sur les corps radio-actifs," Academy of Sciences (Paris). 1902 Jan 13;134:85–7. as translated in Romer, ibid.:121–3.

[20] See, for example, the generally favorable report by White JW. (M. D., Philadelphia) The Röntgen Rays in Surgery. Transactions of the American Surgical Association. 1897;15:59–88.

[21] Codman EA (Surgeon to Out Patients, Massachusetts General Hospital, Skiagrapher to Children's Hospital). No Practical Danger from the X-ray. Boston Medical and Surgical Journal. 1901;144:197.

Germany, and the United States. X-ray and radium therapy were less widely used, but the success of X-ray therapy in treating a number of dermatological ailments was well-established by 1900. Radium emanation during the first few years after the turn of the century was beginning to be administered by bathing, drinking, and inhalation at health spas. X-ray installations appear to have been especially common, as one would expect, in Röntgen's Germany. In the Curies' France, radium was relatively more important to medical radiology. Distinctive national preferences and sentiments would continue to play a role in scientific and medical radiology.

Medicine is in part an economic pursuit. Neither the legitimate medical practitioners nor the considerable number of quacks could have survived, much less thrive as they did, without public support. An initial burst of public enthusiasm and continuing public interest encouraged the adoption of medical techniques that required investments, albeit modest ones, in specialized equipment.[22] New clinics, within hospitals and outside, sprouted quickly. Specialists, alert to new techniques that could establish their competitive edge over general practitioners, were quick to install X-ray apparatus, and health spas vigorously advertised the radium content of their waters. Acceptance of X-rays and radium in medicine was rapid. The vested interest in their continuing use, though small in economic terms, was significant for the individual X-ray practitioners, health spas, and equipment manufacturers.

The growth of medical radiology put strains on the professional mechanisms available, which in any case were not well-suited to the difficulties X-rays and radium posed. Only in Austria, where medicine was tightly professionalized and acutely aware of its prerogatives, did physicians gain immediate and exclusive control of the medical uses of X-rays and radium. In Britain, France, Germany, and the United States, nonphysician practitioners hung out their shingles, primarily for diagnostic work with X-rays. The question of physician control over the medical use of X-rays would

[22] One retrospective account puts the cost of a minimal X-ray installation at 30 pounds sterling in 1896, see Holland CT. X-rays in 1896 in Bruwer AJ Ibid. Similar equipment in Germany cost about 600 marks, which was about the same amount, see the advertisement by the firm of Ferdinand Ernecke in Wunschmann, E. Die Röntgeschen X-Strahlen. Gemeinverständlich dargestellt. Berlin: F. Schmidt; 1896. as reproduced in Glasser, note 1, at 352. Screens for radioscopy, photographic plates, suitable furniture, and a reasonable number of tubes would more than double this minimum. The tube itself was negligible in cost; the induction coil was the most expensive component.

continue to pose problems. Whatever the later merits of the case, the surging demand in the first few years after 1896 permitted nonphysicians with photographic, electrical, and glassblowing skills to compete effectively. The nonphysicians survived in part because physicians referred patients to them, and also because hospitals often employed nonphysicians to run their diagnostic X-ray units. With the exception of physicians who had been using electricity to diagnose and treat their patients before 1896, most physicians were not well-equipped to use X-rays. However important it might be for diagnosing and treating disease, a medical degree hardly testified to the skills required in building and maintaining evacuated electrical discharge tubes and the auxiliary equipment.

While straining the existing professional mechanisms, the use of X-rays in medicine generated new institutions. Often young, the devotees saw in X-rays an opportunity to be first in discovery and to advance rapidly. The intense interest led to the establishment of Röntgen Societies in Britain (1897), Germany (formed initially in Berlin but expanded to a national society in 1905), and the United States (1900). The British and German Röntgen Societies would prove especially important to the history of radiation protection before World War II because they permitted physicians and nonphysicians to participate on an equal footing. Membership in the French Society for Medical Radiology (founded in 1909 by expansion of the Parisian Society for Medical Radiology) was limited to physicians, and the American Röntgen Ray Society restricted nonphysicians to a lower category of membership.

In addition to these professional societies, medical use of X-rays (and later radium) created a new professional literature. The volume of articles on medical applications of X-rays and on the associated equipment was unprecedented. Within two years, the medical radiological literature was outgrowing the capacity of the existing medical journals, and a number of specialty journals were established in the first decade after 1896. In Germany, Advances in the Field of X-rays (*Fortschritte auf dem Gebiete der Röntgenstrahen*) was founded in 1897, and the Proceedings of the German Röntgen Society (*Verhandlungen der Deutschen Röntgengesellschaft*) in 1905. In Britain, there was the *Archives of the Röntgen Ray*, which was founded in 1898 as the Archives of Skiagraphy (shadow-projection), and later also the Journal of the Röntgen Society (first published separately from the Archives starting in 1904). In the United States, the American X-Ray Journal (founded in 1897) gave way as the leading journal to the Transactions of the American Röntgen Ray Society after 1902, which was joined by the American Quarterly of Röntgenology after 1906. In France, the Archives of Medical Electricity (*Archives d'Electricité Médicale*), which had been founded in 1893, became the major outlet for medical X-ray work, and *Le Radium* served both the scientific and medical communities.

With the exception of *Le Radium*, the new journals did not attract original work in physics or chemistry. The scientific radiological community was readily distinguishable from the medical radiological community. The physicists working on X-rays and radioactivity generally used the existing journals like the *Philosophical Magazine* in Britain, the Annals of Physics (*Annalen der Physik*) and the Physics Magazine (*Physikalische Zeitschrift*) in Germany, and the Proceedings of the Academy of Sciences (*Comptes Rendus*) as well as *Le Radium* in France. The material published on physical aspects of X-rays in the medical radiological journals was either derivative or highly practical. The authors were often associated with manufacturers of X-ray tubes and auxiliary equipment. In Germany, where medical radiology showed more interest in scientific developments than elsewhere, most of the "scientific" and "technical" articles in the medical journals were contributed until World War I by Bernhard Walter, a diligent but second-rate physicist, and by Friedrich Dessauer, an X-ray tube manufacturer who would obtain a doctorate in physics only after World War I. The nonphysician members of the Röntgen Society were mostly tube manufacturers, electrical engineers, and interested dilettantes. A series of International Conferences of Medical Radiology and Electrology met seven times between 1900 and 1914. This series was entirely separate from the contemporary international scientific conferences, mostly of physicists, on "Radiology and Ionization" (Liège, 1905) and on "Radiology and Electricity" (Brussels, 1910).

This gap in institutions between medical and physics-focused radiology corresponded to a difference in methodologies. In the scientist's laboratory, experiment and theory are, ideally, tightly linked. The experimenter tries to work within clearly defined theoretical presuppositions that enable him to ask questions about how a small and isolated piece of the natural world behaves. In the medical clinic, the procedure is different. The clinician observes a far broader expanse of nature and tries to bring some sort of recognizable order to it without the experimenter's capacity for controlling the conditions under which observations are made. Delicate and precise instruments may be used in the clinic, but to observe rather than to test. By accumulating ordered experience, and not necessarily scientific understanding, the clinic aims to achieve practical results. Through years of making clinical rounds with more experienced elders, the young physician is trained to recognize a large number of diseases and their appropriate courses of treatment while understanding in scientific detail the causes of only a few.[23] This difference in method would play a role in future debates on radiation protection, where case histories and experiments did not always produce the same results.

There is no question about which of these methods is more precise. The clinical approach leaves a great deal of room for personal judgment, which means both wide scope for individual talent as well as wide scope for error. There is, however, also no question but that the laboratory approach fails to offer solutions to many practical problems. As Wilfred Trotter pointed out in 1932, physiology could then give no explanation of the most common symptoms of which patients complained: feeling ill, pain, sleeplessness, vomiting, loss of appetite, and constipation.[24] Ninety years of effort since has improved the scientific understanding of medical issues, but scientific explanations are still often lacking. A physician can nevertheless learn to recognize and treat hundreds of diseases that cause these symptoms and others. The disadvantage of the laboratory approach is precisely what makes it work so well: "Experiment... isolates the event to be studied from the common order of nature, and causes it to occur in

[23] The methodological distinction between the clinic and the laboratory appears, explicitly or implicitly, in many places. At the risk of attributing a distinction to authors who would not think it valid in the form in which I use it, I would cite the following sources: Bernard C. An Introduction to the Study of Experimental Medicine tr. H. C. Greene. New York: Dover; 1957:9 and 18, where the distinction is made in terms of "experimental" vs. "empirical"; Fleming D. Emigré Physicists and the Biological Revolution. Pers Amer Hist. 1968;2:152–89. where (pp. 160–1) the distinction is made in terms of an instinctual difference between physicists and biologists in responding to evidence; and Levi-Strauss, note 6, where the distinction is made in terms of "the scientist creating events (changing the world) by means of structures and the bricoleur creating structures by means of events," at 22. As noted in Chapter 1, the distinction also appears in Pickstone JV. Ways of Knowing: A New History of Science, Technology and Medicine. Chicago: University of Chicago Press; 2000.

[24] Trotter W. Art and Science in Medicine, an Address Delivered at the Opening of the 1932–1933 Session at the University College Hospital Medical School. In: The Collected Papers. Oxford: Humphrey Milford for the Oxford University Press; 1941:85–101, at 90.

circumstances as far as possible simplified and subject to specification."[25] Even today, this approach has been used on only limited aspects of the vast territory of medical practice, and much of medicine continues to be what Trotter called a "practical art" rather than an applied science.[26] This phenomenon has been all too evident in the COVID-19 epidemic. Even though its viral basis was understood quickly, scientists were initially unable to tell medical practitioners and the public how the virus originated and whether a mask would protect the wearer.[27] The origins of the virus are still in doubt, but most of us long ago reached practical conclusions about whether to wear masks.

The methods of the practical arts are not limited to medicine. In chemistry, the periodic table has survived, despite the discovery of physical laws that make it superfluous in theory. It serves as a device to organize vast experience rather than to explain it. The table permits a great deal of practical work to be done without recourse to what the physicist would regard as a proper explanation of chemical phenomena in quantum mechanical terms. When a chemist said, as she might have until only a few decades ago, "xenon does not react because it belongs to the eighth period, the inert gases" she was stating neither a tautology nor the consequence of a physical law. Rather, she was summarizing the result of a vast quantity of experience, with which she need not have been personally familiar since the position of xenon in the periodic table neatly connotated it. The fact that xenon is now known to react has neither redrawn the periodic table nor limited its usefulness in many other respects.

In the history of radiation protection, mnemonic devices similar to the periodic table, though not so conveniently graphic, were often used. They are the tools of a practical art. One of these was for decades regarded as the foundation of radiation biology, namely the "law" of Bergonié-Tribondeau. This law stated that cells were affected by radiation more strongly the greater their reproductive activity, the longer they took in

[25] Trotter W. Observation and Experiments and Their Use in the Medical Sciences. BMJ. 1930 Jul 26;2(3629):129–34.

[26] Ibid.

[27] Thompson D. Why Are We Still Arguing About Masks? [Internet]. The Atlantic. 2023. Available from: https://www.theatlantic.com/newsletters/archive/2023/03/covid-lab-leak-mask-mandates-science-media-information/673263/?taid=64037a0d28a8a600017ae661&utm_campaign=the-atlantic&utm_content=true-anthem&utm_medium=social&utm_source=twitter, accessed March 27, 2023.

mitotic division, and the less their morphology and functions had been differentiated. This statement summarized, and continues to summarize, many observations, but there were, and are, exceptions to it. Physical laws like Newton's or Maxwell's cannot have exceptions and still remain universally valid. The law of Bergonié-Tribondeau still stands because it is in most cases correct and therefore remains useful. It is closely akin to the engineer's rule of thumb, a "heuristic" that often serves him better in his daily work than Newton's or Einstein's physical laws. In medical radiology, such rules of thumb—concerning which kinds of radiation to use for different purposes, the length and frequency of the exposures required, and the protection measures that were appropriate—grew out of the clinical experience of many practitioners, who would sometimes accord them the status and respect usually reserved for physical laws. The norms associated with radiation protection originated in such rules of thumb, as we shall see.

Scientific and Medical Radiology Remain Separate but Linked

Between the largely separate worlds of laboratory and clinical radiology three important links would prove important to the development of radiation protection. First, the two communities used similar material. Medical radiology in the early years relied directly on scientists to obtain radium. This reliance would keep the medical applications of radium in much closer touch with related experimental work than the medical applications of X-rays, which were developed by a much larger group of often isolated practitioners. Scientists however could purchase X-ray equipment readily because it was produced commercially for the medical radiological market. It took only a few months in the spring of 1896 for glassblowers and for electrical equipment producers, many of whom already manufactured medical electrical equipment, to place on the market a bewildering variety of X-ray tubes, induction coils and interrupters, influence machines, and auxiliary equipment like fluoroscopes, tube stands, and examining tables. Both the scientific and the medical communities took an active interest in innovations in X-ray and radium technology, and although certain items were considered suitable only for the laboratory and not for the clinic or vice versa, there was a common interest in X-ray tubes, the manipulation of radium, and, crucially, the measurement of both.

The second major link between laboratory and medical radiology lies in the goals that the medical radiological community set for itself. Acutely aware of its scientific origins, medical radiology aimed and claimed to be scientific. In retrospect, it is obvious that the discovery of X-rays and radium by scientists did not make their medical use any more certain in its clinical results than if, for example, they had been discovered by a glass-blower, as might well have been the case for X-rays. The image of X-rays and radium as distinctively modern and advanced tools was nevertheless strong. Precisely what it meant to be "scientific" varied considerably. "Scientific" medicine sometimes meant medicine based on scientific theory. Of the people who thought along this line, some were reductionists who wanted explanations of the biological effects of radiation in physical or in chemical terms, but others were satisfied with explanations in terms of cytology or bacteriology. To still other research workers, "scientific" medicine meant the use of measurements or experiments within medicine rather than explanations in scientific terms. Among these people, there were different views of the precision required of measurements and different opinions on what constituted an experiment. The results of research efforts along these different lines were not necessarily consistent with each other, but the goal of scientific medicine was inspirational. It made medical radiology more open to scientific input than many other branches of medicine.

The third link between laboratory and medical radiology was conceptual: they both thought in terms of the "quantity" and "quality" of radiation.[28] It would be decades before the two communities would come to an agreement on their physical basis and how to measure these parameters, but both communities talked of the quantity and quality of X-rays and of radium as if these were self-evident concepts. For X-rays, quantity was the amount of radiation; the term was often used interchangeably with "intensity" (which might also mean quantity per unit of time) and was analogous to the intensity of light. For radium, quantity meant the amount of a substance. Quality, which was analogous to the different colors of light, meant for X-rays the differing ability of radiation to penetrate matter: "harder" rays were more penetrating and

[28] In French, quantité and qualité. In German, quantity was originally Menge but became Quantität with the shift, discussed below, from exposure to dose; quality was Härte, Qualität or sometimes Penetrationsvermögen.

"softer" rays less penetrating.[29] With the discovery of radium, the usage was quickly extended to the radiation it emitted: the softer radiation that could be deviated with a magnet (which we now know as alpha particles consisting of two protons and two neutrons) and the much harder, "gamma" radiation that was not deviable in a magnetic field and was even more penetrating than the hardest X-rays known at the time (which we now know are like electromagnetic waves of shorter wavelengths than the X-rays known in 1900).[30]

X-rays and radium were the great scientific and medical sensations of their time. The communities that dealt with them in the laboratory and in the clinic were distinct, but they shared common material requirements, scientific ambitions, and a common language for describing the newly discovered rays and radioactivity. Those links would eventually provide a scaffolding on which scientists and medical practitioners would construct a common approach to measuring doses and protecting themselves, their patients, and their professions from harmful biological effects. That common approach, rooted in the kind of international, interdisciplinary "epistemic community" mentioned in Chapter 1, would prove remarkably durable and generate universally accepted norms. But it would come to fruition only after years of delay.

The Electrical View Delays X-Protection

While medical applications of X-rays developed rapidly between 1896 and 1900, X-ray protection was at best a minor concern. Lack of knowledge was not the reason for this inattention. Exposure to X-ray tubes was known to have biological effects. These effects were the basis of X-ray therapy. Many operators, however, took no measures to protect themselves or their patients. Of those who did take protective measures, the majority used a grounded aluminum or tin sheet. Lead, though used by some practitioners, was considered unnecessarily inconvenient and even dangerous by others. Many operators assessed the hardness of a tube by

[29] The idea of quality, analogous to the different colors of light, had already been introduced for cathode rays, see Lenard P. Ueber Die Magnetische Ablenkung Der Kathodenstrahlen. Ann Phys. 1894;52:23–33.

[30] For the development of this classification scheme, see Trenn TJ. Rutherford on the Alpha-Beta-Gamma Classification of Radioactive Rays. Isis. 1976 Mar;67(1):61–75.

exposing their own hands and viewing the resulting image on a fluorescent screen. The X-ray tube was, in general, not enclosed. Although physicists in their laboratories routinely recorded some measure of the quantity and quality of X-rays a particular tube produced, measurements were not often made during medical applications in the clinic. Moreover, the bulk of the X-ray practitioners, physicians, and nonphysicians around 1900 were pleased with the situation. The number of cases of harm to patients was, they thought, decreasing rapidly. X-ray therapy was curing a widening range of dermatological ailments. The reddening, scaling, and open sores that had developed on the hands of many X-ray practitioners were usually considered minor ailments. Chronic dermatitis seemed a small price to pay for the benefits obtained from the medical application of X-rays. Even medical professionals did not see a need to protect themselves.

Change would come rapidly after 1900. Measures to protect the patient and the operator would become routine, however inadequate the procedures used appear by today's criteria. By the end of 1902, the weight of professional opinion would shift against the use of aluminum and tin shielding, grounded or not. Methods of measuring the quantity and quality of the rays would come into widespread use. Operators who assessed hardness with their own hands would be considered foolhardy at best. Professional societies and journals would actively promote precautions. While far from the precision it was to acquire in the decades to follow, X-ray protection would by 1903 be a recognized problem for science, medicine, and society.[31] In sharp contrast, radium protection was still unknown.

Why did X-ray practitioners before 1900 use what they themselves would regard by 1903 as grossly inadequate and misdirected methods of protection? What made these practitioners shift gears after 1900, embracing both X-ray measurements and X-ray protection as essential professional concerns? Why did radium protection not become a matter

[31] This early period in the history of X-ray protection has been most accurately discussed in Ratkóczy N. Geschichtliches über Strahlenschädigung und Strahlenschutz. Strahlenth. 1971;141:311–20 and 425–38.

James D. Nauman Provides Some Interesting Excerpts from British and American Materials of this Period in Pioneer Descriptions in the Story of X-ray Protection. In: Bruwer AJ. Classic Descriptions in Diagnostic Röntgenology. Springfield, Illinois: Charles C. Thomas; 1964:311–39. Most other secondary treatments either begin later or fail to take seriously the issue of identifying the agent causing the biological effects.

of concern? We are today all too familiar with a pattern of medical and technological innovation in which the widespread adoption of a technique leads to harmful side effects and subsequent retrenchment. Disinterested expertise seems to offer an obvious solution. We expect professional communities to resolve problems arising from medical and technological innovation. Medicine, in particular, has established self-regulatory mechanisms that should, it can be argued, react automatically to protect both practitioners and patients from harm.

Self-regulation would not suffice for X-rays or radium. Disinterested expertise and professional self-regulation are problematic concepts. The term "expertise" suggests a degree of objectivity that often does not, and sometimes cannot, exist. Those who know a good deal about something by definition have an interest in it. The interest may be intellectual or professional rather than financial, but it is an interest nevertheless and may affect the weighing of evidence. As for the professional self-regulatory mechanisms, they exist, but their operation often depends on pressures from outside the professional community. That was the case for medical radiology. Public concern was necessary to activate the professional mechanisms that are often regarded as automatic.

Although X-ray protection per se was not a concern before 1900, clinical experience had led practitioners to adopt conservative and cautious therapeutic procedures. Patients, it was thought, showed wide variability in their reactions to treatment. This idiosyncrasy contrasted sharply with the presumed invariability of the physical agency, the X-ray tube (which in fact was itself highly variable, though that was not yet recognized). In reporting cases, the practitioner specified the parameters of the tube, such as the equivalent spark gap, the "secondary" current through the tube (or sometimes only the "primary" current flowing into the induction coil), the number of breaks per minute of the interrupter, the distance of the patient from the anticathode, the duration of the exposure, or whatever other parameters had been found by clinical trials to affect the course of treatment. No need arose for measuring the dose of X-rays delivered, and indeed the notion of "dose" did not yet exist. The presumed variability of the biological material made therapy an art. Knowing when sufficient exposure to the X-ray tube had been administered was a matter of clinical judgment, preferably informed by both long experience and, so far as physicians were concerned, a medical degree.

Most physicians solved this matter of judgment simply. They continued exposure until a light skin reaction was visible. The mild erythema was the signal both that the treatment was working, and that the physician should discontinue it. This practical method favored the use of harder tubes, which "burned" less readily, and short, repeated exposures over a period of weeks or even months.[32] Many practitioners administered treatment with little or no concern for the mechanism of the resulting effects, but some X-ray practitioners and medically oriented research workers had their own notions about the nature of X-rays and thereby drew conclusions about how they affected biological materials. These notions were analogies that placed the new discovery within the context of existing biological knowledge.[33] On the one hand, X-rays appeared closely akin to light, and especially to ultraviolet light. Since violet, and ultraviolet, light was known to be a disinfectant, this kinship led to the anticipation of bactericidal effects of X-rays.[34] The analogy to ultraviolet also led to the attempted treatment of lupus vulgaris with X-rays, in imitation of therapeutic successes with ultraviolet lamps.[35]

[32] For a review of this "many sittings" approach, see Möller M. (Docent für Dermatologie und Syphilis in Stockholm). Der Einfluss Des Lichtes Auf Die Haut in Born G. et al. Gesundem Und Krankhaftem Zustande. In: Bibliotheca Medica. Abtheilung DII, Heft 8; 1900. Especially:126–7. For specific instances, see Gasmann A, Schenkel H. Ein Beitrag zur Behandlung der Hautkrankheiten mit Röntgenstrahlen. Fortschr Röntgenstr. 1898;2:121–32; and Hall-Edwards J. The Röntgen Rays in the Treatment of Cancer. Arch Rönt Ray. 1902 Dec;7:45–9. Hall-Edwards believed "that the production of a limited amount of dermatitis is a *sine qua non* to successful treatment... the amount of good done is in direct ratio to the mount of dermatitis produced, so long as this does not exceed the scientific limit," at 46 and 47. See also the editorial, X-ray Dermatitis. Arch Rönt Ray. 1903 Oct;79–82.

[33] This is an approach characteristic of "natural history," see Pickstone JV. Ways of Knowing: A New History of Science, Technology and Medicine. Chicago: University of Chicago Press; 2000.

[34] For the bactericidal effects of violet and ultraviolet light, see for example Downes A (M. D.), Blunt TP (M. A. Oxon.). On the Influence of Light on Protoplasm. Proceedings of the Royal Society. 1878;28:199–212. communicated by J. Marshall (F. R. S., Surgeon to University College Hospital); and Duclaux E. Influence De La Lumière Du Soleil Sur La Vitalité Des Micrococcus. t' C R Soc Biol (Paris). 1885;508–10, séance du 25 juillet 1885.

[35] Niels R. Finsen, 1903 Nobelist in medicine, was the inventor and prime promoter of treatment with electric arc light (often known as Finsen light), see especially "The Treatment of *Lupus Vulgaris* by Concentrated Chemical Rays," tr. from *La Semaine Médicale* of 21 December 1897 by J. H. Sequeira in N. Finsen, *Phototherapy* (London: Edward Arnold, 1901). See also Aggebo, Niels Finsen: *Die Lebensgeschichte eines grossen Arztes und Forschers*, tr. from Danish by M. Backmann-Isler (Zurich: Rascher, 1946).

On the other hand, X-rays appeared closely akin to electricity. Their production in a device excited with an electrical current testified strongly to their "electrical" character, as did their ionization of gases. This latter analogy to electricity, though far from a theory whose implications could be worked out in a scientific fashion, was a step in assimilating X-rays into medical thinking and had profound consequences for work on their biological effects.[36] The biological effects and medical uses of electricity, after falling into disrepute during the 1830s and 1840s, were again the subject of intensive investigation in the late nineteenth century, with interest reviving in the 1860s and probably peaking in the 1880s and early 1890s. Along with other "physical" techniques like baths and massage, electrotherapy played an important role during a period of relative nihilism in chemical therapeutics. Although today much of this tradition is forgotten, electrodiagnosis and electrotherapy were often considered especially modern and promising areas of "scientific" medicine in the 1890s. Medical electricity was also an area in which over-enthusiastic adherents and charlatans put forward excessive claims, as should be expected of a rapidly developing specialty. Because of the similarity in the equipment and skills needed for X-ray therapy, many early X-ray practitioners came from electrotherapy. With his knowledge of batteries, static generators, induction coils, and electrodes, the electrotherapist was far ahead of other physicians in being prepared to set up and maintain an X-ray tube. Moreover, practitioners welcomed X-rays into medical electricity, and until World War I they were often treated as part of that broader and older tradition.[37]

[36] The analogies to light and electricity and the notion that something could be intermediate in character between them was also used by LeBon for his "black light," see Nye MJ. Gustave LeBon's "Black Light: A Study in Physics and Philosophy in France at the Turn of the Century." Historical Studies in the Physical Sciences. 1974;4:163–95, at 173.

[37] Most standard sources fail to make more than passing mention of the electrotherapeutic tradition. For surveys, see Colwell HA. A Sketch of the History of Electrotherapy. Archives of Radiology and Electrotherapy. 1917;21:320–6. and his Essay on the History of Electrotherapy and Diagnosis. London: Heinemann; 1922. See also Coulter JS. Physical Therapy. New York: Paul B. Hoeber; 1932. An interesting account of the Viennese electrotherapists, including one Dr. Sigmund Freud, within the context of physiotherapy can be found in Lesky E. Die Wiener Medizinische Schule Im 19. Jahrhunderts. Graz-Köln: Bohlau; 1965:334–401. For a contemporary review of the effects of high-frequency alternating current and its therapeutic uses, see D't Arsonval. Action Physiologique Et Thérapeutique Des Courants Haute Fréquence. Ann Electro. 1898;1:1–28, communication faite en avril 1897 à la Société internationale des électriciens, and Oudin. Les

The association with medical electricity strongly conditioned the reaction of physicians to the discovery of biological effects of exposure to the X-ray tube. Initially, X-rays themselves were often assumed to be the causal agent, but a variety of other candidates were soon put forward. These included ultraviolet light from the fluorescing tube, ozone produced around the tube or in the skin, metal particles from the anode, and the static electric charges surrounding the tube. Only the last of these suggestions achieved a significant level of acceptance. This electrical view became dominant among medical practitioners through 1900 and persisted for several years thereafter.[38] Attributing the biological effects to the static charges surrounding the tube, which was often placed within inches of the patient, rather than to the X-rays themselves, placed the new technique in the sphere of electrotherapy and avoided the uncertainty concerning the nature of the X-rays. Moreover, there was clinical

Courants De Haute Fréquence Et De Haute Tension Dans Les Maladies De La Peau Et Des Muqueuses. ibid.:86–113. For an important contemporary text, see Erb W. *Electrotherapeutics*, Vol. VI of von Ziemssen TS. Handbook of General Therapeutics, tr. A. de Watteville. New York: William Wood; 1887. Overshadowed by radiotherapy, electrotherapy declined rapidly after World War I because it was unable to establish itself as a creditable specialty with the bulk of physicians, except perhaps in France. Today's radiotherapy and physical therapy can, however, be traced in part to this stillborn branch of medicine.

[38] The best available evidence for the dominance of the electrical view is that contemporary sources on both sides of the issue from 1898 through 1900 treated it as the majority view, see for example the following: Dollinger D. Zweiter Bericht Über Die Arbeiten Auf Dem Gebiete Der Röntgenstrahlen in Frankreich,t' Fortschr. Röntgenstr. 1898;2:36–143 and 73–5; Rodet A, Bertin-Sans H. (laboratoire de Microbiologie et de Physique médicale, Université de Montpellier). Influence Des Rayons X Sur La Tuberculose Expérimentale. Archives of Electronic and Medicine. 1898 Oct 15;6:413–31; Freund S. Rapport Sur l'état Actuel De La radiothérapie, Comptes-rendus Des Séances Du 1 Er Congrès International d' Electrologie Et De Radiologie Médicale, Paris, 27 juillet–1 Er Août 1900. Lille: Bigot Frères; 1900:218–29 with discussion; and R. Kienböck (Röntgen-Institut im Sanatorium Fürth, Vienna), "Über die Einwirkung des Röntgen-Lichtes auf die Haut," originally delivered at the k. k. Gesellschaft der Aerzte (Vienna) 19 October 1900 and printed with revisions in Wien Klin Wschr. 1900 Dec 13;13:1153–66. The electrical view held on even longer in some circles, see the account of a discussion at the Röntgen Society, The Relation Between X Rays and Allied Phenomenae. Arch Rönt Ray. 1902 Jun;7:3–7. and also Williams FR. (M.D. Harvard; graduate of MIT; Visiting Physician at the Boston City Hospital; Fellow of the Massachusetts Medical Society; Member of the Association of American Physicians and of the American Climatological Association; Fellow of the American Association for the Advancement of Science). The Röntgen Rays in Medicine and Surgery. New York: MacMillan; 1901. Williams, whose book was the leading text in the United States, was still recommending the use of a grounded aluminum screen for protection of the patient in the third edition, 1903.

evidence. Practitioners could sometimes see a "brush" discharge of diffuse sparks between the X-ray tube and the skin of the patient.

Experience had taught medical practitioners that increasing the distance between the tube and the patient would often prevent harm. The static electric field around the tube would not extend far, certainly not as far as the X-rays themselves, so this effect of distance favored the electrical view.[39] So, too, did the reports that a grounded aluminum screen would protect the patient.[40] Occasional reports appeared of intensified therapeutic effects when the patient was placed on an insulated platform, a common practice in some electrotherapeutic techniques.[41] Some practitioners claimed that an X-ray tube excited with an influence machine rather than with an induction coil did not cause burns.[42] This claim suggested that it was the electrical means used to excite the tube rather than the X-rays themselves that were responsible. Ungrounded lead, it was said, might be harmful if used for shielding because it would condense the harmful static charges near the skin of the patient.[43]

Experimental evidence against the electrical view was readily obtained. It was a simple matter to expose a finger to the X-ray tube, protecting part of it with ungrounded lead and part of it with grounded aluminum or tin shielding. By 1898 this experiment and comparable ones with other biological materials had been performed. The results were unequivocally against the electrical view. Ungrounded lead protected and grounded aluminum did not.[44] Nonetheless, these results initially had negligible

[39] Destot. Les troubles physiologiques et trophiques dus aux rayons. C R Acad Sci (Paris). 1897 May 17;124:1114–6, présenté par M. Bouchard.

[40] Leonard CL. (Skiagrapher to the University Hospital and Assistant Instructor in Clinical Surgery, University of Pennsylvania). The X-Ray "Burn": Its Productions and Prevention. Has the X-Ray Any Therapeutic Properties?. N Y Med J. 1891 Jul 2;68:18–20. Leonard thought a grounded aluminum sheet provided "absolute protection."

[41] Schürmayer. (Hannover) Die Schädigungen Durch Röntgenstrahlen Und Die Bedeutung Unserer Schutzvorrichtungen. Fortschr Röntgenstr. 1901;5:44–8, delivered at the 73. Versammlung deutscher Naturforscher und Artze in Hamburg (22–29 September 1901).

[42] Frei GA. X-rays Harmless with the Static Machine. Elec Eng. 1896 Dec 23;22:651, as quoted in Nauman, note 31, and Destot in the discussion following Schiff and Freund, note 38, at 228.

[43] Schürmayer, note 41.

[44] For the "finger" experiment, see Thomson E. Röntgen Ray Burns. Amer X-Ray J. 1898 Nov;3:452–3. Thomson had believed from the first that the effects were due to the

effects on medical practice. X-rays were still relatively new, the professional communities were still in the process of formation, and the standards of proof were still uncertain. Moreover, the weight of the clinical evidence was on the side of the electrical view. No matter how decisive the outcome, the experimental evidence was based on a mere case or two, and these occurred in the artificial conditions of the laboratory. The medical practitioner valued the vast experience of the clinic more highly. The recently founded journals turned not to laboratory experiments, but rather to surveys of clinical experience to decide the issue of what caused the injuries. By collecting many cases of injury and studying the conditions under which they occurred, the practitioners hoped to find ways of preventing their recurrence. The surveys, which began in 1897 and were completed by 1899, failed to reach definitive conclusions, and the electrical view continued to dominate in the medical community.[45]

The advocates of the electrical view enhanced their position by shifting the burden of proof. They presumed X-rays were innocent of causing any biological effects. Those who believed the X-rays were the causal agent were asked to demonstrate that none of the other possible agents was

X-rays themselves, see Codman EA. The Cause of Burns from X-rays. Boston Medical and Surgical Journal. 1896 Dec 19;135:610–1. Thomson, it should be noted, had developed an induction coil that was in competition with a static machine developed by Frei, note 39. There may therefore have been vested interests influencing both Thomson's report and Frei's. For experiments comparable to Thomson's with bacteria, see Rieder H. Wirkung der Röntgenstrahlen auf Bakterien, Munchen. Med Wschr. 1898;45:101–4.

[45] For the initiation of the surveys, see X Ray Traumatism. Arch Rönt Ray. 1898;2:61 and Albers-Schönberg. Aufforderung Zu Einer Sammelforschung Über Die Wirkung Der Röntgenstrahlen Auf Den Menschlichen Organismus. Fortschr Röntgenstr. 1898;1:226–7. The inconclusive outcome of the Röntgen Society inquiry is apparent in Payne E. Notes on the Effects of X Rays. Arch Rönt Ray. 1899;3:67–9; and Walsh D. Focus-Tube Dermatitis. Ibid.:69–73. The inconclusive outcome of the German survey, which was mounted in imitation of the English one, is apparent in the report on the 30 July 1900 session of the Congrès International d'Électrologie et de Radiologie médicales in *Fortschr. Röntgenstr.* 4, (1900–1901):99. A similar American inquiry did not attempt to answer the question of what was causing the X-ray injuries, leaving it to "the electricians," see Scott NS. X-Ray Injuries. Amer XRay J. 1897;1:57–66, but the editor of the journal made his position clear, "With all that has been written for the lay press, medical journals and scientific publications, I am unable to find a rational conclusion [sic] for the belief that X-rays ever injured in any instance human tissue," ibid.

responsible.[46] The electrical view was thus bolstered by the demonstration that high-voltage electrical charges could, in the absence of X-rays, cause erythema and epilation.[47] Likewise, a demonstration that electric charges could kill bacteria became evidence for the electrical view since exposure to the X-ray tube was known to have a curative effect in the clinic on a disease like lupus.[48] Since the majority view was that X-rays did not kill bacteria, those who believed X-rays had biological effects also had the burden of accounting for the successful therapy. X-rays might stimulate the body's natural defense mechanisms, but this argument was unconvincing without supporting evidence.

A Decisive Experiment Fails to Decide

Decisive evidence that X-rays themselves caused the biological effects was offered in 1900, but only slowly over the next several years did the proponents of the electrical view give way. With the evidence came a new technique of X-ray therapy, a need for dose measurements, and intensified concern for X-ray protection. The initiator of these changes was a young Viennese physician, not yet habilitated (that is, without a doctorate), who was working at a private clinic.[49] In the course of treating six patients with X-rays in late 1899 and early 1900, Robert Kienböck was forced to switch to a softer tube when his harder one was punctured. All six patients, regardless of how much they had been exposed to the harder tube, quickly developed skin reactions when they used the softer tube. This clinical

[46] For the reversal of the burden of proof, see the reply to Thomson of Leonard CL. (M. D., Assistant Instructor in Clinical Surgery and Instructor in Skiagraphy, University of Pennsylvania) Röntgen-Ray Dermatitis. Amer X-Ray J. 1898 Nov;3:453.: "we must first eliminate all causes that experience has shown are capable of producing like results under different circumstances."

[47] Freund L (aus dem pathologisch-anatomischen Universitäts-institute und dem Institute für Radiographie und Radiotherapie in Wien). Die physiologischen Wirkungen der Polentladungen hochgespannter Inductionsströme und einiger unsichtbaren Strahlungen. Sitzungsber Akad Wiss. *(Wien), 109*, Abtheilung III (1900) 583–65 vorgelegt in der Sitzung 12 July 1900. For a briefer statement of the mature electrical view, see Schiff E, Freund L. (Universitätsdozent in Wien), Der Gegenwärtige Stand Der Radiotherapie. Wien Klin Wschr. 1900;13:827–9, nach einem auf dem XIII internationalen dermatologischen Congresse in Paris gehaltenen Vortrage. Schiff and Freund, who were leading figures in radiology in Vienna, converted to the electrical view around 1898.

[48] Ibid.

[49] For a biography, see Weiss K. Robert Kienböck–80 Jahre. Strahlenth. 1951;84:161–4.

experience suggested to Kienböck that X-rays, which were more intense from the softer tube, caused the burns rather than the static electric charge surrounding the tube, which would be more intense around the harder tube. A series of straightforward experiments decided the issue. Kienböck exposed one side of a living organism to a soft tube and one side to a hard tube. The reaction appeared more rapidly on the side exposed to the softer tube. The point closest to the focus of the cathode rays reacted soonest and most dramatically. Masking with lead showed that shadows were cast from the single point where the X-rays originated rather than from the surroundings of the tube. Rubber, a good electric insulator, did not protect the skin. Biological effects occurred only on the side of the anticathode struck by the cathode rays, the direction in which Kienböck assumed all the X-rays to be emitted.[50]

Replying to the advocates of the electrical view, Kienböck offered explanations for the phenomena they had adduced as evidence. The grounded aluminum or tin foil might delay and lessen the reaction because it absorbed X-rays, but it did not prevent harm altogether. Because the current through the tube excited with an influence machine was lower, it produced a lower intensity of X-rays than a tube excited with an induction coil and therefore burned less readily. Biological effects occurred in close proximity to the tube because the intensity of the X-rays fell off with the square of the distance.[51] Kienböck also offered a new method of X-ray therapy. The idiosyncrasy of the patient, he claimed, was irrelevant. Different tissues reacted differently, but the same tissues in different individuals of the same age reacted in the same way. Instead of irradiating a patient with a hard tube until a reaction appeared, Kienböck suggested fewer and shorter sittings with a soft tube, preferably one

[50] Kienböck, note 38. Kienböck's work was confirmed by W. Scholz (Privatdocent an der Universität Königsberg, frühere Assistenartzt an der dermatolog. Universitätsklinik zu Breslau) in a Habilitationschrift completed in June 1901, Ueber den Einfluss der Röntgenstrahlen auf die Haut in gesundem und krankem Zustande. Arch Derm Syph. 1902;59:87–104, 241–60 and 421–45. See also the experiments in which exposure to an X-ray tube killed guinea pigs protected by a grounded metal cage, as reported by Rollins W. X-Light Kills. Bost Med Surg J. 1901 Feb 14;144:173.

[51] Kienböck, note 38.

whose quality the physician could control. After these sittings, the physician would suspend the treatment and wait for results to appear. The quantity of X-rays to which the tissue was exposed was the key variable in this method, and the notion of dose in medical radiology would begin to develop from its adoption. Kienböck's method required more attention to the tube and its output and less attention to the patient and his idiosyncrasy. Since high doses were given in a few sittings, without waiting for a reaction, there was a compelling need for a means of measuring X-ray dosage.

Kienböck's proofs may in retrospect seem trivial and his new method obvious, but that was not the reaction of his opponents. To them, Kienböck appeared to be making extravagant claims, especially when he advocated the use of fewer exposures and higher doses. He would, they warned, find with further experience that X-ray therapy was more difficult than his mechanical approach suggested. Routinized application of X-rays without regard for the special characteristics of individual patients could only lead to injury. Kienböck's method was inherently dangerous because the reactions only appeared after exposure, while the method in common use fractionated the exposures so that they could be stopped as soon as the first signs of a reaction appeared. One opponent offered an experiment in which the static charges around the cathode section of an X-ray tube appeared to kill a bacterial culture while the X-rays radiating from the anode failed to do so. But the primary argument against Kienböck was the weight of the evidence. So many patients had been treated by so many physicians with hard X-ray tubes surrounded by static electric charges. How could they all be wrong?[52]

The majority electrical view was wrong, but it took more than Kienböck's experiments, and other evidence of the same sort, to turn the tide. These experiments may have been a necessary step, but they were not sufficient to extract X-ray therapy from electrotherapy. The other influences at work lay outside both science and medicine. Popular reaction to

52 Ibid.:1053–5, which gives an account of the discussion following Kienböck's oral presentation of his paper. The flaw in the experiment with bacteria was that the culture exposed to the X-rays was shielded with a grounded aluminum sheet to eliminate the effect of the static charges, while the culture exposed to the static charge around the cathode portion of the tube was not. As Kienböck pointed out, this aluminum sheet kept out sunlight as well, which is presumably what killed the bacteria in the other culture.

cases of X-ray injury, and the fear that popular reaction would bring limitations on the use of X-rays in medicine, were essential to hastening the rejection of the electrical view and acceptance among X-ray practitioners of the need for protection and dosimetry. Also important was the recognition that chronic X-ray dermatitis among practitioners could no longer be considered a minor ailment. Radiation protection was not an automatic response by a professional community to the fact of X-ray injuries. Public concern was essential to activating the supposedly self-regulatory professional mechanisms available in the medical radiological community.

Public Concern Incentivizes X-Ray Measurements and Protection

An initial public outcry over X-ray injuries had occurred in 1897 and 1898 in the lay press. The X-ray burns shocked a public that had greeted the new technology with almost unrestrained enthusiasm less than two years earlier. The X-ray practitioners reacted by mounting surveys of X-ray injuries. Ambiguous though the results of the surveys were on the question of whether X-rays were the causal agent, they in general concluded that dermatitis resulted from idiosyncratic reactions of especially sensitive individuals, and that the risk to most people was small. Public reaction, in other words, brought practitioners together to act jointly in defense of their profession, a pattern that would be repeated. Little professional attention was paid to the presence on the hands of many physicians and nonphysician practitioners of chronic dermatitis, which had been recognized as early as 1897.[53] The public was assured that below a certain level of exposure no harm would be done, and that diagnostic X-rays could be given without any risk. An organizer of the British Röntgen Society survey concluded optimistically:

[53] For photographs of a case of dermatitis on the hands of a physician that began in 1896 and became chronic in 1897, see Hall-Edwards J. Chronic Dermatitis of Both Hands. Arch Rönt Ray. 1905;8:92. Acute and chronic X-ray dermatitis were described in Oudin, Barthelemy, Darier. (Paris) Über Veränderungen an der Haut und den Eingeweiden nach Durchleuchtung mit X-Strahlen. Monat Prak Derm. 1897 Nov 1;25:417–46, vorgetragen auf dem Internat. medizinischen Kongresse zu Moskau (or see their short report, Accidents Cutanés Causés Par Les Rayons X. Gaz Hop. 1897;70:1041–2. The distinction between acute and chronic cases was common thereafter, but apparently no further chronic cases were reported until Unna PG. Die Chronische Röntgendermatitis Der Radiologen. Fortschr Röntgenstr. 1904;8:67–91.

> We may, I think, safely assert that the length of exposure necessary to produce an injury is at least three or four times that required to obtain a radiograph with the improved apparatus now at our disposal, even when the most opaque parts of the body are concerned, and then only when the patient is specially susceptible to the electrical forces which cause the injury.[54]

Indeed, the need for unblurred radiographs and greater efficiency in taking them had led by 1900 to improved photographic plates, intensifying screens, and X-ray tubes whose vacuum could be controlled. These improvements, even without any measures taken for protection, had decreased the reports of acute injury. Practitioners, it appeared, were avoiding the errors of the past, and the future would see even greater results from the medical use of X-rays. The weight of the evidence was substantial: a 1902 survey reported that "only one case in 5000 has been injured, and less than half of these seriously."[55]

A second round of public reaction came in the years 1900–1902 in the courts.[56] Here the problem confronting X-ray practitioners was not to be solved solely by allaying public fears. Harm had been done, and patients were suing for damages. As early as 1898 an unsuccessful lawsuit brought in Germany had led to recommendations for reducing exposures

[54] Payne, note 45.

[55] Codman EA. (Harvard Medical School and Massachusetts General Hospital). A Study of the Cases of Accidental X-Ray Burns Hitherto Recorded. Phila Medical Journal. 1902 Mar 8;9:438–42 and 499–503. Codman, who seems to have been agnostic on the electrical view, had earlier complained in reference to Rollins, note 50, "Such sensational headlines as 'X-Light Kills' are apt to give the wrong impression." The fact that the X-ray is in daily use in the large hospitals without harmful results should be put in blacker type than the death of two guinea pigs, see "No Practical Danger from the X-ray." Boston Medical and Surgical Journal; 1901 Feb 28;144:197.

[56] The most extensive, but by no means complete, survey of these cases is in Holzknecht G. (Sachverständiger für das medizinische Röntgenfahren am Landesgericht in Strafsachen in Wien) Die Forensische Beurteilung Der Sogenannten Röntgen-verbrennungen. Fortschr Röntgenstr. 1902;6:145–50 and 177–84. In Germany, physicians acted as expert advisors to the court in such cases. It is striking that in the United States there were already calls for medical judgments before cases came to court and for medical defense unions "to check the nefarious schemings of those pathogenic bacteria of the body politic, the 'shyster t lawyers, to whom by far the larger proportion of such suits owe their origin, in Actions for Malpractice. N Y Med J. 1898 Jul 2;68:21–2, at 22.

and increasing the distance between the tube and the patient.[57] Beginning in 1900, a series of lawsuits succeeded. A climax of sorts was reached in 1902, when a criminal judgment of "negligent bodily injury" against a German physician resulted in a suit for damages of 36,000 marks. The defendant was a particularly irascible and incoherent advocate of the electrical view who had failed to protect the clothed parts of the patient's body.[58] Reinforcing the intellectual impact of Kienböck's experiments, the lawsuits changed professional standards and clinical practice. Shortly after the suit for 36,000 marks was filed, recommendations appeared in the professional literature that aimed to protect not only the patient but also the operator and the manufacturer. These recommendations assumed that X-rays, not static electric charges, caused observed injuries.

Another factor precipitating this concern for protection was the discovery that chronic X-ray dermatitis was developing into skin cancer (epithelioma in the terminology of the time). X-ray dermatitis had been a painful and debilitating ailment. It had not responded to a wide variety of treatments, and even after healing relapses were frequent. There is an enormous qualitative difference in the reaction to malignant and benign diseases. Physicians, no less than laymen and perhaps more, responded dramatically to the discovery in late 1902 that one of Thomas Edison's assistants was suffering from X-ray-induced skin cancer. Death followed in 1904 after successive amputations aimed at saving him from a malignancy that had spread from his hands up his arm.[59] This death was but one

[57] Gocht H. (Sektmdärarzt der Klinik, aus der chirurgisch-orthopädischen Privatklinik des Prof. A. Hoffa in Würzburg). Anklage wegen "fahrlässige Körperverletzung" nach Anwendung der Röntgenstrahlen (Röntgendermatitis). Fortschr Röntgenstr. 1898;2:110–4.

[58] For the defendant's own indignant view of the proceedings, see Schürmayer B. Röntgentechnik und fahrlässige Körperverletzung. Fortschr Röntgenstr. 1902;6:24–43. Holzknecht, note 56, gives a different view of this case, but Holzknecht, it should be noted, was a strong supporter of Kienböck. Holzknecht himself later paid damages of £1450 for burns inflicted in 1902, see Journal of the Röntgen Society. 1902 Jul;2:22.

[59] The case of Clarence Dally, who had worked with X-rays since 1896, is described in Brown P. American Martyrs to Science Through the Röntgen Rays. Springfield, Illinois: Charles C. Thomas; 1936. Edison himself had this to say: "In the case of our Mr. Dally the damage is serious; but now, when we know just how continued exposure to the rays affects the living tissue, we can go ahead safely. Ample protection can be obtained by using a screen of lead about 1/4 inch thick...I...would continue the experiments myself, but my wife won't let me," from an interview in the *Daily Mail* as quoted in Mr. Edison and the X Rays. Arch Rönt Ray. 1903 Aug;8:45. At about the same time

of several that would generate increased interest in radiation dosimetry and protection during the next few years. Cancer, the dread disease that X-rays were supposed to cure, they also caused. This discovery was once again the result of a clinical accident rather than laboratory experimentation. Laboratory physics and biology still had little to offer in guiding experimenters to the discovery of biological effects.

The protection recommendations that resulted from the concern about lawsuits and about cancer were little more than a wise man's view of the measures that would avoid harm.[60] Physician Heinrich Albers-Schönberg, the wise man, was the editor of the leading German radiological journal, Advances in the Field of X-rays. He would play a continuing role in the development of protection measures until his death from X-ray-induced injuries in 1921.[61] In keeping with the goal of protecting the profession, the first among the precautions that Albers-Schönberg suggested in 1903 was to permit only competent physicians to apply X-rays. The issue of physician control would become a major source of contention in the future. Beyond control of clinical practice by physicians, Albers-Schönberg offered what he considered reasonable exposure times and distances (less than four minutes at 30 centimeters no more than three times per day). He also recommended the use of lead shielding around the tube and between the operator and the tube. Assessing the hardness of the tube with one's own hands he thought highly inadvisable, especially since chronic dermatitis absolutely excluded the physician from surgical or obstetrical practice.

as Dally's carcinoma was reported, another case was demonstrated by Frieben at the Arztliche Verein, Hamburg (21 October 1902), see the report of the ensuing amputation in Sick. Fall von Karzinom der Haut, das auf Boden eines Röntgenulcus entstanden ist. Munchen Med Wschr. 1903;50:1445, from the report of the 23 June 1903 meeting of the Biologische Abteilung des ärztlichen Vereins Hamburg.

[60] Albers-Schönberg H. (in Hamburg). Schutzvorkehrungen für Patientin, Arzte und Frabrikanten gegen Schädigungen durch Röntgenstrahlen. Fortschr Röntgenstr. 1902;6:235–8, reprinted from Zbl. Chir.; 1903; 30:637–41. Recommendations for protection of patients, but with an upper limit of exposure time four times as long at approximately the same distance, had already appeared, see the editorial Dermatitis. Arch Rönt Ray. 1901 May;5:84–5. These recommendations were also explicitly a response to lawsuits for damages.

[61] For biographies, see the obituaries in Fortschr Röntgenstr. 1921;28:197–205. and in Strahlenth. 1922;13:538–48. (including a list of publications).

These recommendations were common sense informed by experience. There was no experimental or theoretical reason to believe that the recommendations were adequate, or that they were not excessive. No one had studied dose–response relationships, as later radiation biologists would. There was nevertheless a good deal of reason to believe that the recommendations would provide a measure of protection to the patient from physical harm and to medical radiology from lawsuits. As Albers-Schönberg put it:

> In order to assure the physician protection from such unfortunate occurrences [as a suit for 36,000 marks] and at the same time to protect the public from the possibility of burns, I have drafted some rules for the radiographic examination of patients, whose observance can guarantee an almost certain protection.[62]

Albers-Schönberg was unquestionably sincere. He was already suffering from chronic X-ray dermatitis himself. To some of his colleagues, the recommendations he proposed seemed overly strict.[63] No one challenged the assumption, implicit in the recommendations, that below a still undetermined threshold, no harm would be done.

More important in the long term than the details of these early recommendations was the introduction of X-ray dose measurements. Kienböck had urged that practitioners keep careful records of more than a dozen parameters while administering therapeutic doses, but this so-called "indirect" method never came into use in the form in which he envisaged it. Instead, several "direct" methods of dose measurement that relied on chemical changes caused by X-rays, as well as some simpler indirect methods, were introduced beginning in 1902. These will be discussed in detail in the next chapter. Here the key point is that the introduction of even the crudest measurement of X-ray quantity in the clinic was not automatic for either physician or nonphysician practitioner, in therapy or in diagnosis. For X-rays, measurement was introduced into medical practice to serve the need for protection, which was not recognized for four or five years after the initial applications of X-rays in medicine, due in part to the erroneous "electrical" theory of their effects. To mark the change,

[62] Albers-Schönberg, note 60.

[63] Levy-Dorn (Berlin) M. Schutzmassregeln gegen Röntgen-strahlen und ihre Dosierung. Deut med Wschr. 1903;29:921–1.

the advocates of X-ray measurements referred to their approach as "more scientific."[64] As we shall see, the methods of measuring clinical dose were in fact highly practical and their connections with contemporary physical science tenuous, but the claim to scientific status was made nevertheless.

Radium Protection Lags

Measurements of the quantity of radium would enter the clinic more readily than X-ray measurements had, but the purpose of radium measurements was not protection. Radium was expensive. Anyone acquiring it would want to know how much was bought. Not until just before World War I would radium protection become even a peripheral professional concern, and not until well after the War would it be treated on a par with X-ray protection.

The lack of radium injuries was not the reason for this delay. Physicists and physicians who worked with radium extensively, foremost among them the Curies, suffered obvious effects on their fingers well before 1903. At worst, raw and itching fingers seemed a small price to pay for working with this wonderful new element, just as a few years earlier chronic X-ray dermatitis had seemed a minor ailment to X-ray practitioners. Marie Curie treated her damaged hands as a badge of honor, and in her laboratory protection measures were not encouraged.[65] Pierre Curie collaborated with two physicians in demonstrating that small quantities of radium emanation (radon) administered by respiration could kill mice and hamsters, but this research on laboratory animals did not lead to calls for radium protection.[66] Emanation was readily detectable in the breath and urine of people who worked with radium, but since they had not suffered any acute symptoms this fact was taken as proof

[64] Belot. De l'importance du dosage et de la méthode dans le traitement röntgenothérapique de quelques affections néoplasiques. Verh Deut Rönt Ges. 1905;1:184–8, at 185: "Les méthodes du premier groupe [which used only a single sitting and measured the dose] sont plus scientifique…".

[65] Robert William Reid. Marie Curie. London: Collins; 1974. especially:121, 125, and 273.

[66] Bouchard C, Curie P, Balthazard V. Action physiologique de l'émanation du radium. C R Acad Sci (Paris). 1904 Jun 6;138:1384–7.

that the amounts of radium emanation involved were harmless.[67] In the absence of severe injuries, lawsuits, and public outcry, the professionals most directly concerned discounted the need for radium protection. That lag would persist, even as X-ray protection progressed, until World War I, as we shall see in the next chapter.

[67] Elster J, Geitel H. Uber die Aufnahme von Radium-emanation durch den menschlichen Körper Phys. Z. 1904;5:729–30. eingegangen 15 Oktober 1904 and Loewenthal S. Uber die Einwirkung von Radiumemanation auf den menschlichen Körper. Phys Z. 1906;7:563–4.

CHAPTER 3

X-Ray Protection Advances, Radium Protection Still Lags, 1902–13

The collaboration of the X-ray physicist and the X-ray technician should enable the X-ray therapist to make the exact fundamentals of research science useful for medical practice. Only with the closest consideration of natural laws will methods be devised that achieve practical value for medical science.

—"Introduction," *Strahlentherapies*, 1 (1912) 2.[1]

Let us not forget…that a series of well-established clinical observations is a solid foundation on which to theorize as are laboratory experiments upon the acceleration of an electroscopic leak…the wise physician, while familiarizing himself in so far as may be with all the advances of physics and chemistry, will regard these sciences not as infallible guides, but as handmaidens to his art. He will remember that there are more things in life than can be weighed in a balance or measured by the micro-millimetre scale.

[1] Zur Einführung. Strahlenth. 1912;1:2.: "Die Mitarbeit der Röntgenphysiker und Röntgentechniker soll den Röntgentherapeuten instand setzen, sich die exakten Grundlagen der forschenden Naturwissenschaft für seine medizinische Praxis nutzbar zu machen. Nur unter genauester Berücksichtigung der Naturgesetze konnen Methoden ersonnen werden, die für die medizinische Wissenschaft praktischen Wert erlangen."

D. Serwer, *Strengthening International Regimes*, Palgrave Studies in International Relations, https://doi.org/10.1007/978-3-031-53724-0_3

—Francis Hernamen-Johnson, M.D., "Theory and Practice in Ray Therapeutics," *Journal of the Röntgen Society* (1912).[2]

The first quotation above reflected a common view, especially in Germany, that medicine is ultimately reducible to physical laws. The occasion for the second requires explication. Following a suggestion from a well-known physicist, British radiologist Hernamen-Johnson had attempted to use the "characteristic" X-rays discovered by C. J. Barkla and C. A. Sadler as a therapeutic agent.[3] Hernamen-Johnson announced success before realizing that his equipment permitted the primary beam as well as the secondary rays to strike the body part being treated. The outburst quoted above came when he realized the error, which he blamed entirely on the physicists. He and many other physicians did not anticipate that measurement techniques would prove at least as important as the physician's art in reconciling the laboratory and the clinic as well as in protecting physicians and patients from harm.

How did measurement and protection gain a strong hold on the medical radiological community in the decade before World War I? How did devices for protection and measurement become widespread, and why were the results so different for X-rays and for radium?

Deep Effects Generate Public Fear

Scattered reports of deep effects after radiation exposure had appeared before 1903, but they had been discounted as isolated events without any general bearing on medical radiological procedures. Symptoms reported as side effects of diagnostic or therapeutic irradiation—including heart palpitations, bellyaches, and nausea—were too obviously subjective to attract sustained attention.[4] Physicians would soon view the reports of illness after irradiation in a different light, and damage to the lining of the

[2] Hernamen-Johnson F (M.D.). Secondary X-radiations: Their Uses and Possibilities in Medicine. Proceedings of the Royal Society of Medicine. 1911;5. Electrotherapeutic Section 87–111, session of 16 February 1912.

[3] Thomson JJ. (Cavendish Professor of Experimental Physics, Cambridge; Professor of Physics, Royal Institution). Röntgen Rays in Therapeutics: A Suggestion from a Physicist. The British Medical Journal 1910;2:512–4 an address to the Section of Radiology and Medical Electricity of the British Medical Association, July 1910.

[4] Oudin B, Darier (Paris). Über Veränderungen an der Haut und den Eingeweiden nach Durchleuchtung mit X-Strahlen. Monat Prak Derm. 1897 Nov 1;25:417–45.

stomach and intestines may account for at least some of the symptoms.[5] Before deeper effects became well-known, however, patients' complaints were for the most part regarded as spurious. They were understandably excited when undergoing X-ray examination for the first time. The noisy clatter of mechanical interrupters, the mysterious glow of the tube and the fluorescent screen, as well as the awesome profusion of electrical apparatus aggravated the natural anxiety accompanying the novel experience. An early published report on a stomach cancer that improved with exposure to X-rays went unnoticed at the time, though it has often been cited since.[6]

Evidence of effects on the deeper layers of the skin likewise failed to attract broad attention. As early as 1898, histological investigation had suggested that the primary lesion in X-ray dermatitis was not the most superficial layer of the skin, the epidermis, but rather in the blood vessels of the lower-lying corium. X-rays appeared to destroy the *tunica intima*, the elastic inner lining of the blood vessels. The resulting expansion of the vessels caused the symptomatic swelling and redness of the skin.[7] This effect on deeper-lying blood vessels was, however, attributed to a special sensitivity of the *tunica intima*. It did not therefore arouse general interest in the possibility of deeper effects. So far as radium was concerned, there were reports of fatigue among laboratory workers before 1903, but this common symptom was usually attributed to long working

[5] Seldin M. (Dr. Med., Bobruisk, Russland). Über die Wirkung der Röntgen und Radiumstrahlen auf innere Organe und den Gesamtorganismus der Tiere. Fortschr Röntgenstr. 1904;7:322–39, submitted as an Inaugural Dissertation in March 1904 for the Medical Faculty at the University of Königsberg. Damage to the stomach and intestines was first demonstrated by Regaud C, Nogier T, Laccasagne A. Sur les effets redoutables des irradiations étendues de l'abdomen et sur les lésions du tube digestif determinées par les rayons de Röntgen. Arch Elec Med. 1912;21:321–34, communication présentée au Congrès de l'Association française pour l'Avancement des Sciences à Nimes, en août 1912. It should be noted, however, that by 1912 much harder X-rays were in use (those of Regaud, et al., were filtered through 2 mm of aluminum) and many of the earlier reports may have been spurious.

[6] Despeignes V. (Ancien chef des travaux à la Faculté de médecine de Lyon). Observation concernant un cas Cancer de l'estomac, traités par les rayons Röntgens. Lyon Medical 1896;82:428–30 and 503–6.

[7] Gasmann A. (aus der dermatologischen Universitätsklinik des Herrn. Prof. Jadassohn in Bern). Zur Histologie der Röntgenulcera. Fortschr Röntgenstr. 1898;2:199–207.

hours.[8] X-rays and gamma rays were known to penetrate the body, but most physicians assumed their biological effects were limited in depth.

This assumption that only superficial effects occurred had some justification in Kienböck's experiments and in contemporary physics. The electrical view was rapidly forgotten, along with the primary purpose of Kienböck's experiments. Thereafter, Kienböck was said to have established that only absorbed radiation could cause biological effects. Rays that passed through biological material without being absorbed were believed to have no effects. Absorption of homogeneous X-rays (that is, X-rays of the same degree of hardness) and of gamma rays obeyed an exponential law. Since intensity according to this law fell off exponentially with depth, it was reasonable to expect biological effects caused by absorbed radiation to be confined to the surface layers of tissue.

The discovery of deep effects stemmed from clinical experience. Albers-Schönberg demonstrated early in 1903 that guinea pigs and hamsters could be sterilized by exposure to X-rays without causing surface lesions.[9] He left no trace of his motivation in looking for sterility, but it appears likely that he had been treating eczema of the scrotum with X-rays.[10] For a physician already concerned with the effects of X-rays, but likely unconcerned with the exponential absorption law, it would be a short step to wonder whether such therapy might cause harm to the reproductive capacity of his patients. At about the same time, an American physician reported that he had cured a case of pseudoleukemia, a disease in which lymphoid tissue proliferates, by irradiating lymph nodes.[11] The physician in question believed pseudoleukemia, which is today known as Hodgkin's disease, to be "microbial" in origin. He was probably working

[8] Fatigue among radium workers was later regarded as the result of effects on the blood, see Gudzent F (Assistent der I.Medizinischen Klinik), Halberstaedter L (Assistenten des Instituts). Über berufliche Schädigungen durch radio aktive Substanzen. Deut med Wschr. 1914;40:633–5. aus dem Radiuminstitut für biologisch-therapeutische. Forschung der Charité in Berlin (Direktor: Geheimrat His).

[9] Albers-Schönberg (Dr. med). Ueber eine bisher unbekannte Wirkung der Röntgenstrahlen auf den Organismus der Tiere. München Med Wschr. 1903 Oct 27;50:1859–60.

[10] The routine character of this procedure is evident from a later statement of Holzknecht. Dieser schweren Schädigung [sterility] müssen auch alle Patienten verfallen, deren Skrotum mit üblichen therapeutischen Dosen (Ekzem) beschickt wird. Discussion at the German Röntgen Society, Verh Deut Rönt Ges. 1905;1 at 239.

[11] Senn N (M. D., surgeon). The Therapeutical Value of the Röntgen Ray in the Treatment of Pseudoleukemia. The New York Medical Journal. 1903 Apr 18;77:665–8.

on the by-then largely discredited assumption that X-rays had a bactericidal effect. This report of clinical success nevertheless raised in the minds of other physicians and biologists the question of whether X-rays affected the hematopoietic, or blood-forming, organs, and blood itself. Affirmative answers were rapidly forthcoming from several quarters.[12] Neither the discovery of sterilization nor the discovery of effects on the blood and blood-forming organs depended on knowledge of contemporary physics, which might even have proved misleading. Clinical trial and error were still proving fruitful in mapping unexplored territory.

These discoveries had far-reaching implications for radiation therapy. No longer was radiation limited to the treatment of dermatological ailments. From 1903 on, deep therapy became the most exciting area for clinical trials. Rather than looking at the exponential absorption of radiation and concluding that the effects would be confined to superficial layers of tissue, practitioners began to ask how greater amounts of radiation could be delivered to deeper tissue without causing dermatitis.[13] More penetrating rays were obviously preferable. Filtering X-rays through leather or metal could remove the softer rays that were absorbed in the skin and caused dermatitis. The gamma rays of radium were soon recognized to be especially useful since they were more penetrating than the hardest rays then available from an X-ray tube. If the X-ray tube or radium were moved farther away from the patient, a greater proportion of the radiation was absorbed in the deeper layers relative to the more superficial layers of tissue. This procedure thus enabled greater doses to be delivered to deeper tissues without causing dermatitis in the overlying skin. Irradiation from several different directions likewise permitted

[12] For effects on the spleen and lymph nodes, see Heineke H (Assistent der chirurgischen Klinik in Leipzig). Ueber die Einwirkung der Röntgenstrahlen auf Tiere. Munchen Med Wschr. 1903;50:2090–2 and Ueber die Einwirkung der Röntgenstrahlen auf innere Organe. 1904;51:785–6. For effects on the blood and on bone marrow, see Aubertin C, Beaujard E. Action des rayons X sur le sang et les organes hématopoiétiques. C R Soc Biol (Paris). 1905 Feb 4;58:217–9, laboratoires de MM. Béclère et Blum.

[13] Perthes G (aus dem chirurgische-poliklinischen Institut der Universität Leipzig). Fortschr. Röntgenstr. Versuch einer Bestimmung der Durchlässigkeit menschlicher Gewebe für Röntgenstrahlen mit Rücksicht auf die Bedeutung der Durchlässigkeit der Gewebe für die Radiotherapie. 1904;8:12–25.

greater doses to be delivered to deeper tissues.[14] Deep therapy was to take a giant step during and after World War I with the invention of high-vacuum, hot-cathode X-ray tubes, but already in the first decade of the twentieth century there was intense interest and widespread debate concerning treatment of leukemia and other blood diseases, of what were then termed uterine fibromas (fibroids today) by irradiation of the ovaries, and deep-lying neoplasia.[15]

X-Ray-Induced Carcinoma Redoubles Concern

In addition to the discovery of deep effects and the advent of deep therapy, 1903 and succeeding years saw confirmation of X-ray-induced carcinoma. Edison's assistant, mentioned in Chapter 2, was not an isolated case. From 1903 to 1911, fifty-four other cases were reported.[16] Of these, twenty-six were physicians, twenty-four were technicians, and four were patients. Twenty-six were reported in the United States, a plurality that probably resulted from the widespread experimentation with X-rays there after 1896. Germany and England each reported thirteen cases. Only two were reported in France, probably because of the continued use there of relatively low-intensity tubes excited by

[14] See, for example, Holzknecht. Die Lösung des Problems in der Tiefe, gleich viel und mehr Röntgenlicht zu applizieren, wie an der Oberfläche (Homogen- und Zentralbestrahlung). Verh Deut Rant Ges. 1903;4:73–4.

[15] For a hint of how quickly deep therapy developed, see the following: on leukemia and other blood diseases, the review by Krause P (Privatdozent, Breslau). Zur Röntgenbestrahlung von Bluterkrankungen (Leukaemie, Pseudoleukaemie, Lymphomatosis, perniciose Anemie, Polycythaemia mit Milztumor). Fortschr Röntgenstr. 1904;8:209–35; on uterine fibromas and other gynecological ailments, see the annual reports by Albers-Schönberg H. Röntgentherapie in der Gynäkologie (the title varies slightly). Verh Deut Rönt Ges. 5 (1909)–8 (1912).

[16] 11. Hesse O (Assistent der Kgl. medizin. Univ.-Poliklinik in Bonn, Direktor Prof. Dr. Paul Krause). Das Röntgenkarzinom. Fortschr Röntgenstr. 1911;17:82–92, which is presumably an abbreviated version of his *Symptomatologie, Pathogenese und Therapie des Röntgenkarzinoms*. Leipzig: J. A. Barth; 1911. Krause reported the same figures in his "Zur Kenntnis der Schädigung der Haut durch Röntgenstrahlen." 3. Beitrag zur Kenntnis des Röntgenkarzinoms. Verb Deut Rönt Ges. 1911;7:101–4. The fifty-four cases did not include malignancies that developed after treatment of *lupus vulgaris*, which was thought to develop frequently into carcinoma, see Belot J (chef du service d'électrothérapie et de radiologie du docteur Brocq à l'hôpital Saint-Louis). La radiothérapie ne donne pas les cancers. Bull Soc Radial Med (Paris). 1910;2:34–44.

static generators rather than by induction coils.[17] The pain of the chronic lesions was "almost unequaled by any other disease." Surgery usually proved incapable of halting the spread of the malignancies, and repeated amputations became the rule.[18] Eleven deaths were unequivocally attributed to X-ray-induced carcinoma between 1904 and 1911, including the deaths of eight physicians.[19] At least one death occurred annually during those years.

X-ray-induced carcinoma, along with deep effects, posed threats not only to the health of individual practitioners and patients, but also to the viability of medical radiology as a professional practice. The effects on the blood and blood-forming organs were at first relatively unimportant in this regard. Only after World War I, when their fatal consequences became known to the public, did blood diseases caused by X-rays begin to play a major role in the history of radiation protection. In the decade before World War I, the confirmation of X-ray-induced carcinoma and the discovery of sterilization had the greatest impact on public and professional perceptions. Within medical radiology, the risk of sterility aroused strong fears for the reproductive capacity of both practitioners and patients. Clinical studies soon confirmed that many radiologists were aspermatic (not producing sperm).[20] Histological investigations on laboratory animals showed that X-rays destroyed the epithelium of the seminiferous canal. The fully developed sperm were not necessarily harmed, but the cells that produced them were destroyed.[21] Laboratory

[17] Walter B (Hamburg). "Bericht über die Röntgenausstellung des 2." Internationalen Kongresses für medizinische Elektrologie und Radiologie in Bern, 1–6 September 1902. Fortschr Röntgenstr. 1902;6:56–8. Italian manufacturers also showed "influence" machines at this exposition.

[18] The quotation is from Charles Allen Porter (M.D.), a surgeon who reported on many operations and skin grafts he had done on 47 cases of chronic dermatitis in The Pathology and Surgical Treatment of Chronic X-Ray Dermatitis. Transactions of the American Roentgen Ray Society 1908;101–70, at 159.

[19] Krause, note 15.

[20] Brown FT (M.D.), Osgood AT (M.D.). X-rays and Sterility. The American Journal of Surgery (New York). 1905;18:179–82. All of those examined who had done extensive X-ray work for more than three years showed no spermatozoa in the seminal fluid, but none had suffered obvious effects on the scrotum.

[21] Bergonié J, Tribondeau L. Actions des rayons X sur le testicule du rat blanc. C R Soc Biol (Paris). 57 (Réunion biologique de Bordeaux, séance du 8 novembre 1904):400–2.; ibid. (séance du 6 décembre 1904) 592–5; and C. R. Soc Biol. (Paris). 58 (Réunion biologique de Bordeaux, séance du 17 janvier 1905) 154–8. See also

experiments also showed that X-rays could cause atrophy of mammalian ovaries.[22] The social implications were regarded as dramatic:

> Thus aspermia in the male, sterilization in the female, these are two of the most fearful discoveries that very recent experiments bring us, and is one not justified in saying that here the use of X-rays in medicine has consequences that extend into the sphere of interests of the individual? that it touches directly on the most serious of social problems, the reproduction of the species?[23]

Some practitioners welcomed X-rays as an ideal tool for birth control.[24] Others thought birth control fundamentally immoral and antisocial, or

Frieben (Dr., aus dem Röntgen-institut und Institut für medizinische Diagnostik von Dr. Albers-Schönberg und Dr. Frieben, Hamburg). Hodenveränderungen bei Tieren nach Röntgenbestrahlungen. München Med Wschr. 1903;502:2295.

[22] Bergonié J, Tribondeau L, Recamier D. Action des rayons X sur l'ovaire de la lapine. C R Soc Biol (Paris). 58 (Réunion biologique de Bordeaux, séance du 17 février 1905):284–6 and Halberstaedter L (Assistenarzt der dermatologischen Universitlitsklinik zu Breslau, Dir. Geheimrat Prof. Dr. Neisser). Die Einwirkung der Röntgenstrahlen auf Ovarien. Berlin Klin Wschr. 1905 Jan 16;421:64–6. Halberstaedter got the same results with radium bromide as with X-rays.

[23] Rapport sur les conditions légales de l'emploi médicale des rayons Röntgen, au nom d'une Commission de MM. Brouardel, Debove, Gariel, Gueniot, Hanriot, Motet, C. Perier, Pouchet et Chauffard, rapporteur. Bull Acad Med (Paris). 1906;55:50–64 and the subsequent discussion, 76–95, at 55: "Ainsi azoospermiechez l'homme, stérilization chez la femme, telles sont deux des plus redoutables revelations que nous apportent des expériences toutes récentes, et n'est-on pas en droit de dire qu'ici la Röntgenisation déborde par ses conséquences le cadres des intérèts individuels? qu'elle touche directement à la plus grave peut-être de toutes ces questions sociales, à la reproduction de l'espèce?" The Commission had been set up in response to a proposal by Debove, who was concerned with the "peril social" posed by the sterility of women, Sur l'emploi des rayons Röntgen. Bull Acad Med (Paris). 1905;53:486, séance du 23 mai 1905.

[24] Philipp (Aus Dr. Philipps Röntgeninstitut in Bonn). Die Röntgenbestrahlung der Hoden des Mannes. Fortschr Röntgenstr. 1904;8:114–9: "Was aber diese Versuche für den Arzt Besonders lockend machen musste, war die Aussicht, eventuell hierdurch ein langersehntes soziales Heilmittel zu gewinnen, in der Form einer bequemen und schmerzlosen Sterilisierungs methode," at 116. Dr. Philipp described two successful male sterilizations.

even unpatriotic.[25] All recognized that the discovery of sterilization signified a new and important impact on society, with which medical radiology as a profession would have to reckon. That would prove prescient.

Pre-World War I, professional fear of the public reaction to sterility was a good deal stronger than the public reaction would appear to justify. Newspapers continued to be more interested in X-ray burns than the reproductive effects the practitioners regarded as the more serious social peril. The continuing interest in X-ray dermatitis was annoying to practitioners, who anxiously assured the public that the greatest danger was to the operator.[26] It was, however, easy for physicians to imagine the concerns the public might express about sterilization and the possibly heightened prospects for government intervention in regulating the use of X-rays. This partly self-generated threat to the profession had profound effects, just as the more tangible threat of lawsuits had had a few years earlier.

So far as X-ray-induced carcinoma was concerned, the medical radiological profession generally viewed the moment of greatest danger as past, but public concern forced the risk of carcinoma to a high priority in protection considerations. The introduction of protection measures would, the professionals thought, avoid burns and chronic dermatitis altogether and reduce the risk of carcinoma to a negligible level. The cases occurring after 1903 were, in this professional view, the unavoidable backlog of the previous lack of caution. In the professional literature, the announcements of death became routine: "He will be long remembered for his skill and kindness, and his name will be forever inscribed

[25] Hennecart (prakt. Arzt). Nécessité d'une législation spéciale pour les Rayons Röntgen. Verh Deut Rant Ges. 1905;1:205–9. Hennecart was especially concerned that women might seek sterilization and that existing laws did not prohibit it:

"N'est-ce pas un de leurs devoirs les plus essentiels de favoriser tout ce qui peut contribuer à la richesse de leur pays, au développement de sa population?....Je suppose le cas suivant, qui serait le plus commun. Une femme saine est soumise sur sa demande ou sur son contentement, a l'action des Rayons Röntgen dans le but de supprimer sa fonction de réproduction. Il ne s'en suit aucun accident (Röntgendermite). Elle devient à jamais stérile. Cette femme, le ou les opérateur (médicins ou non-médicins) sont-ils possibles d'une peine quelconque?" (at 206). Hennecart then surveyed the existing French legislation and concluded that the answer was no.

[26] See Editorials. Archives of the Roentgen Ray. 1903 Sep;8:63–4.

in the scroll of the book of Martyrs to Science."[27] The maudlin imagery of martyrdom became standard. Beneath it lay anxiety not only for the welfare of self and colleagues but also for the profession, which was threatened with government intervention and declining interest among physicians.[28] The attitude of the profession toward the victims was therefore ambivalent, including not only sympathy for their plight but also fear of the effect excessive public reaction might have on medical radiology. The "notes" of the British Röntgen Society observed in 1906:

> One cannot but regret the sensational articles on the subject of burns and other unfortunate accidents that have happened to workers with X-rays. Of course we cannot but sympathize with any who in the pursuit of their profession have received injuries by incautiously exposing themselves to the rays, but by allowing accounts of these misfortunes to appear in the lay press no good is gained, and a great deal of harm is done, people have been alarmed, and many individuals to whom the application of radiations for radiographic or therapeutic purposes would be of great benefit refrain from seeking their aid for fear of the harmful consequences.[29]

This professional disdain and fear of the popular press would remain persistent in coming decades, combined with concern for its impact on medical radiology. By making the victims of X-ray-induced carcinoma martyrs to science, the professional medical radiological community was claiming the loss of life was in a worthy cause and also trying to offset

[27] Mr. Wilson of the London Hospital. Journal of the Röntgen Society. 1911 Apr;7:48–9. Mr. Wilson was a "lay worker," a fact that may have made this announcement more modest than the usual.

[28] For the expectation of government intervention, see for example Levy-Dorn M (Berlin). Schutzmassregeln gegen Röntgenstrahlen und ihre Dosierung. Deut med Wschr. 1903;292:921–4 and Dean AE. Les victimes de la radiodermite en Angleterre. Arch Elec Med. 1908;16:484–7, at 486. For the shortage of personnel, especially in radioscopy, see Reid AD. Presidential Address: Survey of the Year's Work in Electrotherapeutics. Proceedings of the Royal Society of Medicine Electrotherapeutical Section. 1911;51:1–8, at 5: "The inducement at present offered to medical men to take up this work, which under the best conditions is one of danger to health, is at present totally inadequate, and we are conscious of the fact that at present very few names are known to us as entering this branch. Several of the small hospitals find it impossible to get medical men to undertake the charge of their departments, and undoubtedly there will be not only a shortage but a dearth of men who will be willing to run the risk of devoting their lives to radiology."

[29] Notes. Journal of the Röntgen Society. 1906 Dec;III(10):48.

the negative public reaction, which radiologists feared would limit the medical benefits radiology could provide. Not until around 1910 was neoplasia produced in laboratory animals using radiation, well after the clinical discovery had become a major factor in shaping the development of medical radiology and radiation protection.[30]

Physicians Seek Control, Specialists Recognize More Is Needed

Among the physician practitioners, the first line of defense for the patient, and for medical radiology, from deep effects and from X-ray-induced carcinoma seemed obvious: as Albers-Schönberg had urged, diagnostic and therapeutic use of X-rays should be the exclusive preserve of physicians. On this issue, the medical radiological community sought government intervention. The newly formed German Röntgen Society in 1905 passed a resolution urging that the use of X-rays be limited by law to physicians.[31] The French Academy of Medicine followed suit in 1906, rejecting an alternative resolution that would have required physician supervision during the operation of an X-ray tube by a specially trained person.[32] In England, physicians in 1905 urged legal action in a

[30] For one effort that produced hyperplasia but no real·tumor, see Rowntree CW (Hunterian Professor at the Royal College of Surgeons and Surgical Registrar at the Middlesex Hospital). X ray carcinoma, and an experimental inquiry into the conditions which precede its onset (Hunterian Lecture at the Royal College of Surgeons, 17 March. 1909). Lancet. 1909 Mar 20;1:821–4. Experimental success in producing a-neoplasm was first reported by Marie P, Clunet J, Raulot-Lapointe G. Contribution à l'étude du développement des tumeurs malignes sur les ulcères de Röntgen. Bull Ass Franc Cancer. 1910;3:404–26.

[31] "Der Röntgenkongress erklart: Die Untersuchung und Behandlung mit Röntgenstrahlen ist eine rein ärztliche Leistung.Dem muss in der allgemeinen und der Medizinalgesetzgebung Rechnung getragen werden. Auch diejenigen Ärzte, die Röntgenuntersuchungen von anderen machen lassen, müssen dies beachten," see Verh Deut Rönt Ges. 1905;1:240. The proposal for this resolution originated with Hennecart, note 25, who suggested it because he thought that physicians would not perform an immoral act like sterilization: "Le souci de notre dignité professionnelle et de notre bon renom auprès de la clientèle est un frein suffisamment puissant." From the discussion of the resolution, it can be inferred that this view was not unanimously held.

[32] "Considerant:

Que l'emploi médical des rayons Röntgen peut déterminer des accidents graves;
Que certaines pratiques peuvent créer un danger social;

resolution of the Electrotherapeutic Society.[33] They also exerted exclusive control over the Archives of the Röntgen Ray, which had been the official organ of the Röntgen Society, and formed an Electrotherapeutic Section of the British Medical Association, thus creating a forum for medical radiology dominated by physicians.[34] This move forced the Röntgen Society, which aimed to promote cooperation between physicians and nonphysicians, to found its own journal.[35] The Röntgen Ray Society of America, which included nonphysicians, was forced to found

> Que seules les docteurs en médecine, officier de santé ou dentistes diplômés (en ce qui concerne la pratique odontologique) sont capables d'interpréter les résultats obtenus au point de vue diagnostic et du traitement des maladies:
>
> L'Académie est d'avis que
>
> L'application médicale des rayons Röntgen, par des personnes non pourvues des diplômes ci-dessus, constitue

un acte d'exercice illégal de la médecine," note 23, at 64, with approval voted at 95. The alternative resolution, which failed to gain any significant support in the discussion, is at 81:

> "L'Académie est d'avis:
>
> 1. Qu'un enseignement soit institué pour la pratique des rayons Röntgen; .
> 2. Que nul ne puisse, sans un diplôme spécial et san le contrôle médicale, faire l'application des rayons Röntgen;
> 3. Que les positions officielles acquises et justifiées par des travaux antérieurs soient respectées."

Efforts to limit medical radiology to physicians had begun earlier in France, see Béclère A. Antoine Béclère. Paris: J. B. Balliere; 1972:58–60.

[33] See the reference to this resolution, passed unanimously in Hall-Edwards J. On X-ray Dermatitis and Its Prevention. Proceedings of the Royal Society of Medicine, Electrotherapeutical Section. 1908 Nov 20;2:11–34 at 25.

[34] The change in the journal occurred with the November 1903 issue, when a nonphysician (Ernest Payne, M. A. and A. I. E. E.) was dropped as an editor, leaving a physician J. Hall-Edwards (L. R. C. P. (Edinburgh) and F. R. P. S.) in charge. At the same time the title was changed to *Archives of the Röntgen Ray and Allied Phenomena* (namely, phototherapy, electrotherapy, and thermotherapy) and an editorial announced the intention "to safeguard as far as possible the interests of the medical profession," Archives of the Roentgen Ray. 1903;8:95. The Electrotherapeutic Section of the British Medical Association was formed in July 1903, see the Programme of Annual Meeting. A supplement to British Medical Journal. 1903;175.

[35] *The Journal of the Röntgen Society* appeared in July 1904 with the explanation that the Archives, which before November 1903 had been "the only journal in which the transactions of the Röntgen Society of London are officially reported," no longer had a member of the Society as an editor.

its own Transactions when physicians took complete control of the American X-ray Journal, expanding its scope to include electrotherapy.[36] The campaign against nonphysician practitioners appears to have fallen short of establishing any new legal prohibitions in Europe or the United States, but it contributed to a reduction in the number of nonphysicians in clinical practice. The campaign against nonphysicians also caused a split in professional institutions that was only slowly bridged during the next two decades.[37]

While physicians seized the opportunity to exert exclusive control over medical radiology, many practitioners (physician and nonphysician), technicians, and manufacturers thought additional responses to the discovery of deep effects were in order. If reserving the practice of medical radiology to physicians was wise, it was because of their general medical knowledge rather than their knowledge of X-rays. The dermatitis from which so many physician practitioners suffered, and the lawsuits filed against them, showed that physicians were not especially well-equipped for radiation protection.[38] The discovery of deep effects greatly increased the need for

[36] This development had begun before the discovery of deep effects, as physician electrotherapists sought control of the *American X-ray Journal*. In 1902, a "publisher's announcement" declared that the journal would "devote its columns to the education of the medical profession in X-Ray and ElectroTherapeutical Practice." This announcement followed the sale of the journal by its founder, Heber Robarts (M. D., M. E.) to T. Proctor Hall (Ph. D., M. D.), see The American X-Ray Journal. 11(1902):1114–5. The official version of this story, told in the anonymous The American Röntgen Ray Society, 1900–1950. Springfield, Illinois: Charles C. Thomas, 1964:5–6 and sanctioned in Ruth and Edward Brecher. The Rays: A History of Radiology in the United States and Canada. Baltimore: Williams and Wilkins, 1969, at 304, would have it that Robarts was "euchred" out of his journal by the electrotherapists, but the contemporary evidence indicates that Robarts himself would have been counted among the electrotherapists, see H. R. Injurious Forces from X-ray Tubes. The American X-Ray Journal. 1902;1049–50. The Transactions of the American Röntgen Ray Society first appeared in 1903 with a report of the third annual meeting (10 and 11 December 1902).

[37] In 1908, the English physician who had proposed the resolution for physician control at the Electrotherapeutic Society commented on the failure to obtain a legal prohibition, "Parliament as a whole is not at all friendly to the medical profession, and it considers that profession is capable of taking care of itself." At the same time, he admitted, "the X-rays, at any rate in the provinces, are not very much used by the quacks. I think that quacks have been frightened by them," see Hall-Edwards, note 33, at 25.

[38] This point was made forcefully by Paul Reynier during the debate on medical control at the French Academy of Medicine. In introducing the alternative resolution quoted in note 32, he exclaimed: "Croyez-vous qu'il suffise de dire que la radiologie sera du ressort exclusivement médical pour éviter [les accidents]? Hélas! trop de procès où des médecins

specialized knowledge of radiation, dosage measurements, and protection devices. Physicians were active in meeting these new demands, but so too were nonphysicians.

The protective devices introduced after the discovery of deep effects and X-ray-induced carcinoma generally aimed to avoid exposure of the operator of the X-ray tube and those parts of the patient's body that were not being treated or diagnosed. In principle, all unnecessary exposure was to be avoided, a principle that would prove fundamental thereafter (and up to the present). Albers-Schönberg and others advocated that the operator stand in a double-lined lead box while using an X-ray tube, which was also enclosed in a lead box that allowed only a narrow pencil of rays to escape.[39] Lead-impregnated glass and rubber appeared on the market.[40] The glass was used to line fluoroscopic screens and in "X-ray proof" spectacles (in order to protect the practitioner during radioscopic examinations) and also to manufacture X-ray tubes with unleaded windows through which only the X-rays that were to be used could pass. Lead-impregnated rubber was preferable to lead sheets for protecting the patient's body because it was more flexible and durable as well as easier to disinfect. An English observer reported as early as 1905, after attending the founding session of the German Röntgen Society:

> A wonderful collection of shields, or 'Schutz-Apparatus' was exhibited. Gloves, aprons and spectacles were universally worn. A mannikin was exhibited clothed in armour of X-ray proof, from eyes to boots, not forgetting the mustache, the most cherished ornament of the German physician.[41]

ont été condamnés à des dommages et intérêts pour brûlures sont là pour démontrer qu'il ne suffit pas d'être médecin pour manier sans accident ces terribles rayons!" Generally, the reply was that physicians should nevertheless be in charge because they had diplomas and licenses, see Debove, note 23, at 92 and "Dangers of X Rays," reprinted from The Family Doctor of 5 September 1903 in Archives of the Roentgen Ray. 1903 Oct;8:84.

[39] Albers-Schönberg H. Technische Neuerungen. Fortschr Röntgenstr. 1903;7:137–49.

[40] For the introduction of lead-impregnated rubber, see Holzknecht G, Grünfeld R (aus dem Röntgenlaboratorium des k. k. allgemeinen Krankenhauses in Wien). Ein neues Material zum Schutz der gesunden Haut gegen Röntgenlicht und über radiologische Schutzmassnahmen im Allgemeinen. München Med Wschr. 1903 Jul 14;502:1202–5.

[41] Butcher, WD. The Röntgen Congress at Berlin. Journal of the Röntgen Society. 1905 Jul;2:6–10.

German manufacturers continued to lead the field, but protection devices also spread rapidly to other countries.

Though protection in the first decade of the twentieth century aimed to avoid all unnecessary exposure, clinical practice entailed compromises. Few operators used the lead-lined boxes.[42] Radioscopy, which necessarily exposed the operator during his viewing of the fluorescent screen, remained in widespread use, both because some diagnoses required it and because it allowed more patients to be examined in less time.[43] Many practitioners took care to avoid the primary beam of X-rays leaving the tube, but they often paid no attention to the scattered X-rays arising from material struck by the primary beam.[44] Some practitioners thought it sufficient merely to stand behind or above the anticathode, because they mistakenly assumed, as Kienböck had, that X-rays were emitted only on the side of the anticathode struck by the cathode rays.[45] The need for protection after 1903 was not in dispute, but under the actual conditions of practice in the clinic the degree of protection achieved varied widely. The individual practitioner had to consider the need for speed, convenience, and simplicity as well.

Nonphysicians Prompt Professional Reaction

Protection measures were not, however, left entirely up to individual practitioners. Public reaction threatened the profession. The profession responded by discussing protection at its meetings, appointing special committees, and subjecting protection to normative decisions of the medical radiological community. Recommendations with professional community endorsement replaced the recommendations of a single wise

[42] Levy-Dorn, note 28.

[43] See the French Academy's report, note 23, at 52: "l'examen radioscopique est le plus économique des procédés (et pour la pratique hospitalière un tel avantage est capital)."

[44] Walter B (Hamburg). Über den Schutz des Untersuchers gegen sekundäre Röntgenstrahlen. Verh Deut Rönt Ges. 1910;6:51–7.

[45] For evidence of this assumption, see the drawings in Kienböck R (aus dem Röntgen-Institut im Sanatorium Fürth in Wien). Ueber die Einwirkung des Röntgen-Lichtes auf die Haut. Wien Klin Wschr. 1900 Dec 13;13:1153–66 and the comments on the dangers of secondary radiation from the glass walls of the tube in B. Walter, note 44. Many tube boxes before World War I appear to have been built without backs, probably to facilitate cooling and to avoid what was considered an unnecessary expenditure.

man. The German Röntgen Society played the leading role in these developments. The issue of physician control had not led to a serious split in this Society. Nonphysicians who specialized in using X-rays continued to play a major role. In Britain, an attempt to establish professional standards through the physician-controlled Electrotherapeutic Society of the Royal Society of Medicine failed.[46] The British Röntgen Society, in which both physicians and nonphysicians continued to participate, was the primary forum for discussion of protection measures, including dosage measurements. In France, Austria, and the United States, countries that had active medical radiological communities but no organizations in which physicians and nonphysicians participated on an equal footing, there were few signs of organized promotion of radiation protection. Interdisciplinary institutions were more amenable to ensuring protection.

This pattern is one we shall see repeated. There were two reasons for this. Though the biological effects of radiation were of medical interest, the choice of protection and measurement methods involved physical and engineering issues beyond the ken of most physicians. In addition, the nonphysicians, including many associated with the manufacturers of X-ray tubes, were readier to act than the physicians, whose economic interests were more directly at stake. Physicians were prepared to maintain the professional equilibrium with which they had been trained to observe disease. Like the general public, the nonphysicians in the medical radiological community were more readily shocked. In a sense, they represented the public reaction in an attenuated form, though with the advantage of being in a position to prevent harmful effects.

From its founding in 1905 until World War I, the German Röntgen Society formed several committees concerned with aspects of radiation protection. Generally, these committees originated in discussions after relevant papers presented at the annual conferences of the Society. The papers were often grouped together in such a way to make the formation of a committee the natural outcome of their presentation, so it is likely that the committees reflected the interests of the Society's leadership. In 1905, at the first congress, a group of papers on dosage measurements led

[46] The Section passed a resolution in 1908 calling for a committee to consider protection measures and to formulate rules, see the discussion following Hall-Edwards, note 33, at 31. This proposal was to be brought before the council of the Royal Society of Medicine at its next meeting, but there is no indication in the succeeding Proceedings of the Section that the committee was created.

to the formation of a Commission for the Determination of Permanent Standards for the Measurement of X-Ray Intensity (later scaled down in its objective and renamed the Special Committee for Scientific and Practical Measurement Methods). It reported its findings in 1907 and ceased to exist in 1912. In 1909, two papers offered evidence of damage to bone during rapid growth, a danger that aroused public and professional concerns because X-rays were being used to treat ringworm in school children by epilating their scalps.[47] These papers led to a Special Committee for the Survey of the Influence of Röntgen Rays on Body Growth, which reported in 1910 that such injuries occurred in men very infrequently, but it also averred that

> ...their possibility is nevertheless present; thus X-ray therapy shall only be engaged in by physicians, and generally by those sufficiently trained; in the hands of every layman and incompetent it is a very dangerous affair that can cause irreparable injury.[48]

[47] Forsterling (Mars, Niederrhein). Wachtumsstarungen nach Röntgenbestrahlung and Krukenberg (Elberfeld). Gehirnschädigung durch Röntgenbestrahlung. Verh Deut Rönt Ges. 1909;5:68–75. In England, there were similar concerns, precipitated by a decision of the Education Committee of the London County Council requiring X-ray treatment of ringworm in school children, see Dawson Turner (M. D.), letter to The Times (30 March 1909); "The Röntgen Ray Treatment of Ringworm," Lancet. 15 1909 May 15;1:1399–1400; J. M. H. Macleod (M. A. St. And; M. D. Aberd; M. R. C. P. Lond; Physician for Diseases of the Skin, Victoria Hospital for Sick Children, Chelsea; Assistant Physician for Skin Diseases, Charing Cross Hospital; Lecturer on Dermatology, London School of Tropical Medicine), "The X Ray Treatment of Ringworm of the Scalp With Special Reference to the Risks of Dermatitis and the Suggested Injury to the Brain," ibid.:1373–7; H. G. Adamson (M. D. Lond; M. R. C. P. Lond; Physician for Diseases of the Skin, St. Bartholomew's Hospital), "A Simplified Method of X Ray Application for the Cure of Ringworm of the Scalp: Kienböck's Method," ibid.:1378–1; Dawson F. D. Turner (B. A., M. D., F. R. C. P. Edin., F. R. S. E., Lecturer on Medical Physics, Surgeons' Hall, Edin.; Examiner in Physics, R. C. P. Edin. and R. C. P. Lond. and University of Edinburgh) and George TJ (L. R. C. P., L. R. C. S. Edin., Carnegie Assistant to Lecturer in Physics, School of Medicine, Royal Colleges, Edin.). Some Experiments on the Effects of X Rays in Therapeutic Doses on the Growing Brains of Rabbits. British Medical Journal 1910;2:524–6, from the Section of Radiology and Medical Electricity, British Medical Association, July 1910.

[48] Bericht des Sonderausschusses für die Sammelforschung über den Einfluss der Röntgenstrahlen auf das Körperwachstum. Verh Deut Rönt Ges. 1910;6:16–17: "ihre Möglichkeit ist doch vorhanden; deshalb darf Röntgentherapie nur von Ärtze, und zwar von genügend hierfür vorgebildeten, getrieben werden; in der Hand eines jedes Laien und Unkundigen ist sie ein sehr gefährliches Wagnis, das irreparable Schädigungen stiften kann."

When in doubt, the medical radiological community reverted to reiterating the need for physician control.

The German Röntgen Society, however, went farther than the issue of physician control in pressing the need for radiation protection. The Society adopted in 1910 a set of "Theses" concerning radiation damage that had been recommended to it by a physician who had frequently acted as an expert in court cases.[49] These theses established general standards of professional conduct, including obligations to provide and use protective apparatus and dosage measurement, to obtain liability insurance, and to permit only experienced personnel to work in X-ray clinics. The implication was that a physician who abided by the theses would be better off in any legal action taken against him. Three years later, in 1913, the German Röntgen Society reinforced the general obligations of the Theses with an "Instruction Sheet" of protection rules, which was to be posted in X-ray clinics and in workshops where tubes were made and tested.[50]

The rules established 2 mm of lead, or its equivalent in other materials, as the minimum protection during lengthy irradiations. The Instruction Sheet also authorized workers in X-ray clinics and employees of tube manufacturers to refuse to work if adequate protection was not provided. Otherwise, compliance was voluntary, though abiding by the rules might prove useful in defending against lawsuits. Compliance might have also made it easier to obtain insurance to cover liability for injuries to patients and practitioners.[51] The 2 mm of lead was a practical compromise that did

[49] For the proposal of the theses, see Gocht (Halle a. S.). Röntgenschädigungen. Verh Deut Rant Ges. 1909;5:72–3. For their adoption, see the Bericht der Kommission zur Beratung der Thesen Bezüglich Röntgenverbrennungen. Verh Deut Rönt Ges. 1910;6:15–16.

[50] The "Sonderausschuss zur Schaffung eines Merkblattes für Schutzregeln" distributed a draft Merkblatt to the 1912 Congress of the German Röntgen Society, but no discussion was held because the committee had not yet reached full agreement, see the report of the Chairman (A. Kohler), Verh Deut Rönt Ges. 1912;8:16. The Instruction Sheet was complete by 1913, when it was decided to print 10,000 copies, suitable for posting, that would be distributed free to manufacturers, see Verh Deut Rönt Ges. 1913;9:14. I am indebted to Mr. A. Hilpert, Geschaftsführer of the Fachnormenausschuss Radiologie, for providing a transcription of this Instruction Sheet from the original in his files.

[51] Albers-Schönberg reported in 1913 that the Stuttgart Allgemeine Versicherungsgesellschaft had reclassified X-ray injuries to physicians and technicians as accidents (for which insurance would be made available) instead of treating them as occupational diseases (for which insurance would not have been available). The Council of the German Röntgen Society responded with approval and suggested that the premiums should be determined

not interfere unduly with clinical manipulations. The specific figure had little, if any, support from laboratory experimentation. Clearly, however, important developments had taken place in the wake of the discovery of deep effects and X-ray-induced cancer. Professional discussion of protection measures had gone far beyond the issue of physician control toward establishing norms for professionals, physicians, or nonphysicians. The German radiological community was reaching consensus on measures that aimed to limit exposure of both patients and practitioners. An interdisciplinary epistemic community concerned with radiation protection norms was beginning to emerge at the national level, though governments were not yet involved.

The approach the German medical radiological community was taking to radiation protection is known today as "command-and-control" regulation, which dictates specific methods, materials, and processes.[52] It is easy to determine whether the practitioner is using the particular practices identified in "command-and-control" regulation. It is less clear that they provide adequate protection. They may even over-protect. Nor is there any guarantee that they will optimize protection with respect to practitioner costs or social cost and benefit. It is far easier to tell people what to do than to require that what they do achieve a particular outcome. But it is also less likely that "command-and-control" regulation will be appropriate to all circumstances, diverse equipment, and different countries. Radiation protection began with "command and control," but it would not remain there.

by considering radiology in the same danger class as surgery, see Verh Deut Rönt Ges. 1913;9:15. During the War, AlbersSchönberg emphasized the importance of carrying liability insurance for damage to patients, see Albers-Schönberg (Prof.), Lorenz (Dr.) (aus dem Röntgeninstitut des Allgemeinen Krankenhauses St. Georg in Hamburg). Die Schutzmittel für Aerzte und Personal bei der Arbeit mit Röntgenstrahlen. Deut med Wschr. 1915;411:301–5.

52 Review TR. Types of Regulation | The Regulatory Review [Internet]. www.theregreview.org. 2016 [cited 2023 Jun 23]. Available from: https://www.theregreview.org/2016/04/05/pritchett-types-of-regulation/.

Practical Clinical Measurements Become Common

The discussion of radiation protection in Germany included X-ray measurement techniques, which came into use more slowly than protection devices.[53] Dose measures, as discussed in Chapter 2, became in an with Kienbock's demonstration that X-rays themselves caused biological effects and with his biological effects suggestion that therapy should be administered in fewer and shorter sittings without awaiting a skin reaction. One of Kienböck's supporters, Guido Holzknecht, introduced the first dosimeter designed for clinical use, a device termed a "chromoradiometer."[54] It was simply a yellow disk of unspecified composition that turned darker on exposure to X-rays. The unit of dose, H (after the inventor of the device), was one-third of the dose required to produce a slight erythema on normal adult skin. The chromoradiometer was supposed to be, above all, a practical device that any physician could utilize without unduly complicating his clinical procedures. The disk was simply placed on the part of the body to be exposed and compared with a standard scale of three shades of yellow, each corresponding to 1 H. Minimum knowledge and manipulation were required, there was no need for the operator to understand how the color change came about, and the device could be read directly without any calculation.

The discovery of deep effects and the confirmation of X-ray-induced carcinoma in 1903 vastly increased the incentive to use X-ray measurements and led to the introduction of other dosimeters as well. Holzknecht's chromoradiometer, though it remained in use in modified form at least until World War I, failed to attain universal acceptance. It was difficult to read because of small differences in the shades of yellow and the variability of the available light. Holzknecht's colleagues resented

[53] Butcher, note 41, reported (at 10): "In only one of the Röntgen-ray institutions which I visited did I see any instruments used for therapeutic dosage." Similarly, an American physician who had visited Germany reported in 1906, "they do not pay so much attention to the dosage of the ray," M. K. Kassabian in the discussion following Williams EG (M. D., Richmond, Virginia). The Regulation and Measurement of the Therapeutic Dose of the Röntgen Ray. Transmission of American Roentgen Ray Society. 1906:84–95.

[54] Holzknecht G. Eine neue einfache Dosierungsmethode in der Röntgentherapie. Wien Klin Wschr. 1902;15:1180–1 with discussion, or Eine neue, einfache Dosierungsmethode in der Radiotherapie (Das Chromoradiometer). Wien Klin Rund. 1902;16:685–7. For a biography of Holzknecht, who died of radiation injuries in 1931, see Kienböck R. Holzknecht semper vivus. Strahlenth. 1937;58:497–8.

his decision to keep the composition of the salts used in the chromoradiometer a secret.[55] Two French physicians designed a "pastille" made of barium platinocyanide.[56] This device was similar to Holzknecht's but it was easier to compare with a standard scale as dehydration of the barium platinocyanide caused a color change from the bright green tint to a dark yellow tint with exposure to a quantity of X-rays supposedly equivalent to 3 H. Designed initially for measuring dosage in the treatment of ringworm, this "Sabouraud-Noire" pastille became the most commonly used clinical dosage device for all therapeutic procedures before World War I, despite the dependence of the pastille readings on the light available and on the ambient temperature and humidity, and despite the requirement that it be placed halfway between the anticathode and the part of the body to be exposed.[57] Also popular was Bordier's variant of the Sabouraud-Noire pastille, which was placed directly on the body and compared with a standard scale of four tints, corresponding to the "principal reactions required in radiotherapeutic treatment."[58] Kienböck proposed a photographic "quantimeter" based on the comparison of exposure of exposed silver bromide with a standard scale. His unit, K, was originally equal to one-half of Holzknecht's H, though both were later changed.[59]

[55] One source says the chromoradiometer was a fused mixture of hydrogen chloride and sodium carbonate, see Hudson JC. Röntgen-Ray Dosimetry. In: Glasser O. The Science of Radiology. Springfield, Illinois: Charles C. Thomas; 1933.

[56] Sabouraud R (Chef du laboratoire de la Ville de Paris à l'hôpital Saint-Louis), Noiré H (adjoint au laboratoire). Traitements des teignes tondantes par les rayons X à l'École Lailler (Hôpital Saint-Louis). Presse Med. 1904;12:825–7.

[57] For the dependence on temperature and humidity, see Bordier H (Professeur agrégé à la Faculté de médecine de Lyon), Galimard J (Préparateur de chimie à la Faculté de médecine de Lyon). Actions des rayons X sur les platino cyanures et en particuliers sur celui de baryum. Cause de leur régénération. Conséquences pratiques de cette étude. Arch Elec Med. 1905;13:323–6. For the effect of the available light, see Regaud, Nogier T. Estimation différente des doses de rayons X suivant les divers modes d'éclairage du chromoradiometre. Arch Elec Med. 1911;19:458–60, Communication au Congrès de l'A. F. A. S., Section d' Électricité Médicale, août, 1911.

[58] Bordier H (Lyon). Radiometric Methods. Arch Rönt Ray. 1906;11:4–13 at 9. The four Bordier tints corresponded to the following: (1) epilation after twenty days; (2) erythema; (3) true dermatitis; (4) ulceration and necrosis.

[59] Kienböck R (Privatdozent, aus dem Radiologischen Institut der Allgemeinen Poliklinik in Wien). Über Dosimeter und das Quantimetrische Verfahren. Fortschr Röntgenstr. 1905;9:276–95.

These "direct" methods of measuring X-ray quantity were the most commonly used in the decade after 1903, but almost any physical or chemical effect of X-rays could be made the basis of a new method. The release of iodine gas from a solution of iodine in chloroform, the precipitation of calomel (mercurous chloride) from a solution of ammonium oxalate and mercuric chloride, the decrease of electrical resistance of selenium, and many other X-ray effects were used to design measurement devices for the clinic.[60] Also available were a number of "indirect" methods based on the parameters of the X-ray tube rather than the measurement of its output. The quantity of X-rays produced was thought to be proportional to the current through the tube. This high-voltage "secondary" current depended on the type of interrupter used and the frequency of the interruption, so it was not related in a simple way to the low-voltage "primary" current used to excite an induction coil. The secondary current had to be measured either by a milliammeter or by the heat generated in the anticathode or in the wall of the tube behind the anticathode. Of the various milliammeters available, the "Deprez-D'Arsonval" instrument, which had a small pivoting coil in the field of a fixed electromagnet, seems to have been most commonly used.[61] Special tubes equipped to measure the heat generated by secondary cathode rays in the wall behind the anticathode were available in Germany, but they do not appear to have been widely used even there.[62]

With some important exceptions mentioned below, both the "direct" and "indirect" measurements of X-ray quantity were assumed before World War I to be independent of X-ray quality, which was not yet understood to refer to wavelength but merely to the penetrating capacity of the

[60] For iodine in chloroform, see Freund L. Ein neues radiometrisches Verfahren (Vorläufige Mitteilung). Wien Klin Wschr. 1904;17:417–8. vorgetragen in der Sitzung der k. k. Gesellschaft der Aerzte in Wien am 8 April 1904; for the precipitation of calomel, see G. Schwarz, *Fortschr. Röntgenstr., 10* (1906–07) 251, in a report on the 25 May 1907 session of the k. k. Gesellschaft der Artze in Wien; for the decrease of selenium resistance, see Athanasiadis G (Athen, Physik. Laboratorium d. Univers.). Wirkung der Röntgenstrahlen auf den elektrischen Widerstand des Selens. Ann Phys. 1908;27:890–6.

[61] D'Arsonval. Dispositif permettant de se rendre identiques les tubes à rayons X. C R Acad Sci (Paris). 1904;138:1142–5 and Walter (Assistent a. Physkal. Staats-Labor. Hamburg). Über die Messung der Intensität der Röntgen strahlen. Verh Deut Rönt Ges. 1905;1:126–34.

[62] Köhler A (Wiesbaden). Über Dosierung in der Röntgentherapie und Vorgänge im Innern der Röntgenrohre. Fortschr Röntgenstr. 1907;11:1–12.

rays. The term "dose" was used loosely, sometimes referring only to quantity and sometimes encompassing measurements of quality as well. The precise relationship between these parameters was undefined. Practitioners measured quantity and quality separately and used the results to specify clinical conditions. The effects of quality differences on measurements of a quantity were generally not considered. The clinical measurement devices were mainly used to observe and characterize, not to experiment and test hypotheses.

Since quality determined the sharpness of an image on the photographic plate, clinical methods of measuring this parameter had been in use before 1900, and the introduction of quality measurements cannot be linked directly with the need for radiation protection. Interest in quality measurements did, however, increase markedly after Kienböck's work and the discovery of deeper effects. "Hardness" of X-rays was originally associated with the degree of evacuation of the tube. It soon became apparent, however, that the essential factor was the voltage across the tube. The length of a gap in parallel with that at which sparks would begin to jump was the simplest method of measuring voltage, and various "spintermeters" of this sort came into clinical use.[63] The sparking potential measured with a parallel spark gap, however, was many times the potential at which most of the current actually flowed through the tube, so several voltmeters were introduced to measure this lower, effective potential.[64] More difficult to use than the parallel spark gap, these voltmeters were less common in the clinic.

In addition to these "indirect" methods of measuring X-ray quality, there were also a number of "direct" methods. The simplest of these was the "phantom hand" which was nothing more than a pasteboard replacement for the practitioner's own hand with which to test the image

[63] For the earliest of these clinical devices, see Béclère A (Médecin de l'hôpital Saint-Antoine). La mesure indirecte du pouvoir de pénétration des rayons de Röntgen à l'aide du spintermètre. Arch Elec Med. 1900 Apr 15;8:153–7.

[64] Klingelfuss (Basel). Die Einrichtung zur Messung der Röntgenstrahlen mit de Sklermoter. Fortschr Röntgenst. 1910;16:64–65; Bergonié J. Mesure du degré radiochromomètrique par le voltmetre électrostatique dans l'utilisations en médicine des rayons de Röntgen. Acad Soc (Paris). 1907;144:28–9, presentée par M. d'Arsonval; and Bauer H. Über einige konstruktive Neuerungen. Verh Deut Rönt Ges. 1909;2:122–6, especially 125–26 and Das Qualimeter. Verh Deut Rönt Ges. 1911;7:137–9 with discussion.

on a fluorescent screen.[65] Such devices were in common use during the first decade of the twentieth century, though they were mentioned only occasionally in the medical literature. More frequently mentioned, though likely less commonly used, were the direct methods that gave a numerical reading. Several of these were based on the same phenomenon: the difference in the absorption of a given output of X-rays in two materials. In one common version, aluminum disks of various thicknesses were mounted with a single disk of silver. The X-rays passed through this "penetrometer" and struck a fluorescent screen. By comparing the brightness of the spots on the screen, the thickness of aluminum that reduced the intensity of the X-rays by the same fraction as the silver could be chosen. The thicker the aluminum disk, the harder the X-rays. The results were specified according to one of a number of arbitrary scales (Benoist, Benoist-Walter, or Wehnelt), depending on the particular instrument used.[66]

For the practitioner, choosing among these different methods of measuring X-ray quantity and quality was perplexing. Each method had an advocate, if only its inventor or manufacturer, and different clinics developed their own preferences. Reviews of the methods available became standard in the medical radiological literature, and both the British and German Röntgen Societies in 1906 and 1907 mounted efforts to compare and evaluate measurement techniques.[67] The results were inconclusive. The English survey, based on experiments undertaken by two nonphysicians, pinpointed the shortcomings of some of the methods of measuring

[65] Beck. Zum Selbstschutz bei der Röntgenuntersuchung. Fortschr Röntgenstr. 1902;6:268.

[66] For the aluminum/silver instrument described, see Benoist L. Définition expérimentale des diverses sortes de rayons X par le radiochromomètre. C R Acad Sci (Paris). 1902;134:225–7, presentée par M. Lippmann; for other versions, see Walter B. Zwei Härteskalen für Röntgenröhren. 6. 1902;68–74 and Wehnelt A. Über eine Röntgenröhre mit veränderlichem Härtegrad und über einen neuen Härtemesser. Fortschr Röntgenstr. 1903;7:221–2.

[67] The best of the pre-war reviews of clinical measurement techniques, discussed below, was Th. Christen (Dr. med. et phil., Privatdozent an der Univ. Bern), *Messung und Dosierung*, Ergänzungsband 28 of *Fortschr. Röntgenstr.* in a series that comprised the *Archiv und Atlas der normalen und pathologischen Anatomie in typischen Röntgenbildern*. Hamburg: Lucas Gräfe und Sillem, 1913.

quantity, but it failed to propose a practical solution.[68] One physician commented, "...to measure a Rontgen ray tube is very much like measuring a will o' the wisp; it is one of the most freakish and capricious things which it is possible to deal with."[69] The German survey, undertaken by a commission of physicians and nonphysicians on the basis of their collective experience, concluded that there was not enough information for a definitive choice on the basis of accuracy or on the basis of theoretical considerations. Practical considerations could therefore be overriding.[70]

This emphasis on practical considerations in selecting a measurement method contrasted sharply with emphasis on the scientific character of a medical procedure that relied on measurements. Especially in therapy, the

[68] Lord Blythswood, Scoble W. A Test of Kienböck's Quantimeter. J Rönt Soc. 1906;3:36–8 and The Relation Between the Measurements from a Focus Tube, with a View to Determine Which are Proportional to the Intensity of the Röntgen Rays. J Rönt Soc. 1907;3:53–67, with discussion. Scoble concluded that ionization methods were best, see his X-Ray Measurement: the Present Position. J Rönt, Soc. 1907;3:99–102, but this solution was not considered practical for the clinic, as discussed below.

[69] Butcher WD. J Rönt Soc. 1907;3 at 62.

[70] Kommission zur Festsetzung fester Normen für die Messung der Intensität der Röntgenstrahlen, Bericht. Verh Deut Ront Ges. 1907;3:15–26 read by the Rapporteur, Wertheim Salomonson (Professor of Radiography and Neuropathology at the University of Amsterdam), at the session of 31 March 1907. The report led to a proposed resolution, at 33 (it is not clear whether it passed): "Bei jeder Messung sollen Daten angegeben werden, die die Stärke der Röntgenstrahlen charakterisieren."

> Die Intensität soll in der Weise angegeben werden, dass die Dosis reproduzierbar sei.
>
> Alle gangbaren Messmethoden, sowohl die direkten als auch die indirekten können dafür gebraucht werden.
>
> Eine bestimmte Methode lässt sich zur Zeit noch nicht empfehlen.
>
> Falls eine photographische, photometrische oder ähnliche Methode benutzt wird, so sollen die Messungsergebnisse womöglich mit der Wirkung einer Hefnerkerze verglichen werden."

This last point, which referred to the standard amyl acetate lamp used in measuring illumination, went unheeded, the Commission was renamed the Sonderausschuss für wissenschaftliche und praktische Messmethoden, and it was disbanded, without reporting again, at the eighth congress (1912). The Commission had been created at the first congress in 1905 in response to a proposal by Friedrich Dessauer, see Verh Deut Rönt Ges. 1905;1:238.

introduction of measurements of quantity and quality brought a claim to scientific precision that only a physician could properly exercise:

> The current great progress that radiotherapy makes each day is to learn to dose with more and more precise rigor the quantity and the quality of the rays used. Just as there is a medicamentous posology [dosage measurement], there exists today a genuine radiologic posology. Is it not obvious that only the physician can examine and settle such delicate questions, and that it is only in this condition that radiotherapy can be a method that is scientific in its procedures, and effective in its results?[71]

Those were rhetorical questions. The answers were intended to be obvious. The public was repeatedly assured that with these new scientific methods, the mistakes of the past could not be repeated.[72] To be sure, new techniques had made both diagnosis and therapy easier and faster: self-regulating tubes that eliminated the widest variations in X-ray quality; transformers that used both phases of alternating current to produce stronger and more continuous high-voltage currents; and water-cooled anticathodes that could withstand the more intense bombardment

[71] See the "Rapport sur les conditions légales...," note 23, at 60: "Le grand progrès actuel que fait chaque jour la radiothérapie, c'est d'apprendre à doser avec une rigueur de plus en plus précise la quantité et la qualité des rayons employés. De même qu'il y a une posologie médicamenteuse, il existe aujourd'hui une véritable posologie *radiologique.*
N'est-il pas évident que seul le médecin peut examiner et trancher ces questions si délicates, et que ce n'est qu'à cette condition que la radiothérapie peut être une méthode scientifique dans ses procédés, efficace dans ces résultats."

[72] See, for example, Holland CT (M. R. C. S., L. R. C. P.). Presidential Address. J Rönt Soc. 1904 Dec;1:25–37, at 36: "At the same time these articles in the daily press are calculated to do harm, as many of the general public reading them may be led to conclude that there is a danger of chronic dermatitis and cancer being caused by having an X-ray examination made, or by being treated with X-rays....It may be definitely stated that no harm whatever can follow from a properly conducted examination, and I think one is justified in saying that the treatment by X-rays in skilled hands is also harmless" Or, see Phillips GES. Presidential Address. J Rönt Soc. 1910 Jan;6:1–14, at 4: "The public are still a little nervous as to X-ray burn. Apart from the fact that a satisfactory remedy seems to have been found, I take it we are agreed that 'burning', in these days, is due either to the ignorance or carelessness of the operator. It would perhaps be well, therefore, if an authoritative and reassuring statement upon the matter were issued by the Council of this Society."

of cathode rays.[73] None of these inventions nor the methods of measuring X-ray quantity and quality, however, owed much to scientific knowledge or the laboratory. Within their own professional organizations, out of sight of the newspapers, the courts, and the public, practitioners agreed that the methods the laboratory physicist used to measure X-ray quantity and quality, to be described shortly, were unsuitable for use in the clinic.[74]

How good, or bad, were the clinical measurements? The answer depended on the needs of their users. X-ray practitioners were generally satisfied with the techniques available for measuring quality directly. Only an occasional voice of concern was raised over the known inhomogeneity of the rays from most tubes and the consequent ambiguity in a specification like "Benoist 5," a reading that could result from X-ray beams that differed significantly in the quality of the rays of which they were composed. There were anomalies in the readings of quality when X-rays were filtered through one of the materials of which a penetrometer was made, since the secondary rays arising from a given material were known to be readily transmitted through that same material. Practitioners did not, however, acknowledge this difficulty.[75] Many physicians doing superficial therapy were also satisfied before World War I with the most commonly used devices for direct measurement of X-ray quantity, or with devices of their own design. As one English physician put it, "I have always three or four means of measurement at hand. I have been working with Kienböck's method, as well as with those of Bordier and Sabouraud, and with the meter I have described to you, and they all work very exactly together."[76]

[73] For these technical developments, see Knox R (M.D.). Recent Improvements in Radiographic Technique. J Rönt Soc. 1910 Oct;6:110–3 and Butcher WD. The Amsterdam Congress, Presidential Address. J Ront Soc. 1909 Jan;5:1–8.

[74] See, for example, the "Bericht," note 70.

[75] This problem had been pointed out even before the discovery of characteristic X-rays, see Walter B. Über das Röntgensche Absorptionsgesetz und seine Erklärung. Fortschr Röntgenstr. 1904;8:297–303.

[76] Pirie H (M. D., B. Sc.). Practical Observations on Everyday X-ray and Electrical Work. J Rönt Soc. 1910 Oct;6:105–10. Or see c. Phillips ES (F. R. S. E.). The Measurement of Radioactivity and X-Rays. J Rönt Soc. 1907 Apr;3:89–99., at 93: "...I gather that the need for a very precise method of comparing X-rays is not so pressing as some appear to think. At least one medical practitioner has pointed out that the errors due to matching the tint of a Sabouraud disc are small relatively [sic] to those arising from the idiosyncracy of the patient. Cases of X ray burn are now happily rare and it therefore

It was among the practitioners doing deep therapy that serious practical and conceptual problems arose. Working at the limits of contemporary capabilities, deep therapists posed questions that would prove of interest to physics as well as to medicine. They had two practical problems. First, they had to choose a filter that would enable them to deliver higher doses to deeper-lying tissues without causing damage to the patient's skin. Aluminum and leather were most commonly used, but some physicians claimed that very thin silver filters were preferable.[77] The advocates of aluminum, and of filters generally, believed that the filter raised the average hardness of the X-ray beam by absorbing more of the softer than of the harder rays, while the advocates of silver claimed that it selectively removed only those rays that caused skin burns.[78] Secondly, deep therapists had to measure doses and compare them with doses measured by colleagues, who used different X-ray tubes and filters and therefore rays of different quality. Such comparisons made it apparent that the existing techniques of measuring X-ray quantity did not give comparable results when quality changed. In France, it appeared that barium platinocyanide varied widely in its response to X-rays of different qualities. As a result, the H units measured in Lyons were "very different from those measured by our colleagues in Paris," perhaps different by a multiplicative factor of four or five.[79] In Germany, deep therapists at Freiburg who used Kienböck's silver bromide strips to measure doses reported delivering safely as much as 200 times the dose normally required to produce erythema to

seems that added to a good practical experience, the methods of Kienböck and others are accurate as far as they go. While I agree that more convenient means should be looked for, a greater degree of accuracy does not appear to be required than is already attainable at the present time."

[77] Von Jaksch R (Hofrat, Professor, Prague). Über Metallfilter. Verh Deut Rönt Ges. 1912;8:71–6, with discussion.

[78] Belot J (chef du service d' Électrologie et de Radiologie à l'Hôpital Saint-Louis). La Filtration En Radiothérapie. Arch Elec Med. 1910;18:648–61.

[79] Regaud C, Nogier T (Agrégés à la Faculté de Médecine de Lyon). Les effets produits sur la peau par les hautes doses de rayons x selectionnées par filtration à travers 3 et 4 millimètres d'aluminium. Applications à la Röntgentherapie. Arch Elec Med. 1913;22:49–66 and 97–128, at 103: "Il est donc évident que les unités H que nous mesurons à Lyon sont très différentes de celles que mesurent nos confrères à Paris."

the skin of women whose ovaries were being irradiated.[80] Most deep therapists did not believe that such high doses were possible without causing harm.[81]

Related to both the filtration problem and the problem of measuring doses was a question that began to attract experimental attention around 1910: did the harder rays used in deep therapy have the same biological effects as the softer rays used for superficial therapy? Many practitioners believed that softer rays were more efficacious since softer tubes often caused epilation and erythema more quickly during diagnosis and brought about more rapid results in superficial therapy, but this clinical observation failed to consider the different absorption of the harder and softer rays in the skin. The experiments undertaken to resolve the question of the variation of biological effects with quality yielded ambiguous answers.[82] At the same time, these experiments would help to clarify the concept of dose, to separate it from the notion of quantity, and to reveal the shortcomings of the clinical measurement methods in use.

Laboratory Concepts and Measurements Fail to Gain Traction in the Clinic

The clearest pre-war statement of these developments was a review of measurement techniques prepared in 1913 by Theophil Christen, a Swiss physician who had obtained a doctorate in mathematics before turning

[80] Gauss CJ, Lembcke H (Freiburg i. B.). Röntgentiefentherapie, ihre theoretischen Grundlagen, ihre praktischen Anwendung und ihre klinischen Erfolge an der Freiburger Universitätsfrauenklinik, 1. Sonderband zu Strahlenth., mit einem Vorwort von Prof. Dr. B. Krönig. Berlin/Wien: Urban and Schwarzenberg; 1912.

[81] See the discussion of dosimeters in Verh Deut Rönt Ges. 1914;10:187–91 and Rundschreiben der Sonderkommission für Dosimetervergleich. Fortschr Röntgenstr. 1915;23:69–70 and the comments of Meyer, at 75–76.

[82] Some experiments showed no effect of quality so long as the absorbed doses were the same, see for example Guilleminot, "Actions biologiques comparées des radiations du radium et des radiations de Röntgen. Loi d'efficacité biochimique des radiations," Comptes Rendus Et Communications IIIe Congres International De La Physiotherapie. Paris: Masson; 1911:674–84. Others showed that the harder rays had greater effect for equal absorbed doses, see for example Meyer H, Ritter H. Experimentelle Untersuchungen zur biologischen Strahlenwirkung. Verh Deut Rönt Ges. 1912;8:126–35, with discussion. Still others thought that different cells reacted differently to radiation of different qualities, see Regaud and Nogier, note 79.

to medicine.[83] To Christen, it was essential to distinguish between the quantity or intensity of the X-rays, which he identified as the energy passing through a given surface, and the dose, which he defined as the energy absorbed in a given volume. This physical dose, which was not necessarily equivalent to the biologically effective dose, was proportional to intensity and, since the harder rays were less absorbed, inversely proportional to hardness. With this distinction in mind, the usefulness of existing direct clinical techniques became dubious. As instruments to measure the quantity of X-rays moving through a given surface, they were inadequate because their readings depended on the absorption in a test body like barium platinocyanide; this absorption varied with hardness. As instruments to measure the dose of X-rays absorbed, they were inadequate because there was no guarantee that absorption in the test body was similar to absorption in a human body. The measurement of absorbed dose would, as we shall see, provide the occasion for much further discussion and lead to the adoption of a less practical dosimetry based on ionization methods, which were virtually unknown in medical clinics before World War I. For the moment, however, Christen's 1913 definition of absorbed dose was a purely theoretical statement, with no instrumental means of entering clinical practice. Despite efforts to design more convenient devices for measuring the ionization of air caused by X-rays, ionization methods continued to be considered suitable apparatus for the laboratory, but not for the clinic.[84]

There were several reasons for this lack of acceptance of ionization methods among X-ray practitioners. Ionization methods were more precise, but they required calculations. Practitioners preferred instruments that would provide an immediate reading. Medical practitioners also needed measurements that were comparable among different clinics. Ionization measurements were comparable only when made with the same instrument, and there was no means yet of comparing X-ray quantity as determined by ionization in different laboratories. Moreover, many practitioners considered the chemical changes they used to measure X-ray

[83] Christen, note 67. For an obituary of Christen by Bernhard Walter, see Fortschr Röntgenstr. 1921;28:391–2.

[84] See especially the instruments designed by Villard P. Instruments de mesure à lecture directe pour les rayons X. Arch Elec Med. 1908;16:692–9 and his "Radiosclérométre," ibid.:236–35.

quantity more appropriate for producing biological effects than ionization. The prevailing assumption was that biological effects were basically chemical, not physical. There was continuing hope that one of the chemical methods of measurement would parallel the desired therapeutic effects. Ionization was eventually to become the focus of reductionist thinking among physicians and biologists, but to the X-ray practitioner before World War I the word still meant little.

Physicists had generally preferred ionization as the basis for their measurements of X-ray quantity and quality since the discovery in 1896 that X-rays ionized air. If air exposed to X-rays was placed in an electric field, there was a "leakage" current that could be used to measure the ionization, which physicists assumed to be a measure of X-ray quantity or intensity. Two types of devices were used to measure the amount of charge produced. In an electroscope, two pieces of gold leaf or other conductor were hinged to an insulator so that they diverged when charged to a high voltage. The rate of fall of the gold leaf was proportional to the leakage current and therefore provided a measure of the ionization of the air. Alternatively, the ionization could be produced between the plates of a condenser charged to a high voltage, and any one of a number of sensitive electrometers could be used to measure the leakage current. Generally, the smaller capacity of the electroscope made it preferable for measuring smaller amounts of ionization. In both devices, it was essential that the voltage be above a certain minimum, the saturation voltage, at which the rate of the discharge of the electroscope or the current measured by the electrometer became independent of the applied voltage. As Ernest Rutherford and J. J. Thomson had explained, the saturation voltage was the voltage required to prevent recombination of the ions before they reached the gold leaf of the electroscope or the parallel plates of the condenser.[85] For specifying X-ray quality, the physicist used the absorption coefficient or sometimes the thickness of a material required to reduce the X-ray intensity to half its original value (the "half-value layer"). To determine the absorption coefficient or the half-value layer, the physicist generally used ionization measurements of X-ray intensity

[85] Thomson JJ (M. A, F. R. S., Cavendish Professor of Experimental Physics, Cambridge), Rutherford E (M. A., Trinity College, Cambridge, 1851 Exhibition Scholar, New Zealand University). On the Passage of Electricity through Gases Exposed to Röntgen Rays. Phil Mag. 1896 Nov;11:392–407, read before Section A of the British Association, 1896.

after passage through aluminum. None of these laboratory techniques, or the concept of ionization on which they were based, made their way into the clinic before World War I.

Commerce Makes Radium Measurements Essential, But Protection Still Lags

Therapy with radium and radium emanation enjoyed an initial period of almost unqualified enthusiasm from about 1903 to about 1906. Thereafter it survived a period of skepticism among physicians who thought exaggerated claims had been made. By 1910 radium therapy was recovering with a more realistic estimate of its potential, which seemed high in the treatment of some dermatological ailments, cancerous growths, and arthritis. The public had remained enthusiastic throughout, with many people "trying radium" for almost any ailment that could not be treated in some other way.[86] After 1910, enthusiasts and skeptics, laymen or physicians, were happy to see the establishment of medical radium institutes.[87] To enthusiasts, these institutes appeared to offer readier availability of radium treatments. To the skeptics, the radium institutes meant more rigorous control of clinical trials. Radium emanation by 1910 was widely available in Continental Europe at health spas.

Radium protection lagged. Few patients suffered acute clinical harm from radium and radium emanation, due to the small quantities available and the frugality of their application. There had been at least one death of a laboratory worker due to a burn caused by radium "imprudently carried in his pocket," but this isolated incident does not appear to have aroused

[86] See the complaints about this public attitude in Moulin CM (Consulting Surgeon to the London Hospital, Vice President of the Royal College of Surgeons). The Treatment of Malignant Growths by Radium. J Rönt Soc. 1911 Jul;7:67–75. In the discussion, J. MacKenzie Davidson, a medical radiologist who was knighted in 1911, commented (at 73): "It is very unfortunate that the public have an idea that radium does cure cancer. I think by 'trying' radium people often end their existence a little sooner than they would otherwise do."

[87] The London Radium Institute began operations in 1911, see its First Report, 14 August 1911–31 December 1912. Brit Med J. 1913 Jan 25. The Pasteur Institute and the University of Paris agreed to build the Curie Institute in 1912, but it was not operational until after World War I. The Radiumhemmet in Stockholm opened before the War.

public concern.[88] Rutherford, Britain's leading researcher on radioactivity, told the Röntgen Society in 1911 that radium had never affected him and that his assistant simply wore rubber gloves to avoid damage to his hands.[89] Without public protest, radium protection continued to lag behind X-ray protection as a subject of professional concern.

Ionization methods were however used in radium clinics. The reasons were largely practical. The sources of radium were few. After 1903, when the Curies won the Nobel Prize and the therapeutic effects of radium started to be widely discussed, the price rose to about $100 per milligram, where it stayed until the opening of the Congo uranium mines around 1922.[90] At this astronomical price, precise measurements of the purity and amount of radium being sold or loaned were an obvious commercial necessity. For the ordinary practitioner, the price of radium was so high that it was entirely out of reach. A few biologists and research-oriented physicians were, however, able to borrow radium from the Curies, from the Viennese Academy of Science, from the German manufacturer Giesel, from the French manufacturer Armet de Lisle, or from individual physical laboratories. With the radium generally came instruction in ionization measurements.[91]

There was no difficulty obtaining radium emanation (radon), since it occurred naturally in mineral waters, but in concentrations that could only be detected by ionization techniques. The sensitive electroscopes

[88] This death is mentioned, without a name or further reference, in the report to the French Academy of Medicine, note 23.

[89] Rutherford E. The Radioactivity of Thorium. J Rönt Soc. 1911 Apr;7:23–30.

[90] "At last supplies of pure radium salts are coming to hand both of home manufacturers and from abroad; the price is high, about £20 per milligramme, but it is something that it is obtainable at any price...," J Rönt Soc. 1911 Jan;7:16. In 1923, the price fell to around £15 per milligramme, see the *South African Mining and Engineering Journal*, 17 February 1923, BARP Clipping File IV at the Library of the British Institute of Radiology. See also Thomson, note 3, who indicated that the price in 1903 had been 8s. per milligram, and said of the subsequent rise to £20 per milligram, "there is no doubt that this enormous rise in price has been due to the widespread belief that radium had been found to be a cure for cancer...".

[91] For reviews of radium therapy, see Oudin P (Paris). État actuel de la radiumthérapie. Comptes rendus des séances du 3e Congrès International d' Électrologie et de Radiologie Médicale, Milan, 5–9 September 1906. 1906; Lille: Camille Robbe:113–27; Loewenthal, S. ed. Grundriss der Radiumthérapie und der biologischen Radiumforschung. Wiesbaden: J. F. Bergmann; 1912; and Lazarus P. Handbuch der Radium-Biologie und Therapie, einschliesslich der anderen Radioaktiven Elemente. Wiesbaden: J. F. Bergmann; 1913.

required were readily available. Physicists had been using them extensively before 1898, and also thereafter, for the study of atmospheric electricity.[92] With the discovery of radium emanation in mineral springs, physicians and nonphysician practitioners at health spas learned quickly how to use electroscopes, though not without making serious errors.[93] By 1910, ionization measurements of radium emanation for medical purposes were common. In Germany and Austria, the results were most often expressed in the "Mache-unit," which was the amount of emanation that would produce a charge of one one-thousandth of an electrostatic unit in a given electroscope.[94] In France, the unit in which amounts of radium emanation were expressed was usually the milligram-second, which was the amount of emanation produced by a one milligram sample of radium in one second.[95] In England and the United States, both units were used, as was the amount of ionization produced by a given amount of uranium.

The ionization measurements used in scientific radiology and in radium work were much more precise than the clinical X-ray dosage techniques physicians continued to regard as "scientific." By 1913, radium measurements would be comparable on an international basis to one part in

[92] See, for examples of this vast literature, Elster J, Geitel H. Beobachtungen des atmosphärischen Potentialgefälles und der ultravioletten Sonnenstrahlung. Ann Phys. 1893;48:338–73, and Mache H. Beiträge zur Kenntnis der atmosphärischen Elektrizität XXI: Über die Genesis der Ionen in der Atmosphäre,. Sitzungsber Akad Wiss (Wien), Abt IIa. 1905;114:1377–88. Elster, Geitel and Mache turned their electroscopes to use in measuring radioactivity as well.

[93] Errors occurred, for example, when practitioners introduced a sample into an electroscope without taking account of the consequent change of the electroscope's capacity, see for example the criticism of Herr Saubermann (an advocate of radium emanation in therapy) in Mache H, Meyer S. Über die Radioaktivität der Quellen der böhmischen Bädergruppe: Karlsbad, Marienbad, Teplitz-Schönau-Dux, Franzensbad sowie von St. Joachimsthal. Sitzungsber Acad Wiss (Wien), Abt IIa,. 1905;114:355–85., vorgelegt in der Sitzung am 16 Februar 1905, at 376; and also S. Russ' criticism of W. S. Lazarus-Barlow's (M. D., F. R. C. P.) claim to have discovered substances that would retard the leak of an electroscope, in the discussion following the latter's Radioactivity and Animal Tissues. J Rönt Soc. 1910 Apr;6:33–51, at 40. For reviews of the therapeutic uses of radium emanation, see Lowenthal and Lazarus, note 91, and also Lachmann (Bad Landeck i. Schl.). Die Radiumemanation in der Balneologie. Strahlenth. 1913;2:153–69.

[94] The unit was introduced by Mache H (aus dem II. physikalischen Institute der k. k. Universität in Wien). Über die Radioaktivität der Gasteiner Thermen. Sitzungsber Acad Wiss (Wien), Abt IIa. 1904;113:1329–52.

[95] Curie P, Laborde A. Sur la radioactivité des gaz, qui se dégagent de l'eau des sources thermales. C R Acad Sci (Paris). 1904;138:1150–3, transmise par M. Potier.

a hundred. Physicists nevertheless emphasized the practical character of ionization methods. The physicist knew only too well that the process of ionization was not one he understood. By 1906, it was clear that the prevailing theory of X-rays and gamma rays, the pulse theory described briefly in Chapter 2, could not account readily for the expulsion of an electron from an atom. The pulse, which spread as it left the source of X-rays or gamma rays, would decrease in intensity with the square of the distance. No single pulse would have enough energy localized in a given direction to cause ionization and to give the secondary electrons as much energy as they were known to have.[96] For the physicist, the "scientific" way of measuring the energy of X-rays or gamma rays was to measure the heat produced when they were absorbed. But the physicist's attitude toward this procedure was similar to the X-ray practitioner's attitude toward ionization measurements: theoretically desirable, but impractical. Only occasionally was the heat produced by X-rays and gamma rays measured directly, sometimes producing inexplicable results.[97] For most purposes ionization measurements sufficed, despite their lack of scientific grounding.

For a decade after the discovery of radium, physicists and chemists had managed without any formal international cooperation in standardizing

[96] This "spreading difficulty" would generate many proposals and debates over the next twenty years, but for one of its earlier manifestations see Wien W (Physikalische Institut, Würzburg). Über die Energie der Kathodenstrahlen im Verhältnis zur Energie der Röntgen und Sekundärstrahlen. aus der Willner Festschrift mit einigen Zusätzen, Ann Phys. 1905;18:991–1007, received 27 November 1905. Wien suggested that the pulses were stored up in an atom until there was sufficient energy to trigger the expulsion of an electron, and that the secondary electron got some of its energy from the atom rather than from the X-ray pulse.

[97] The earliest of the efforts to measure the heating effect of absorbed X-rays was Dorn E. Ueber die erwärmende Wirkung der Röntgenstrahlen. Ann Phys. 1897;63:160–76, Halle, 8 August 1897 (Die Ergebnisse sind der Naturforschenden Gesellschaft zu Halle am 8. Mai d.J. mitgetheilt). Especially well-known and often-cited was Rutherford E (M. A., B. Sc., Macdonald Professor of Physics, McGill University, Montreal). Energy of Röntgen and Becquerel Rays, and the Energy required to produce an Ion in Gases. Phil Trans. 1901;196A:25–59, communicated by Professor J. J. Thomson, received 15 June 1900 and read 21 June 1900. Others, however, had difficulty finding any heating, see Leininger F (Würzburg, Physikal.-Institut). Notiz fiber Energiemessungen der Röntgenstrahlen. Phys Z. 1900;2:691–3., eingegangen 3 August 1901. Moreover, the notion of a "trigger" effect, as in Wien, note 96, cast doubt on using the heating effect as a measure of the energy of X-rays since some of the heat would have been due to energy originating in the atom.

measurements. Each laboratory kept a small radium standard of its own in order to determine the radioactivity of samples in terms of the activity of a given weight of radium. If problems arose, standards were exchanged among laboratories and checked against each other. If a new research group needed to establish a standard, a member of the group went to a leading laboratory and compared a highly purified sample of radium salt with the sample kept as a standard there. In Britain, this decentralized system had become more formal than elsewhere after an effort to establish an X-ray standard by comparison with a given amount of radium led a Standards' Committee of the Röntgen Society in 1908 to define the ionization produced by the gamma rays from a pure one milligram sample of radium bromide after passage through a one-centimeter-thick lead shield as the "Unit of Radioactivity."[98] This unit never served the initial purpose of X-ray standardization. It was used only in radium work. Radium standards were prepared, compared with the standard of Rutherford and Boltwood, and deposited in the National Physical Laboratory. There was, however, still no formal means of establishing whether the British standards were the same as those used in other countries.

The informal system of radium standardization started fraying in 1909 when Otto Brill, an Austrian working in the laboratory of Sir William Ramsay, one of the leading English radium chemists, challenged Marie Curie's 1907 determination of the atomic weight of radium. Criticizing Curie for not checking for impurities other than barium, Brill claimed that with improved purification he had determined an atomic weight of 228.5

[98] "Interim Report of the Standards' Committee" presented in January 1908. Journal of the Röntgen Society. 1908 Feb;4:27–36. The suggestion that X-rays be standardized by comparison with radium had been made by Phillips CES. The Need for a Radioactive Standard. Journal of the Röntgen Society. 1906 Apr;2:79–90 and 92–102. The Council of the Röntgen Society formed a committee "of men sufficiently well known in the scientific world to carry weight," including ten people from the scientific community, four from the medical community and two who are not readily identifiable, see Journal of the Röntgen Society. 3 (1906) 16 and 48. The suggestion for the Committee had been made originally by Butcher WD. The Means of Accurate Measurement in X-ray Work. Journal of the Röntgen Society. 1905 Apr;1:74–87 with discussion. For the deposit of the-standard at the National Physical Laboratory, see Journal of the Röntgen Society. 1909 Jan;5:20 and W. Deane Butcher's comments during the session "Radiometrie, Terminologie," 13 September 1910 at the Congrès International pour l' Étude de la Radiologie et d'Electricité, *Comptes rendus*, volume 1.

rather than Curie's 226.[99] Her figure, it would turn out, was correct for the most common isotope of radium. But Rutherford, who had participated in the Röntgen Society Standards' Committee, was sufficiently concerned to compare his own standard with samples obtained from other countries. He found a sample Curie sent 9 percent lower in activity than his own, and other samples were low by as much as 20 percent.[100] The purity of a radium sample reflected directly on the skills of its producer and the value of the product, so at stake was the national and professional pride and reputation of radium research workers in Britain, Britain, Austria, and probably other countries as well.

Also at stake was the capacity to continue scientific and medical research with radium on an international basis. The purity and atomic weight of radium had a direct impact on scientific questions like determining the charge of an alpha particle, on medical questions like the amount of radium to use in reproducing the therapeutic results of other clinics, and on commercial questions like the value of radium from different sources. Physicists had faced difficulties of this sort before. They had been solved by establishing international standards like the meter and kilogram kept at the International Bureau of Weights and Measures at Sèvres or by carefully defining the precise conditions under which a physical unit should be measured, as in the international definitions of the unit of electrical resistance (the ohm) adopted in the 1880s and 1890s.[101]

[99] Curie. Sur le poids atomique du radium. C R Acad Sci (Paris). 1907;145:422–5 and Brill O. Über die Fortschritte der chemischen Forschung auf dem Gebiete der Radioactivität,. Verh Ges Deut Naturf Artz. 1909;81:124–49, at 132ff.

[100] The 20 percent figure is mentioned in E. Rutherford, *Radiumnormalmasse und deren Verwendung bei radioaktiven Messungen*, tr. B. Finkelstein. Leipzig: Akademische Verlagsgesellschaft, 1911, at 13. This booklet apparently never appeared in English and is not included in Chadwick J. The Collected Papers of Lord Rutherford of Nelson. London: George Allen and Unwin; 1962. Curie's sample is mentioned in a Rutherford letter to Stefan Meyer, 25 April 1911 (Rutherford Correspondence microfilms): "I forgot whether I told you that a small standard which Mme Curie sent me last year was about 9 per cent lower than my standard. She was cautious, however, in committing herself to its correctness on account of the uncertainty of weighing such small quantities." The Rutherford Correspondence microfilms are on deposit with the Sources for the History of Quantum Physics at the American Institute of Physics (New York); the American Philosophical Society (Philadelphia); the University of California (Berkeley); and the Niels Bohr Institute (Copenhagen). The material contained in these microfilms is listed in Badash L. Rutherford Correspondence Catalogue. New York: American Institute of Physics; 1974.

[101] Isaachsen D. Introduction Historique. In: Ch-Ed Guillaume, La Création du Bureau International des Poids et Mesures et Son Oeuvre. Paris: Gauthiers-Villars; 1927:1–31;

Taking the lead in promoting international standardization, Rutherford was careful to avoid any reference to Curie's sample and any identification of the others that had not agreed with his own. Publicly, he agreed with the view "that no one else should be called on for the important work of furnishing a radium standard than Mme. Curie, the discoverer of radium."[102] Rutherford also emphasized that the needs of science, medicine, and commerce converged, leaving to the imagination of his readers the difficulties in continuing competitive efforts in all three fields if agreement were not reached on a radium standard.[103]

Agreement was reached by 1912, though not without manifestation of the strong national feelings that the question of standardization aroused. At the International Congress of Radiology and Electricity, a meeting of the scientific radiological community in Brussels in 1910, there were proposals for standards and comparison methods from England, France, and Germany.[104] Amid the chaos of the poorly organized and high-spirited meeting, there emerged under Rutherford's guidance an agreement that Curie would prepare a radium standard to be certified by an International Radium Standards Committee with a maximum of two physicists representing each country. The amount of radium emanation in equilibrium with one gram of radium was defined as the "curie."[105] Unsure of the health and competence of Curie, Rutherford encouraged

British Association for the Advancement of Science. Reports of the Committee on Electrical Standards: A Record of the History of "Absolute Units" and of Lord Kelvin's Work in Connexion with Cambridge: University Press; 1913.

[102] Rutherford, note 100, at 44: "...dass niemand anders zu der wichtigen Arbeit, ein Radiumnormalmass herzustellen berufen sei, als Mme Curie, die Entdeckerin des Radiums ...".

[103] Ibid.

[104] Rutherford E (Manchester). Rapport sur les étalons de Radium; Danne J (Paris), Sur la nécessité de créer un étalon international de Radium; Lenard P (Heidelberg), Sur les mesures et les unités radioactives and Becker A (Heidelberg), Sur l'émanomètr; all in the 380. Résumés des communications, Congrès international de Radiologie et d'Électricité, Bruxelles, 13, 14 and 15 September 1910. Radium. 1910;7:221–47.

[105] Statuts de la Commission de étalon. Radium. 1910;7:65 (feuilles de couverture). The members of the International Radium Standards Committee were M. Curie and A. Debierne for France, H. Geitel and O. Hahn for Germany, St. Meyer and E. von Schweidler for Austria, B. Boltwood for the United States, E. Rutherford and F. Soddy for Britain, and A. S. Eve for Canada. Geitel's appeal to include Elster, his constant collaborator, on the basis "dass er sich als Hälfte von Elster und Geitel fühle," was rejected on the grounds that only two from each country were permitted, see Stefan

the Viennese physicist Stefan Meyer to prepare an additional standard. Curie's work was delayed, less by her chronic illness than by the scandal over her alleged affair with the married physicist Paul Langevin.[106] Early in 1912, however, the standardization was completed to everyone's satisfaction: Curie's standard and Meyer's were found to be in very close agreement using a comparison method invented by Rutherford and his student James Chadwick.[107] Competition in scientific and medical work with radium, as well as commerce in the radioactive material, could continue on firm ground.

By 1913 the contrasts between X-ray and radium dosimetry and protection were striking. X-ray medical practitioners used a bewildering array of devices to measure doses and to protect both themselves and their profession. They emphasized the scientific character of the therapy they administered. In fact, however, clinical X-ray measurement techniques and protection devices were unknown in scientific laboratories and were designed to meet practical requirements. Medical users of radium, disregarding the issue of protection, nevertheless used the more precise ionization techniques familiar to the scientific laboratory, where they were regarded as practical. What was "scientific" depended on which community you belonged to. Despite medical radiology's claims of "scientific" status, there was still no understanding, even in contemporary terms, of the physical, chemical, and biological phenomena underlying the impact of X-rays and radium on living organisms. That did not prevent medical applications in the clinic.

Meyer to Rutherford, 29 September 1910 (Rutherford Correspondence microfilms), note 100, though this requirement does not appear in the statutes.

[106] See Reid R. Marie Curie. New York: New American Library; 1974. The encouragement to Meyer is in the letter quoted in note 100: "In case Mme Curie is unable to complete her work, it will be of great importance to have another standard ready to put in its place."

[107] Hahn, St. Meyer, v. Schweidler E. Bericht über die Versammlung der internationalen Radiumstandardkomission in Paris vom 25. bis 28. März 1912. Radium Biol Heilk. 1912;1:354–6 and Rutherford E (F. R. S.), Chadwick J. (B. Sc.) A Balance Method for Comparison of Quantities of Radium and Some of Its Applications. Proceedings of the Physical Society. 1912;24:141–51, received 21 February 1912, read 23 February 1912.

CHAPTER 4

War Enlarges and Enriches Medical Radiology, 1912–18

In the history of physics, the demonstration of X-ray diffraction in 1912 by three German physicists was a critical event. It might seem reasonable to assume that this experimental breakthrough was critical for medical radiology as well. In fact, two other events in physics proved more significant: the 1907 discovery of characteristic secondary X-rays by the English physicists C. G. Barkla and B. A. Sadler; and the 1911 cloud-chamber photographs showing the paths of secondary cathode rays taken by another English physicist, C. T. R. Wilson. This work in physics was closely tied to the question of the nature of X-rays. Barkla was a leading exponent of the pulse theory, which held that X-rays were pulses of no single wavelength generated in the deceleration of charged particles. Wilson's cloud-chamber photographs supported the views of W. H. Bragg, who from 1907 to 1912 advocated a particle theory of X-rays and gamma rays. Bragg and Barkla were enmeshed in these years in a complex controversy over the nature of X-rays and gamma rays that was resolved by the experimental work of Max Laue, Paul Knipping, and

D. Serwer, *Strengthening International Regimes*, Palgrave Studies in International Relations, https://doi.org/10.1007/978-3-031-53724-0_4

Walter Friedrich.[1] Their X-ray diffraction patterns demonstrated that X-rays behaved neither like Barkla's pulses nor Bragg's particles, but rather like ordinary electromagnetic waves like light.

The Physicists Understand More but Still Have Little to Offer Medical Radiology

What would a physicist in 1914 have known about the interaction of X-rays with matter? Today we regard X-rays and gamma rays as having a dual character that enables them to behave both like particles and like waves, but that apparently contradictory notion would not find general acceptance until quantum theory provided a theoretical basis after World War I. The detailed story of the X-ray diffraction experiments and their interpretation is a complex one. Physicists did not accept Laue's original explanation of the diffraction patterns, and that explanation is not the one in use today.[2] To those outside physics, however, it appeared that the nature of X-rays had been unequivocally elucidated. They were not electromagnetic pulses. Instead, X-rays were electromagnetic waves like light but with much shorter wavelengths. The "softer" X-rays had longer wavelengths closer to ultraviolet light and the "harder" X-rays had shorter wavelengths. Crystals diffracted X-rays just as a sufficiently fine slit or grating diffracted light. Using the interference patterns, it was possible to determine X-ray wavelengths, and by 1914 it was also possible to calculate them from the known absorption coefficients of homogeneous X-rays.[3]

As fundamental as the discovery of the nature of X-rays was to physics, it failed to solve other important problems and had little immediate effect on medical radiological research or practice. Medical radiologists knew the results of the X-ray diffraction experiments and they increasingly

[1] For an account of the Bragg-Barkla controversy, see Stuewer RH. William H. Bragg's Corpuscular Theory of X-Rays and γ-Rays. The British Journal for the History of Science. 1971 Jun;5(3):258–81.

[2] On the lead-up to the diffraction experiments, see Forman P. The Discovery of the Diffraction of X-rays by Crystals; a Critique of the Myths. Archive for History of Exact Sciences. 1969 Jan 1;6(1):38–71. On the different treatments of the results, see Chapter 5 of Heilbron JL. H. G. J. Moseley: The Life and Letters of an English Physicist, 1887–1915. University of California Press; 2022.

[3] Siegbahn M. Über den Zusammenhang zwischen Absorption und Wellenlänge bei Röntgenstrahlen. Phys Z. 1914;15:753–6, eingegangen 11 Juli 1911.

talked of "wavelengths" rather than "hardness" and "penetrating power" in referring to X-ray quality. Interference measurement of X-ray wavelengths remained, however, a laboratory technique and did not enter the clinic.[4] Moreover, the nature of X-rays was only one of the three interrelated problems physicists had faced since 1896. The other two were the nature of the processes generating X-rays and the mechanism of the interaction of X-rays with matter. The diffraction experiments and the theory that accounted for them failed to solve these problems. The notion that X-rays were produced by the deceleration of cathode rays remained much as it had on the pulse theory. In 1915, when it was discovered that the maximum frequency of the X-rays produced by Coolidge's tube was proportional to the voltage across the tube, the electromagnetic wave theory could provide no better explanation than the pulse theory.[5] Moreover, the electromagnetic wave theory did nothing to solve the "spreading difficulty." Like pulses, waves would spread from their point of origin and have insufficient energy to cause the observed ionization when they were absorbed in air.

It was partly to solve the spreading difficulty that Bragg had proposed a particle theory of X-rays. In his theory, ionization produced by the absorption of X-rays was due to secondary cathode particles. Bragg regarded an X-ray or gamma corpuscle as a "neutral pair," which he described as a cathode particle combined with enough positive electricity to neutralize its negative charge. In passing through matter, the neutral pairs would occasionally be torn apart by collisions with atoms, and releasing more cathode rays. These "secondary" cathode rays would then cause the ionization usually attributed to the X-rays themselves.[6]

[4] For reference to spectrometers as scientific instruments unsuitable in the clinic, see Glocker R (D. phil.). Eine neue Methode zur Intensitäts- und Härtebestimmung von Röntgenstrahlen (besonders für Zwecke der Tiefentherapie). Fortschr Röntgenstr. 1916;24:91–101.

[5] Duane W, Hunt DL. On X-ray Wave-Length. Physical Review. 1915 Jan 1;6:166–77. This relationship was readily explicable on Einstein's light quantum hypothesis, which was not yet generally accepted, see Stuewer RH. The Compton Effect: Turning Point in Physics. Science History Publications; 1975.

[6] Bragg WH. On the Properties and Natures of Various Electric Radiations. Philosophical Magazine. 1907 Oct 1;14(82):429–49, read before the Royal Society of South Australia, 7 May 1907 and 4 June 1907, and Bragg WL. The Consequence of the Corpuscular Hypothesis of the γ and X rays, and the Range of β rays. Philosophical Magazine 20. 1910 Sep 1;20(117):385–416.

In 1911, C. T. R. Wilson had succeeded in making the paths of the charged particles involved in the ionization of a gas visible and thereby lent strong support to Bragg's view of this process. By triggering a lamp with a mechanism that also caused the expansion of a chamber saturated with water vapor and exposed to X-rays, Wilson photographed the water droplets that condensed along the paths of the charged particles immediately after the expansion. These "cloud-chamber" photographs clearly showed the short paths of the secondary cathode rays. The ionization was not spread uniformly throughout the gas, as would have been expected if it were caused by either electromagnetic pulses or waves. As Wilson said, the pictures agreed with Bragg's view that cathode or β rays caused the ionization attributed to X-rays.[7] Bragg's particle theory of X-rays fell victim after 1912 to the diffraction experiments, but the cloud-chamber photographs remained. Physicists could no longer view the cathode rays as coming from Bragg's neutral pairs and instead thought absorbed X-rays ejected them from an atom, a process termed "ionization." Moving at high velocities through a gas, or through living tissue, these secondary cathode rays collided with atoms and caused the bulk of the observed ionization.

Physicists had observed secondary cathode rays from the absorption of X-rays in metal sheets before Wilson's cloud-chamber photographs of their paths in a gas. Their velocities, like those of electrons produced from metal surfaces by ultraviolet light (the "photoelectric effect"), were independent of the intensity of the radiation and depended only on the hardness of the X-rays.[8] When in 1912 the diffraction experiments showed that X-rays were electromagnetic waves, physicists assumed that the velocities of the secondary cathode rays could be calculated from the

[7] Wilson C. On a Method of Making Visible the Paths of Ionising Particles Through a Gas. Proceedings of the Royal Society of London. 1911 Jun 9;85(578):285–8.

[8] Cooksey CD (Sheffield Scientific School of Yale University). On Corpuscular Rays Produced in Different Metals by Roentgen Rays. American Journal of Science. 1907 Oct 1;(142):285–304. and, Innes P. (M. A., B. Sc., 1851 Exhibition-Scholar of the University of Edinburgh, Trinity College, Cambridge). On the Velocity of the Cathode Particles Emitted by Various Metals under the Influence of Röntgen rays, and Its Bearing on the Theory of Atomic Disintegration. Proceedings of the Royal Society of London. 1907 Aug 2;79(532):442–62.

same "Planck-Einstein" relation that governed the photoelectric effect.[9] Today, we associate the Planck-Einstein relation with a particle theory of light and X-rays, which are regarded as "photons" or light quanta. Before the early 1920s, however, physicists did not regard this relation as a statement concerning the energy of light particles. They viewed the Planck-Einstein relation as governing the transformation of the energy of an electromagnetic wave into the kinetic energy of cathode rays. Applied to the secondary cathode rays revealed in the cloud-chamber photographs, the Planck-Einstein relation would play an important role in the development of X-ray dosimetry.

The cathode rays were not the only "secondary" rays produced by X-rays when they were absorbed in matter. Röntgen himself had been among the discoverers of scattered X-rays.[10] These appeared to be equivalent in hardness to the primary beam, but they radiated in all directions from the place where the primary beam was absorbed. A great deal of experimental research had been conducted on scattered X-rays during the first decade of the twentieth century. Barkla, using the pulse theory as a guide, had been a major contributor to this work. In 1907, he and Sadler discovered that on exposure to a heterogeneous beam of primary X-rays, the element nickel produced not only scattered radiation but also homogeneous secondary rays softer than the primary beam. Further investigation showed that these homogeneous X-rays were characteristic of the element exposed to the primary beam, that they were softer the lower the atomic weight of the material, and that they could only be

[9] On the origins in Einstein's work on the "Planck-Einstein" relation, see Klein MJ. Einstein's First Paper on Quanta. Natural Philosophy. 1963;2:59–86. See also Stuewer, note 5.

[10] Even in his "preliminary communication," Röntgen concluded that solid bodies scatter X-rays just as turbid media scatter light, see paragraph 8 of Eine neue Art von Strahlen (Vorläufige Mitteilung). Sitzungsber Phys-Med Ges (Würzburg). 1895;132–41, at 137–8. In his third (1897) communication, Röntgen demonstrated the scattering of X-rays by air, see paragraph 1 of "Weitere Beobachtunger über die Eigenschaften der X-Strahlen," *Math. Naturwiss. Mitt. Sitzungsber. Preuss. Acad. Wiss.*, Physik.-math. Kl., 189,7 as translated in Glasser O. Wilhelm Conrad Röntgen and the Early History of the Roentgen Rays. Springfield, Illinois: Charles C. Thomas; 1934:401–18. Stuewer, note 5 above, mistakenly calls J. J. Thomson's 1903 suggestion that X-rays would be scattered "an extremely bold conjecture, since no scattering experiments of any kind had been carried out as yet," at 3. In fact, however, scattered X-rays, or S (for secondary) rays as they were sometimes called, were well-known before Thomson's theoretical explanation for them on the basis of the pulse theory.

excited by a primary beam containing X-rays of equal or greater degree of hardness.[11]

By 1914, physicists were focused on Barkla's characteristic X-rays, which would prove critical to the development of a quantum theory of the atom.[12] For practical purposes, however, the most important aspects of the characteristic rays were experimental. Corresponding to the emission of characteristic secondary X-rays were absorption edges: as the hardness of the primary beam was increased, its·absorption in a given material increased sharply at the same degree of hardness as the characteristic secondary X-rays and then declined gradually. As a result of this selective absorption, materials absorbed X-rays of different quality differently, and the exponential law for the decrease in X-ray intensity did not hold in the region of the absorption "edges." Moreover, every material appeared to be especially transparent to X-rays corresponding to the hardness of its own characteristic X-rays, since these would be selectively absorbed and reemitted. By the beginning of World War I, characteristic secondary X-rays had been observed in all elements down to the atomic weight of aluminum.

With these details in the background, we can summarize the immediate pre-war situation in physics from the point of view of someone interested in the interaction of radiation with matter. The simple picture of exponential absorption of X-rays or gamma rays of any given hardness held ten years earlier had changed considerably. X-rays produced several different kinds of secondary radiation: the scattered X-rays of approximately the same quality as the primary X-rays; the characteristic X-rays of equal or lesser hardness than the primary beam; and the cathode rays that were directly responsible for the ionization caused by exposure to the primary beam. Gamma rays from radium were also scattered and produced secondary cathode rays. With increasing hardness, X-rays showed selective absorption edges characteristic of a given element. The proportion of X-rays or gamma rays that was scattered increased with the

[11] Barkla CG, Sadler CA. Secondary X-rays and the Atomic Weight of Nickel. Philosophical Magazine. 1907 Sep 1;14(81):408–22 and the general review, Barkla CG, Sadler CA. Homogeneous Secondary Radiations. Philosophical Magazine. 1908 Oct 1;16(94):550–84.

[12] Heilbron JL. The Kassel-Sommerfeld Theory and the Ring Atom. Isis. 1967;58:450–85 and Forman P. The Doublet Riddle and Atomic Physics Circa 1924. Isis. 1968 Jul;59(2):156–74.

hardness of the rays, and this proportion was also greater for elements of lower atomic weight. The velocity of the secondary cathode rays produced in the absorption of X-rays or gamma rays increased with the hardness of the radiation in accordance with the Planck-Einstein relation, and this velocity was independent of the intensity of the radiation. The interaction of X-rays with matter was a complex process, and these phenomena were not readily explicable on the generally accepted theory that X-rays and gamma rays were electromagnetic waves. The physicist understood far more than a decade earlier, but little of this knowledge was readily applicable in medical radiology.

Biologists and Physicists Find Some Common Ground

While this anomalous situation was developing in theoretical and laboratory physics, the use of radiation as a research tool in biology was expanding rapidly nevertheless. The effects of radiation on germ cells and radiation-induced carcinoma excited the interest of biologists and research-oriented physicians working on embryology, heredity, and cell development. In the decade before World War I, they began to regard radiation as an elegant means of disturbing the normal course of development and reproduction. If they could identify the primary lesion in such a disturbance, the biologists would have a hint of which structures in the cell controlled these processes. Biological laboratories used radium more than X-rays, but this preference was due to the constant attention required in operating an X-ray tube rather than to scientific considerations. If radium could be obtained, it was easier to use than an X-ray tube. Biologists assumed the gamma rays of radium would produce biological effects similar to those of X-rays.

Exposing a variety of experimental samples—molds, fertilized eggs of sea urchins and of worms found in horse saliva, tadpoles, and plant cells as well as various tissues from higher species—biological investigations produced a significant volume of descriptive material concerning radiation damage on the cellular and subcellular levels.[13] In 1905, two

[13] Hertwig 0. Das Radium als Hilfsmittel für Entwicklungphysiologische Experimente,. Deut Meu Wschr. 1911;373:2209–12; also Bohn G. Influence des rayons du radium sur les animaux en voie de croissance. C R Acad Sci (Paris). 1903;136:1012–3, présentée par Alfred Giard, séance du 27 mil 1903 and Influence des rayons du radium sur les

French physicians had summarized their investigations of the differential effects of X-rays on the various cells of the rat testicle: "X-rays act with greater intensity on cells the greater their reproductive activity, the longer they take in cell division, and the less their morphology and functions are definitively determined."[14] This rule of thumb, known as the "law" of Bergonié-Tribondeau, stood up remarkably well during the next ten years. There were exceptions to the generalization, but it nevertheless summarized a vast amount of experience and came to be regarded as the cornerstone of radiation biology.

To biologists who believed the chromosomes were essential to cell reproduction and heredity, the law of Bergonié-Tribondeau suggested that the strings of highly staining material in the nucleus might be the site of the primary lesion in radiation effects. The chromosome theory of heredity was not, however, a dominant view before World War I. Radiation had other biochemical effects that might account for the damage to tissue. It affected a number of enzymes and also cleaved the phospholipid lecithin (which seemed to be present in all cells), producing toxins.[15]

oeufs vièrges et fécondés, et sur les premiers stades du développement, ibid., 1085–86, presentée par Alfred Giard, séance du 4 mai 1903; Dauphin J. Influence des rayons du radium sur le développement et la croissance des champignons inférieurs. C R Acad Sci (Paris). 1904;138:154–6; Perthes (aus dem Chirurgisch-poliklinischen Institut der Univ. Leipzig). Versuche über den Einfluss der Röntgenstrahlen auf die Zellteilung. Deut Med, Wschr. 1904;301:632–5 and 668–70; and Gager CS (New York Botanical Garden), Effects of Exposing Germ Cells to the Rays of Radium and Effects of Radium Rays on Mitoses. Science. 1908;27:335–6.

[14] Bergonié J, Tribondeau L. Interprétation de quelques résultats de la radiothérapie et essai de fixation d'une technique rationnelle. C R Acad Sci (Paris). 1906;143:983–5, présentée par M. d'Arsonval, at 983: "les rayons X agissent avec d'autant plus d'intensité sur les cellules que l'activité reproductrice de ces cellules est plus grandes, que leur devenir karyokinetique est plus long, que leur morphologie et leurs fonctions sont moins définitivement fixées."

[15] The lecithin hypothesis was originally proposed by Schwarz G (cand. med., aus dem Röntgen-Laboratorium des k. k. Wiener allg. Krankenhauses). Ueber die Wirkung der Radiumstrahlen (Eine physiologisch-chemische Studie am Hühnerei). Arch Physiol Mensch Thier. 1903;100:532–46. See also Schaper A (Prof., aus der Entwicklungsgeschichtlichen Abteilung des Anatomischen Institutes in Breslau). Experimentelle Untersuchungen über die Wirkung des Radiums auf embryonale und regenerative Entwicklungsvorgänge. Deut Med Wschr. 1904;302:1434–7 and 1465–8; and Werner R (Assistenten der Chirurgischen Klinik der Universität Heidelberg. Direktor: Geh.Rat Professor Dr. V. Czerny Exzellenz). Zur Kenntnis und Verwertung der Rolle des Lecithins bei der biologischen Wirkung der Radium- und Röntgenstrahlen. Deut Med Wschr. 1905;311:61–3. A report to the tenth Röntgen Congress favored the lecithin hypothesis, see Krause P (Prof. Dr., Bonn). Die

Foremost among the advocates of the chromosomes as the site of the primary lesion in radiation effects before the War was the German embryologist Oscar Hertwig who, with his daughter Paula, produced extensive experiments to demonstrate that radiation affected the chromatin directly (that is, not indirectly as a result of other biochemical effects) and that the effects on the unfertilized sperm or egg manifested themselves after fertilization in the development of the individual.[16] Indeed, there were several claims to the experimental demonstration that characteristics acquired by exposure to radiation were inherited, but these claims did not gain general recognition.[17]

Beginning around 1910, and accelerating rapidly thereafter, the chromosomal view of radiation damage gained ground, becoming the plurality if not a majority view during and after World War I. There were two important factors in this change: the chromosome theory of heredity was gaining wider acceptance from 1910 on, and the colloidal aggregate theory of proteins appeared to offer a general account of how radiation might affect the chromosomes, which were then thought to consist primarily of many small protein molecules (only forty years later were they demonstrated to be the long double helix DNA molecules familiar today).[18] According to the colloidal aggregate theory, proteins

biologischen Wirkungen der Röntgenstrahlen auf tierisches und menschliches Gewebe,. Verh Deut Rönt Ges. 1914;10:24–45. For effects on enzymes, see the summary in Loewenthal S. Grundriss der Radiumtherapie und der biologischen Radiumforschung. Wiesbaden: J. F. Bergmann; 1912.

[16] Hertwig O (aus dem anatomisch-biologischen Institut zu Berlin). Die Radiumkrankheit tierischer Keimzellen. Ein Beitrag zur experimentellen Zeugungs- und Vererbungslehre. Arch Mikro Anat, 77, Abt II. 1911;1–164; Hertwig, P. Durch Radiumbestrahlung hervorgerufene Veränderungen in den Kernteilungsfiguren der Eier von Ascaris megalocephala. ibid.:301–11; and Hertwig O. Versuche an Tritoneiern über die Einwirkung bestrahlter Samenfäden auf die tierische Entwicklung. Zweiter Beitrag zur experimentellen Zeugungs- und Vererbungslehre. Arch Mikro Anat, 82, Abt II. 1913;1–63. For Oscar Hertwig's advocacy of the chromosome theory of heredity, see Der Kampf um Kernfragen der Entwicklungs- und Vererbungslehre. Jena: Gustav Fischer; 1909.

[17] Fraenkel M (Charlottenburg). Die "Vererbung erworbener Eigenschaften" mittels Röntgenbestrahlen nachgewiesen. Verh Deut Rönt Ges. 1911;7:91–9 with discussion, and Marie P, Clunet J, Raulot-Lapointe G. Hérédité des caractères acquis, chez les cellules néoplastiques. Bull Ass Franc Cancer. 1911;4:166–72.

[18] On the acceptance of the chromosome theory of heredity, see the brief discussion in Allen GE. Life Science in the Twentieth Century. New York: Wiley; 1978:56–68. For the colloidal aggregate theory of proteins, see Loeb J. Proteins and the Theory of Colloidal Behavior. 2nd edition. New York: McGraw Hill; 1924, the tendentious denigration in

were colloids held in suspension by electric charges on their surfaces. Discharge of the colloidal particles would cause precipitation. Beta rays from radium had been shown to cause the precipitation of inorganic colloids as early as 1904.[19] X-rays apparently also caused the precipitation of organic colloidal protein in the formation of cataracts in the eye, an effect that had been observed in laboratory animals as early as 1905.[20] A French physician reviewed the relevant medical and biological literature and drew a straightforward conclusion shortly before the War: radiation precipitated the colloidal proteins that he thought constituted the chromosomes and thus affected the hereditary material.[21] In some cases, the cells might be so damaged that they could not reproduce at all, thus resulting in the destruction of tissue after a latency period that depended on the life span of the cells.[22] With smaller doses, biologists thought the precipitation of colloidal protein could stimulate cell growth, leading to cancer.

Florkin M, Stotz, EM. The Dark Age of Biocolloidology. In: Chapter 14 of A History of Biochemistry. Amsterdam: Elsevier; 1972, the brief description in Olby R. The Path to the Double Helix: The Discovery of DNA. London: Macmillan; 1974:6–7, and the references to the important role of the colloidal aggregate theory in studies of the antigen-antibody reaction between 1900 and 1920 in Mazumdar PMH. The Antigen-Antibody Reaction and the Physics and Chemistry of Life. Bulletin of the History of Medicine. 1974 Jan 1;48(1):1–21.

[19] Henri V, Mayer A (laboratoire de physiologie de la Sorbonne). Action des radiations du radium sur les colloïdes. C R Soc Biol (Paris). 1904;56:229–30 and Précipitation des colloïdes positifs par les radiations β du radium 57. Soc Biol (Paris). 1904;57:33–4.

[20] Tribondeau, Récamier. Altérations des yeux et du squelette facial d'un chat nouveau-né par röntgenisation. C R Soc Biol (Paris). 58 (Réunion biologique de Bordeaux, séance du 6 juin 1905):1031–2.

[21] Bordier H. Actions biochimiques des radiations et en particulier des radiations de Röntgen. Arch Elec Med, presented to the Fourth International Congress of Physiotherapy (Berlin, 23–30 March 1913). 1913;22:289–314, and in German. Biochemische Wirkung der Strahlen, insbesondere der Röntgenstrahlen. Strahlenth. 1913;2:367–95. Bordier had suggested earlier that radiation precipitated colloidal proteins in causing damage to the fingernails of radiologists, see Bordier H (Professeur agrégé à la Faculté de médecine de Lyon). Actions des rayons X sur les ongles: essai d'interprétation des effets de ces rayons sur les tissus vivants. Congrès International pour l' Étude de la Radiologie et de l'Ionisation (tenu à Liège du 12 au 14 septembre 1905), Comptes rendus. Paris: H. Dunod; 1906:86–8.

[22] Reineke H. Zur Theorie der Strahlenwirkung, insbesondere über die Latenzzeit. München Med Wschr. 1914;61:807–14.

In addition to its plausible links to the chromosome theory of heredity and to the colloidal aggregate theory of proteins, this view of radiation effects had the advantage of being comprehensible from the point of view of the physicist. Ionization was precisely the physical process required to discharge the colloidal proteins. Not until the early 1920s would the "point-heat" theory (discussed in Chapter 5) provide a mathematical link between the secondary cathode rays in Wilson's cloud-chamber photographs and biological effects, but already on the eve of World War I there appeared to be a loose articulation between the physicist's view of the interaction of radiation with matter, a view he could admittedly not account for on the prevailing electromagnetic wave theory of X-rays, and the biologist's view of the interaction of radiation with colloidal proteins, including chromosomes. The physics and biology of radiological effects appeared to be more unified, but scientific radiology still had little to offer medical radiology.

Technology Offers More Than Physics or Biology to Medical Radiology

The invention just before World War I of a high-vacuum, hotcathode X-ray tube by William David Coolidge would be a major factor in bringing about post-war integration of scientific and medical radiology.[23] At least since Rutherford's comment that the Coolidge tube was "a triumph of the application of the latest scientific knowledge and technique," it has been traditional to stress the scientific component of this invention, and even to suggest that it stemmed from a program of "pure," as opposed to "applied," research.[24] Coolidge was an American working at the newly founded General Electric Research Laboratory in Schenectady. With a bachelor's degree from MIT in electrical engineering and a

[23] Coolidge WD (Research Laboratory of the General Electric Company, Schenectady, New York). A Powerful Röntgen Ray Tube with a Pure Electron Discharge. Physical Review. 1913 Dec 1;2(6):409–30. For a biography of Coolidge, see Miller JA. Yankee Scientist. Mohawk Development Service; 1963.

[24] For Rutherford's comment, see his Silvanus P. Thomson Memorial Lecture. Journal of the Röntgen Society. 1918;14:75–86, at 83. For the notion that the General Electric research program was "pure," see Trout ED. Tubes and Generators. In: Classic Descriptions in Diagnostic Röntgenology. Springfield, Illinois: Charles C. Thomas; 1964:213–23 at 217: "From a program of pure research, three men, Coolidge, Langmuir and Dushman reported on work that would bring significant changes in X-ray technology."

doctorate from the University of Leipzig in physics, Coolidge belonged to a growing group of academically trained physicists doing industrial research. The scientific component of his invention was unquestionably strong. Coolidge knew the relationship between the temperature of a filament and the charge it emitted from the work of the English physicist O. W. Richardson.[25] Irving Langmuir, Coolidge's colleague at General Electric, had worked with these "thermionic" currents in high-vacuum tubes.[26] To evacuate his tubes, Coolidge used a so-called "molecular" pump designed in 1913 by the German physicist W. Gaede. This pump worked on physical principles that had been discovered in the previous decade.[27] Neither the heated cathode nor the high vacuum was entirely new to X-ray tube technology, but the combination was a unique one. Coolidge understood from Langmuir's work that the residual gas in the ordinary X-ray tube was the source of rapid variations in X-ray hardness, and that a tube could operate without this gas if a sufficient flow of electrons could be generated from the cathode.

The scientific input was not, however, the entire story of the Coolidge tube. Coolidge began his research in the mundane world of product improvement by working on the production of ductile tungsten for use as a filament in electric light bulbs. With a melting point of well over 3000° centigrade, tungsten was well-suited to this use, but because it was hard and brittle at ordinary temperatures it could not be easily "worked," as required in a mass production process. By mechanically manipulating tungsten at temperatures well below its melting point and removing small trace impurities, Coolidge managed to produce flexible tungsten

[25] Richardson OW. On the Negative Radiation from Hot Platinum. Mathematical Proceedings of the Cambridge Philosophical Society. 1902;11 and Richardson OW. The Electrical Conductivity Imparted to a Vacuum by Hot Conductors. Proceedings of the Royal Society. 1903;71:415–18, communicated by Professor J. J. Thomson (F. R. S.), received 28 February and read 26 March 1903. Thomas Edison was the discoverer of the emission of "negative radiation" from hot filaments, which was generally known as the Edison effect.

[26] Langmuir I. The Effect of Space Charge and Residual Gases on Thermionic Currents in High Vacuum. Physical Review. 1913 Dec 1;2(6):450–86.

[27] Gaede W. Die Molekularluftpumpe. Ann Phys. 1913;41:337–80. For this and other developments, see Dushman S. Scientific Foundations of Vacuum Technique. Wiley; 1949:126–7, 136–59 and 176–90.

wire.[28] Having succeeded in making this refractory element workable, Coolidge looked for other applications. General Electric was a major producer of X-ray tubes. The use of alternating current transformers to produce high-voltage discharges had increased the amount of current that could be passed through an X-ray tube. The resulting increased bombardment of anticathode targets by cathode rays generated much more heat. For this and other reasons, the problem of choosing a material for the anticathode was a common subject of discussion among manufacturers around 1910.[29] In his 1912 patent application, Coolidge noted the use of ductile tungsten not only as a filament in incandescent lamps, but also as a covering for the anticathodes of X-ray tubes.[30]

This part of Coolidge's work cannot be described as "pure" research. Far from transforming technology by the application of scientific principles, Coolidge reported that his work on ductile tungsten required

> ...twenty trained research chemists, with a large body of assistants, in the research laboratory. These men were of course given, from the factory organization, all of the mechanical and electrical assistance they could use, and were assisted in no small measure by the staff of the incandescent lamp factory.[31]

The methods were essentially trial and error, especially in the purification of tungsten. There were no fundamental principles of physics involved. There were even reasons to believe, as Coolidge pointed out, that tungsten, because of its relationship to other metals in the periodic table, would not become more ductile with further purification. Coolidge's success in producing ductile tungsten cannot, then, be viewed solely as a scientific contribution to technology. When in 1913 he used his ductile tungsten as a hot-cathode in a high-vacuum X-ray tube, Coolidge was again responding to a commercial imperative, not a scientific one.

[28] Coolidge WD. Ductile Tungsten. Transactions of the American Institute of Electrical Engineers. 1910;29:961–5 as reproduced in A. J. Bruwer, note 24 above, 247–9, at 249.

[29] See, for example, Gardiner JH. Quantitative Measurements of the Conversion of Kathode Rays into Röntgen Rays by Anti Kathodes of Different Metals. Journal of the Röntgen Society. 1910;6:83–97 with discussion.

[30] Coolidge WD. Tungsten and Method of Making Same for Use as Filaments of Incandescent Lamps and for Other Purposes. 1930. U.S. Patent 1,082,933 as described by Trout, note 24 above.

[31] Coolidge, note 28 above, at 249.

Rapid variations in hardness made it difficult to use X-rays for either diagnostic or therapeutic purposes. A great deal of ingenuity had gone into inventing regulators that would automatically adjust the gas pressure in the tube, and easy control of X-ray quantity and quality had been a major selling point for General Electric and other tube manufacturers.

The Coolidge tube had significant advantages over earlier models when it came to controlling X-ray output. Because cathode rays (or as Coolidge said, electrons) rather than ions of the gas in the tube carried the bulk of the current, the quantity of X-rays produced was more nearly proportional to the current through the tube and their quality was more nearly proportional to the voltage across the tube. These two parameters could be adjusted independently, with the current depending on the temperature of the cathode. Easy regulation of output, along with spectacular reliability in continuous use, incentivized the rapid adoption of the Coolidge tube in medical practice. Less obvious to Coolidge in 1913, but just as important for medical radiology in the next decade, were the high voltages that could be used across a Coolidge tube. Before World War I, the voltages in use were almost entirely in the range of 20,000 to 50,000 volts. By the end of the War, a few clinics were using up to 200,000 volts. Higher voltages meant more penetrating X-rays. Medical practitioners would double and triple the thickness of the aluminum filters they used, and they would then turn to copper filters. In the physicist's terms, the wavelengths of the X-rays available decreased from a minimum of around 0.4 angstrom to a minimum of around 0.04 angstrom. Medical radiology, and especially deep therapy, had a new and powerful tool at its disposal.

Thus, on the eve of World War I, X-ray technology more than radiation biology, and radiation biology more than radiation physics, offered contributions to medical radiology. Clinicians, however, were just beginning to absorb them. The first reports on the clinical use of Coolidge tubes had just appeared, the medical radiological literature was beginning to mention secondary rays, and physicians were slowly becoming familiar with ionization. No major impact from these developments was yet detectable. Coolidge tubes were only one of several sorts being tested, including the hot-cathode but lower-vacuum Lilienfeld tube.[32]

[32] Lilienfeld JE, Rosenthal WJ (aus dem physikalischen Institut (Direktor: Prof. Dr. O. Wiener) und dem chirurgisch poliklinischen Institut (Direktor: Prof. Dr. H. Reineke) der Universität Leipzig). Eine Röntgenröhre van beliebig und momentan einstellbarem, vom

The importance of secondary rays in X-ray dosimetry and protection was still uncertain. Kienböck's silver bromide paper and the barium platinocyanide pastilles were the most commonly used clinical dosage devices, with ionization methods still limited to the physics laboratory and to clinical work with radium.

War Expands the Profession and Its Resources

The War disrupted many professional institutions and the easy international discourse among scientists and physicians that had previously prevailed. It may seem plausible to suggest that it simply delayed inevitable developments. Thus, Derek de Solla Price's notion that war shifts the exponential growth curves of a scientific field might have proven true for both scientific and medical radiology.[33] International conferences of scientific radiologists (scheduled to be held in Vienna in 1915) and of the medical radiologists (which would normally have been held in 1916) were postponed.[34] The German Röntgen Society did not hold its annual congress between 1914 and 1920. Journals on both sides suffered delays in publication.[35] A leading French practitioner completed a report on the radiotherapy of uterine fibromas that he had begun in 1913 with a continuation published in 1918.[36] British radiologists, who had been

Vakuum unabhängigem Härtegrad. Fortschr Röntgenstr. 1912;18:256–63. Lilienfeld and Rosenthal used an auxiliary hot cathode to increase the flow of current through the tube.

[33] De Solla Price DJ. Science since Babylon. New Haven, CT: Yale University Press; 1961:102–4.

[34] For the plans for the Vienna "Congress for Radioactivity and Electronics," see the letters between E. Rutherford and Stefan Meyer (Rutherford Correspondence microfilms), 25 October 1913 to 29 June 1914. I have been unable to find a clear reference to a 1916 International Conference of Medical Electrology and Radiology. Such conferences had been held until then every two years from 1906 to 1914, see Antoinette Béclère. Antoine Béclère. Paris: J. B. Bailliere; 1972 at 420.

[35] For mention of war-time delays, see 391. Förtschr Röntgenstr. 1916;24:516 and Journal of the Röntgen Society. 1919;15:94.

[36] Béclère (Physician to the Hospital of Saint Antoine, Member of the Academy of Medicine), Communication on the Radiotherapy of Uterine Fibroids, With the Results of 400 Cases, personally observed, the Mode of Action of the Treatment, and the Indications for its Adoption. Archives of Radiology and Electrotherapy. 1919;24:254–61, translated from Journal of Radiology and Electrotherapy. 1918–19;3:433–9. Béclère regarded this as a sequel to his August 1913 report to the 27th International Congress of Medicine (London), "Le traitement des fibro-myomes utérins par les rayons de Röntgen."

assured by their government that X-ray tubes would not "be considered as contraband in the event of a war with a Continental Power" because they "would be used for the relief of the wounded," found themselves cut off from essential German suppliers of both the tubes and the glass used in their manufacture.[37] The Prussian Ministry of War in 1915 prohibited the export of medical journals, including to Neutral Powers.[38] Even informal communications between the German medical radiological community and non-German counterparts were disrupted, and it was not until the early 1920s that communication was re-established. The War, in short, redirected resources and personnel, limited supplies of equipment, and cut professional communities off from their colleagues in other countries.

All that is consistent with Price's curves, but other things were happening as well. The disruptions affected medical research work with X-rays and with radium differently, and the net results varied markedly from country to country. In the short term, radium research suffered more than X-ray research, though the longer-term effect was highly favorable to expanding the use of radium in medicine. In France, where work with radium had been relatively more important than in other countries, the war seriously disrupted research. The volume of the medical radiological literature fell dramatically. A large portion of the papers published were devoted to localization of bullets and shrapnel by X-rays and other work directly related to the War.[39] In Britain, medical radiological research and the number of original contributions to the Archives of Radiology and Electrotherapy increased dramatically between 1914 and 1917.[40] There was, however, a severe shortage of X-ray tubes in Britain that hampered this intense research work. Only four small British firms were making tubes in 1914, and all of them depended on glass imported from

[37] Mr. Haldane (Haddington) gave this reply in response to a question raised in the House of Commons by Mr. Weir (Ross and Cromarty), see Notes. Journal of the Röntgen Society. 1907;15(94).

[38] Interdiction de sortie des publications médicales. Arch Elec Med. 1915;25(88 (feuilles de garde)).

[39] The *Archives d'Electricité médicale*, a large portion of which was devoted to radiological research, published over 1200 pages in 1913 and shrank to a mere 391 pages in 1915. The *Journal de Radiologie et d'Electrologie* (which was founded in 1914) published 751 pages in the year 1914–15, the same number of pages in the two-year period 1915–17 and only 576 pages in 1918 and 1919 combined. The Journal had still not recovered its initial size in 1920.

[40] Editorial, Archives of Radiology and Electrotherapy. 1918;23:1–2.

Germany.[41] About half the pre-war tubes used in England were manufactured abroad, mostly in Germany, and part of the remaining half was manufactured by German firms in England.[42]

The German medical X-ray community, which for most practical purposes included the German-speaking medical radiologists of Austria-Hungary and Switzerland, was the largest in the world before the War, and non-Germans considered it the most advanced.[43] Dependent almost entirely on domestic manufacture, with a large part of the market dominated by subsidiaries of large electrical firms, German research thrived even without the Röntgen Society congresses. Only after the War, in the midst of political and economic upheavals, was there a noticeable effect on the volume of the medical radiological literature, and even then the effect was slight.[44] Research in the United States continued at something like its pre-war level, with American radium and X-ray equipment manufacturers filling the gap left by the Germans. In addition, there was a striking rise in the quality of work done in the United States, so that by the early 1920s what had been a provincial community that reacted to European developments was contributing to major advances in both X-ray technology and medical applications.

Delay of inevitable developments was not, then, the only, or even the primary effect of World War I on medical radiological research. We would miss several effects of major importance if we looked only at the shift in Price's exponential growth curves. Looking beyond research to the impact of the War on medical radiological practice and on the social institutions

[41] The Shortage of X-Ray Tubes. Archives of the Roentgen Ray. 1914 Oct;19:159–60 and the letter of A. E. Dean at p. 197.

[42] Pearce G. The Future of the British X-Ray Industry. Journal of the Röntgen Society. 1917;13:60–87, 91–106.

[43] In 1913, the German Röntgen Society had 655 members and the British Röntgen Society had 188 members, see Verh Deut Ges Rönt. 1913;9 and Journal of the Röntgen Society. 1913;9:114–8; in 1914 the American Röntgen Ray Society had 170 members, see American Journal of Roentgenology. 1913;394–7. See also Archives of the Roentgen Ray. 1913;18:317, where *Strahlentherapie* is described as "by far the most important periodical devoted to Röntgen- and Radio-therapy."

[44] Volumes 23 (1915–16), 24 (1916–17) and 25 (1917–18) of *Fortschritte auf dem Gebiete der Röntgenstrahlen*, averaged 567 pages. Volume 25 was printed on noticeably lower quality paper, and volume 26 (1918–19) was 482 pages, smaller than each of the previous three volumes. But by the early 1920s, the journal had grown beyond its previous size, despite the resumption of the German Röntgen Society congresses and the publication of their *Verhandlungen* in 1920.

that supported it, there were other important changes. While medical radiology was suffering in some respects from the inevitable disruption of civilian activities in wartime economies, the rechanneling of resources to meet military needs was also benefiting the profession. X-rays had proved their usefulness in military medicine even before 1900. Used primarily to locate bullets and shrapnel, X-ray machines had seen service in the British army's 1897 Sudan expedition, in the Greco-Turkish War of the same year, in the Spanish-American War, and in the Boer War. Meeting military demands for mobility and reliability had called for innovations in basic equipment, simplified and accelerated techniques, and intensive training of both physicians and nonphysicians.[45] In all these respects, the demands of World War I far exceeded those of the previous campaigns in which X-rays had been used. The vast armies of the Allies and the Central Powers by the end of the War included among their support operations thousands of diagnostic X-ray installations.

The most important direct effect on medical radiology was the demand for personnel to staff these units. In 1914, the French Army had fewer than two dozen X-ray installations. By 1918, it had 400. Staffing these installations were 840 physicians and almost 1200 nonphysician operators, including 175 women trained by Marie Curie.[46] The U.S. Army, which before the War had only five mobile X-ray units mounted on four-mule escort wagons, sent more than 700 installations, many of them automobile-mounted, to Europe before the Armistice.[47] In the second

[45] Battersby J (M. B., Major, R. A. M. C.). The Present Position of the Röntgen Rays in Military Surgery. Archives of the Roentgen Ray. 1899;3:74–80; Küttner H (Assistenarzt der Tübinger Chirurgischen Klinik). Ueber die Bedeutung der Röntgenstrahlen für die Kriegschirurgie nach Erfahrungen im Griechisch-TUrkischen Krieg 1897. Beit Klin Chir. 1898;20:167–230; Abbott FC. Surgery in the Graeco-Turkish War. Lancet. 1899:30 and 152; Borden WC (Captain and Assistant Surgeon, U.S. Army). The Use of the Röntgen Ray by the Medical Department of the United States Army in the War with Spain a report to Brigadier General G. M. Sternberg, Surgeon-General, U.S. Army. Washington: U.S. Government Printing Office; 1900; and Hall-Edwards J. Bullets and Their Billets: Experiences with X-Rays in South Africa. Archives of the Roentgen Ray. 1902 Jan;6:31–9.

[46] Haret (Paris). La radiologie dans le Service de Santé de l'armée française pendant la guerre 1914–18. Bull Acad Med (Paris). 1919 May 27;81:718–20.

[47] Duncan WA. The X-Ray Equipment and Work in the Army at the Present Time. American Journal of Roentgenology. 1913;1:275–85, read by invitation at the Boston meeting of the American Röntgen Ray Society and Ashburn PM. A History of the Medical Department of the United States Army. Boston New York, Houghton Mifflin Company; 1929.

half of 1917, Army schools in Boston, New York, Philadelphia, Pittsburgh, Baltimore, Richmond, Chicago, Kansas City, and Los Angeles trained 200 physicians in X-ray diagnosis. Radiology was second only to surgery in getting the pick of the physicians available to the U.S. Army.[48] In Britain, there was also extensive training of physicians and nonphysicians for the Army. One estimate placed the number of X-ray operators in 1916 at six times the pre-war level, and it was presumably this increase that led to the increased number of original contributions to the Archives.[49] Despite the disruptions of war and because of its requirements, medical radiology grew as it had never grown before.

This greatly enlarged profession had to be supplied with X-ray tubes, high-voltage generators, protective devices, and other auxiliary equipment. Before 1914 artisans blew X-ray tubes by hand, but by 1918, they were mass-produced.[50] However new and untried, Coolidge tubes were so much more regular in their output and reliable in their operation that they were greatly preferable for use under military conditions. Coolidge himself designed an automobile-mounted model for the U.S. Army.[51] By the end of the War, Coolidge tubes were common in both the United States and Germany. They came into use more slowly in France and England.[52] Even cut off from a large portion of their export

[48] Manges WF. Military Röntgenology. In: The Science of Radiology. Springfield, Illinois: Charles C. Thomas; 1933:187–97. Physicians who claimed to be Röntgenologists had a relatively low rejection rate (4.6%, compared to 70% for otolaryngology) on United States Army tests, see Munson EL. "The Needs of Medical Education as Revealed by the War." Journal of the American Medical Association. 1919 Apr 12;72(15):1050–55, read before the 15th Annual Conference of the Council on Medical Education of the American Medical Association, Chicago, 3 March 1919.

[49] Batten GB. The Injurious Effects Produced by X-Rays. Journal of the Röntgen Society. 1916 Apr 1;12(47):38–56.

[50] Robinson RC, Moore CN. Manufacture of the Coolidge X-Ray Tube. American Journal of Roentgenology? 1920;7:254–60. A few glass-blowing operations still had to be done by hand, but Robinson and Moore do not say which ones.

[51] Coolidge WD, Moore CN. A Portable Röntgen-Ray Generating Outfit. General Electric Review. 1918;21:60–7.

[52] Coolidge had first demonstrated his tube in December 1913, when there were reportedly "...no arrangements...yet...made for its commercial manufacture," see the Editorial. American Journal of Roentgenology. 1923;1:90–1 at 91. But in April 1914, the Coolidge tube was the sensation of the 10th congress of the German Röntgen Society, see Fortsch Röntgenstr. 1914;142, where a German-made model was described, see Levy-Dorn (Berlin). Über die neue Coolidgeröhre der A. E. G. Verh Deut Ges Rönt.

market, German manufacturers of X-ray tubes did well during the War. The firm of Siemens and Halske, which had patented the tungsten anticathode before the invention of the Coolidge tube, arranged with AEG, the German firm licensed to produce Coolidge tubes by General Electric, to exchange rights and to produce the high-vacuum, hot-cathode tube jointly. Siemens and Halske, which had previously assigned X-ray tubes and other medical electrical equipment to its Division for Measuring Instruments, established a separate Sales Division for Electromedical Apparatus. In 1916, the firm of Reiniger, Gebbert and Schall acquired control of Veifawerke by buying the shares of Friedrich Dessauer, one of the pioneer tube manufacturers.[53] At about the same time, Reiniger, Gebbert and Schall, which two decades earlier had provided Röntgen with his Ruhmkorff coil, brought Theophil Christen from his university post in Bern to lead an enlarged research unit in Munich.[54]

The War also increased the demand for radium. Medical use was not the major factor, though after the War medicine benefited from the increased supply. During the War, radium was needed primarily in self-luminescent paints, which were used for gun sights and dials (especially in airplanes) and also for warning signs on the backs of military vehicles. Dial-painting was destined to cause a major post-war incident in the history of radiation injuries. In addition, radium recovered from gunsights and dials was distributed to British hospitals for therapeutic trials after the War.[55] The United States was also successful in increasing its supplies of

1914;10:156–7 with discussion, 158–60. In France, the Coolidge tube was described by Belot J, Vignal W. A propos d'un nouveau tube de Röntgen à vide de Hittorf (tube Coolidge). Journal of Radiology and Electrotherapy. 1914;1:227–32, but Béclère, note 36 above, was just beginning to use a Coolidge tube in 1918. The British Thomson-Houston Company owned the British patents (Notes, Journal of the Röntgen Society. 1914;11:50), but an English visitor to the 1923 congress of the German Röntgen Society reported, "One was struck by the state of hot cathode tube production in Germany and Austria, which appears to be far in advance of England," see Schall WE. The German Röntgen Society. Journal of the Röntgen Society. 1923;19:172–4.

[53] Siemens G. Der Weg der Elektrotechnik., 2 volumes. Freiburg/München: Karl Alber, 1966, II, 112ff.

[54] See the obituary of Christen by Walter B. Fortschr Röntgenstr. 1921;28:391–2.

[55] Radium and Clinical Research. Journal of the Röntgen Society. 1920;16:83, where the initial loan of five grams to the Middlesex Hospital was reported. For a later report on the use of this war-generated supply of radium, see the U.K. Medical Research Council. Medical Uses of Radium, Summary of Reports from Research Centres for 1923, Special

radium, and by the end of the War it had more than any other country: a total of about 50 grams.[56]

With the rapid increases in personnel and equipment came a need for controlling quality and standardizing procedures. Quality control of military purchases fell in part to national standards laboratories. The German Royal Physical-Technical Institute at Charlottenburg, the British National Physical Laboratory, and the U.S. Bureau of Standards would become especially important for radiation protection and measurement. Created as a result of nineteenth-century increases in trade and manufacturing, these laboratories were responsible for maintaining reference standards and comparing them with commercial standards or products. Much of this work was routine. The British National Physical Laboratory in the early years tested a large number of clinical thermometers.[57] Before the War, the standards laboratories had played only peripheral roles in radiology. They acted as depositories for radium standards, but they had played little or no role in their development. The standards laboratories had, however, one important feature that repeatedly led them beyond routine testing activities: they used academically trained scientists to work on technological problems, a practice that was still new in industry. During the War, the national standards laboratories were called on to test X-ray equipment, protection devices, and self-luminescent paints.[58] After the War,

Report Series no. 60. London: His Majesty's Stationery Office; 1924. An earlier report received only limited circulation and is not readily available.

[56] The figure is from Reid RW. Marie Curie. New American Library; 1974 at 216. See also Radium by the Gramme. Journal of the Röntgen Society 1920;16:83, where it was reported that three new radium factories had been established in the United States since 1913. The Standard Chemical Company of Pittsburgh alone produced 18 grams per year, which was said to be as much as all the French producers combined.

[57] National Physical Laboratory. Report for the Year 1902. London: Harrison; 1903:7.

[58] United States. War Work of the Bureau of Standards. Washington: Government Printing Office; 1921:251–55, 298–99. The National Physical Laboratory in 1916 began issuing certificates specifying the percentage of hard, medium and soft X-rays absorbed by protective materials, see J. H. Gardiner in the discussion at the Röntgen Society, note 49 above, at 56. A proposal that protection materials be tested was made at the April 1914 German Röntgen Society Congress, see David Halle. Verh. Deut. Ges. Rönt. 1914;10:19. The Royal Physical-Technical Institute began work with X-rays at the beginning of the War and established a special Röntgenstrahlenlaboratorium in 1919, at the behest of industry (especially the Osram-Kommanditgesellschaft), see Behnken (Berlin). Die Eichung von Dosismessern in absolutem Masse in der Physikalisch-technischen Reichsanstalt. Verh Deut Ges Rönt. 1924;15:92–4.

the staff turned in part to work on radiation measurement and protection. Physicists interested in these problems thus gained a much stronger institutional basis than they had had before, and medical radiology was provided with a level of applied scientific expertise that had not been so readily available to it previously.

In addition to quality control of equipment, there were problems in controlling the quality of the procedures used in military radiology, and especially in ensuring that the newly trained operators were adequately protected. Civilian radiological practice might permit wide variations in clinical technique, but the military required standardization, especially when hundreds of new X-ray operators had to be trained and sent immediately into the field. The single most successful effort in this regard was the U.S. Army X-ray Manual, which was prepared by a Cornell physics professor.[59] Without being innovative, it gave considerable weight to both protection and measurement techniques. The British Röntgen Society, following the pre-war lead of its German counterpart, prepared "Recommendations for the Protection of X-ray Operators."[60] The War Office was sent 250 copies for distribution to military hospitals.[61] The 2 millimeters of lead protection that the Germans had decided on in 1913 was included in the original British draft, but it was eliminated in the final version.[62] The British recommendations emphasized enclosing both the tube and the operator in protective boxes, but unlike the U.S. Army

[59] John Sandford Shearer, see the obituary in American Journal of Roentgenology. 1922;9:520–4.

[60] The proposal for these protection recommendations originated in a "Discussion on Protective Devices for X-ray Operators," at the 1 June 1915 Annual General Meeting of the Röntgen Society, Journal of the Röntgen Society. 1914;11:110–13, at 113: "...in view of the recent large increase in the number of X-ray installations, this Society considers it a matter of the greatest importance that the personal safety of the operators conducting the X-ray examinations should be secured by the universal adoption of stringent rules..." In response to this resolution, the Council of the Röntgen Society decided in September 1915 "that a set of rules should be prepared for the protection of X ray operators," see the circular letter dated 18 September 1915 signed by Robert Knox (M. D., Honorary Secretary) in a box of Röntgen Society documents in the library of the British Institute of Radiology referred to below as RS (BIR). The rules, ibid., were dated November 1915. A proposal to purchase for the War Office a model X-ray installation apparently went unfulfilled, see the Annual Report. Journal of the Röntgen Society. 1914;11:92–102.

[61] See the letter of acknowledgement dated 7 February 1916 on War Office stationery from a Lieutenant Colonel whose signature is illegible, RS (BIR), ibid.

[62] See the draft attached to Knox's letter, note 60 above.

manual they failed to recommend dosage measurements (beyond the use of a penetrometer to test hardness).

The War, then, strengthened the medical radiological community in a number of ways: the body of practitioners was enlarged, the capacity to produce improved X-ray tubes and larger quantities of radium was increased, the national standards laboratories became involved, and national measurement and protection procedures were standardized.

War Also Narrows the Gap Between Physicists and Physicians, Especially in Germany

In addition to these impacts, the War also affected the career patterns of individuals. Many physicians entered radiology who would not otherwise have done so. The status of the profession within medicine rose, and the first efforts at making radiology a separate specialty requiring postgraduate training began during the War.[63] The War also brought to medical radiology an influx of academically trained physicists beyond those in the national standards laboratories. Most famous of these was Marie Curie, who deposited her radium with the physician Bergonié in Bordeaux at the beginning of the War and devoted herself and her daughter, the future Nobelist Irène, to medical X-ray work for the duration. Marie and Irène Curie initially went into the field as radiographers, but they later returned to Paris to train women as X-ray operators.[64]

More important than the Curies for later developments in medical radiology were German physicists who turned to research in medical radiology during the War.[65] Walter Friedrich, who had performed the diffraction experiments with Knipping in 1912, went during the War to the University of Freiburg, where he collaborated with the gynecologist

[63] The British Association for the Advancement of Radiology and Physiotherapy, whose primary object was the establishment of a post-graduate diploma, was established in 1917. See also Shearer JS. Graduate Instruction in Röntgenology. American Journal of Roentgenology. 1922;9:459–64.

[64] For a description of Marie Curie's work during the War, see Chapter 19 of Reid, note 56. For Curie's own story, see Curie M. La Radiologie et la guerre. Paris: Librairie Flix Alcan; 1921. Curie's figures on the numbers of X-ray installations, physicians and operators differ from those of Haret, note 46.

[65] Unless otherwise noted below, biographical details are taken from various volumes of Poggendorff JC, Biographisch-literarisches Handwörterbuch.

Bernhard Krönig on research that was critical to the development of X-ray deep therapy. In 1923, Friedrich, as *Ordinarius* for medical physics and scientific radiology, founded the Institute for Radiation Research at Berlin, where he remained for the rest of his long career.[66] At Freiburg, Friedrich had trained the physicist Otto Glasser, who would emigrate to the United States in the early 1920s and in 1924 settle at the Cleveland Clinic Foundation. Leonard Grebe, an experimental physicist who had failed to obtain a professorship after habilitating at Bonn in 1910, began working in medical radiology shortly after the War with Heinrich Martius, a younger *Privatdozent*. They both had successful careers in medical radiological research. Richard Glocker, who had been a student of Röntgen's at Munich with Friedrich, began working on radiation dosimetry during the War, as did Gustav Grossmann, who had obtained a doctorate from the Zurich Polytechnique in 1903 and who later pursued a career in the X-ray industry. Hermann Behnken, who received his doctorate in physics at Berlin in 1913, was by the end of the War in charge of X-ray work at the Royal Physical-Technical Institute.[67]

The precise reasons for these shifts of interest among German physicists are obscure, but speculation is possible. In part, the physicists may have wanted to contribute toward work that they saw as beneficial to the War effort. That was a major motive for Marie Curie. The German physicists did not, however, go into the field, as she did. Their motives may have been less patriotic and more personal. Even before the War, there had been signs of worsening career prospects for academic physicists. Despite substantial increases in the resources available to the academic physics community as a whole, the age at which physicists entered their first professorship in the decade before 1910 had risen throughout Europe compared to the 1880s. A significant percentage of the German physicists who habilitated between 1890 and 1910 had never received a professorship.[68] The War aggravated this pre-existing condition. With research funds and academic posts in short supply, recent doctoral recipients and *Privatdozenten* found themselves unable to continue the basic research in which they had been trained. A desire to stay out of the army and far from

[66] The obituary in Strahlenth. 1968;136:765–6.

[67] Jaeger, RG. In memoriam Hermann Behnken. Strahlenth. 1970;139:113–5.

[68] Forman P, Heilbron JL, Weart S. Physics circa 1900: Personnel, Funding, and Productivity of the Academic Establishments. Historical Studies in the Physical Sciences. 1975 Jan 1;5:1–185.

the front was likely a factor for some. Whatever their individual motives, Friedrich, Glasser, Glocker, Grebe, Martius, Grossmann, and Behnken were only a few of the German physicists whose careers took turns toward more practical work during the War.

Not only medical radiology, but also fields like metallurgy, chemical and electrical engineering, shipbuilding, and airplane design benefited from increased interest among academically trained physicists and chemists. For German physicists, the founding of the Society, and *Journal*, for Technical Physics in 1920 institutionalized these new interests.[69] By 1924, the Society would have 1600 members.[70] The physicists who entered medical radiology did not play a major role in the new Journal and Society, preferring to participate in the German Röntgen Society (which continued to permit participation by nonphysicians) and to publish primarily in the medical radiological journals. The influx of physicists into medical radiology should, however, be viewed as parallel to a broader movement among German physicists and German scientists into fields of applied science.

In addition to the flow from physics into medical radiology, there was a small, but highly significant, flow in the other direction, from medical radiology into physics. Friedrich Dessauer, the manufacturer of X-ray tubes who had been involved in medical radiology for over a decade, sold his interest in Veifawerke, retired from industry, and obtained a doctorate in physics from the University of Frankfurt in 1917 at the age of thirty-six. In 1922, Dessauer became director of the newly founded Institute for the Physical Foundations of Medicine in Frankfurt, where both physicists and biologists found facilities for research.[71] There were also two physicians destined to play important roles in radiation protection who obtained advanced training in physics. Hermann Holthusen, who even

[69] Ibid., at 53.

[70] On the founding of the Society for Technical Physics, see Forman P. The Environment and Practice of Atomic Physics in Weimar Germany: A Study in the History of Science [University of California at Berkeley]; 1967. University Microfilms, 1968:139 ff.

[71] Dessauer's interesting biography is among those of several others mentioned here in Del Regato JA. Radiological Oncologists: The Unfolding of a Medical Specialty [Internet]. Radiation Oncology Institute (ROI)—Radiological Oncologists—ROI Juan A. del Regato Fund. 2023. Available from: https://www.roinstitute.org/About-the-ROI/The-ROI-Juan-A-del-Regato-Fund/Radiological-Oncologists, accessed August 30, 2023.

before the War had studied with Philipp Lenard at Heidelberg, habilitated there in 1918. He then began a research career in medical radiology that relied heavily on both the use of the physicist's laboratory tools and competence in contemporary physical theory.[72] He would eventually be a member of the ICRP's main commission from 1953 to 62. Another young physician, Hermann Wintz, began his work in medical radiology at Erlangen during the War in collaboration with Ludwig Seitz, *Ordinarius* and director of the University Women's Hospital, with assistance from the firm of Reiniger, Gebbert and Schall. In 1920, Wintz obtained a doctorate in physics from the University of Erlangen. When Seitz went to Frankfurt in the same year, Wintz succeeded to his posts, becoming at age 33 the youngest *Ordinarius* in gynecology in the country.[73] Theophil Christen, the Swiss physician with a doctorate in mathematics who worked for Reiniger, Gebbert and Schall during the War, would probably have proved another important contributor to later developments, but he committed suicide in 1920 after an unsuccessful electoral campaign as a Social Democratic candidate for the Swiss National Council.

Dessauer, Holthusen, Wintz, and Christen, along with the physicists who were orienting their research toward medical radiology, belonged to a small but growing group of German-language research workers who would be difficult to classify as belonging exclusively to either the scientific or the medical radiological communities. From their efforts during and after the War to apply contemporary physics to medical radiological problems would develop a new style of deep therapy, a physical theory of radiation effects, a much more thorough understanding of radiation dosimetry, and a commitment to radiation protection, as we shall see in Chapter 5.

[72] Gehloff G. Fünf Jahre Deutsche Gesellschaft für technische Physik. Z Tech Phys. 1924;5:201–4.

[73] For some autobiographical comments by Holthusen, see the 23 January 1971 lecture he gave at Würzburg reproduced in Braunbehrens HV, Frommhold W. Hermann Holthusen. Fortschr Röntgenstr. 1971;1151:141–6. Holthusen's contact with physics appears to have begun not with X-rays but with a study of the absorption of radium emanation by blood, see Ramsauer C, Holthusen H (aus dem Radiologischen Institut und der Medizinischen Klinik der Universität Heidelberg), Über die Aufnahme der Radiumenataion durch das Blut, *Sitzungsber. Akad. Wiss. (Heidelberg)*, Math.-naturwiss. Kl., Abt. B (Biol. Wiss.), Jahrgang 1913, 2. Abh. vorgelegt von P. Lenard, eingegangen 25. Februar 1913.

CHAPTER 5

X-Ray Measurements and Radium Protection Catch Up, 1914–22

In the question of practical dosimetry the physicist has for the present given the word; here it is the duty of the clinician to carry the work further on the available basis.

—W. Friedrich (Ph. D.) and O. A. Glasser (Ph. D.), 1922[1]

The question of radium protection is now in the midst of development, and comparable to the state in which the question of X-ray protection was fifteen years ago.

—Thibonneau (M. D.), 1921[2]

The shift to ionization measurements in medical radiology initially took place in Germany among people capable in physics. Their work again raises the issue of the relationship between practical concerns in medical

[1] Untersuchungen und Betrachtungen über das Problem der Dosimetrie. Strahlentherapie. 1922;14:362–88, at 388.

[2] In the discussion following Laquerrière, Des dangers des installations de Radio et de Radiumologie. Rapport à une compagnie d'assurance sur le "risque" du personnel et des visiteurs dans un institut de Radio et de Radiumologie. Bull Off Soc Franc Electroth Radial. 1921 May;132–7.

D. Serwer, *Strengthening International Regimes*,
Palgrave Studies in International Relations,
https://doi.org/10.1007/978-3-031-53724-0_5

radiology and contemporary scientific knowledge. It would be reasonable to suppose that the shift to ionization measurements was based on theoretical understanding of the mechanisms underlying the biological effects of radiation. As it turned out, however, even within the small group of research workers directly involved there would be no agreement before 1925 on the physical and chemical mechanisms of radiation effects. Instead, the reason for the shift to ionization measurements in clinical X-ray work would be the practical requirements of a new type of therapy reaching deeper into the human body. Despite many advances, scientific theory still failed to offer a firm basis for medical practice.

The development of radium protection raises again the issue of the relationship between professional "self-regulation" and public pressure. The risks of radium exposure would become a subject of concern in the early 1920s, except in Germany. As with the previous development of X-ray protection, radium protection would be a professional response to public outcry, not automatic professional self-regulation. This time the public pressure would come primarily in newspapers rather than in the courts.

Ionization Measurements Enter the Clinic

The shift to ionization measurements for clinical X-ray work originated in the radiation therapy German clinicians were already applying deep in the human body before World War I. Therapists at Freiburg had reported delivering high doses to the skin without causing harm. The doses had been measured with Kienböck's silver bromide strips. The Freiburg claims were greeted with disbelief at other clinics, where much lower doses had often been observed to cause severe skin reactions. The problem of comparing the Freiburg results with results in other gynecological clinics inspired in the German medical radiological community a practical proposal: to compare the most commonly used measuring devices (dosimeters) and to draw up tables that would enable their readings to be interconverted. Responding to an appeal by its President, the German Röntgen Society established a new subsidiary group, the Special Commission for Comparison of Dosimeters.[3] Despite the War and the suspension

[3] For the President's appeal, see Levy-Dorn's opening address to the Society's congress, Verh Deut Rönt Ges. 1914;10, at 16, and for the creation of the Commission see the business meeting, at 18: "Der Zweck dieser Kommission soll sein, die Dosimeter, die

of the Röntgen Society congresses, the Commission remained nominally active until 1918, with nine of its sixteen members indicating that they could participate.[4]

The most important conclusion of the Special Commission was reached, however, in 1915, after eight of the members had replied to a request for suggestions as to how to proceed. Their views on the heterogeneity of the X-rays in use and on the usefulness of the available clinical dosimeters in comparing quantities of X-rays of different qualities varied widely. Austrian physician Guido Holzknecht, who had introduced the "chromoradiometer" more than a decade earlier and suffered radiation injuries to his skin that would eventually require amputation of a hand and part of a leg, reported in his capacity as Chairman of the Commission:

> The simple comparison of the dosimeters was expressly or implicitly characterized by most of the committee members as impossible. It is therefore necessary that, first of all, some sort of exact measurement procedure be created, and that would be a very complicated laboratory task.... For this, all those who have done and can do physics and mathematics should be called upon.[5]

landläufig sind und sich irgendwie bewährt haben, untereinander zu vergleichen, damit so feste Daten bekannt werden, auf die Sie sich einigermassen verlassen können; denn wie Sie ja wissen, geben die verschiedenen Dosimeter ganz verschiedene Auskünfte." Of the sixteen original members, seven are readily identifiable as physicians (including Christen), five as nonphysicians and the remaining four are not readily classifiable.

[4] For the decision to continue the work of the ·commission, see the II. Rundschreiben des Vorsitzenden. Fortschr Röntgenstr. 1915;23:72: "Es wäre recht erfreulich, wenn die Dosimeterkommission nach dem Kriege mit den erreichbaren Resultaten hervortreten würde, die wir Daheimgebliebenen unter dem Schutze unserer mächtigen Heeresorganisation fast wie im Frieden leisten könnten."

[5] Fortschr Röntgenstr. 1915;23, at 213: "Der einfache Vergleich der Dosimeter ist von den meisten Arbeitern ausdrücklich oder implizite als unlösbar bezeichnet worden und es hat sich die Notwendigkeit ergeben, zuerst irgendein exaktes Verfahren der Messung der Röntgenstrahlen zu schaffen, und wäre es eine noch so komplizierte Laboratoriumanordnung ....Dazu sollte alles, was Physik und Mathematik geleistet haben und leisten können, herangezogen werden." Holzknecht's biography is at Radiation Oncology Institute, Radiological Oncologists: The Unfolding of a Medical Specialty [Internet]. RO Institute. 2023. Available from: https://www.roinstitute.org/About-the-ROI/The-ROI-Juan-A-del-Regato-Fund/Radiological-Oncologists, accessed October 22, 2023.

Many papers were published as Proceedings of the Commission, but its name was changed to the Special Committee for Röntgen Ray Measurement and its initial purpose remained unfulfilled.[6] A similar British group, created by the Röntgen Society, also failed in 1915 to come to definitive recommendations on X-ray measurements, and in France it was concluded that the problem was "too complex for the construction of measuring instruments giving precise readings that were always intercomparable."[7]

Within the German medical radiological community, the response to Holzknecht's call for "all those who have done and can do physics and mathematics" was quick. Already in 1914, the physicist Gustav Grossmann had pointed out that the silver bromide in Kienböck's quantimeter was not suitable for measurements of X-ray quantity over a wide range of qualities because silver had a selective absorption edge within the range of X-ray wavelengths used for deep therapy. Selective absorption would cause the Kienböck strips to darken more rapidly at some wavelengths than at others, leading to dosage readings that were much higher than the doses actually delivered to the tissue being irradiated. Barium and platinum, constituents of other widely used clinical measuring devices, were also known to have selective absorption edges, but for the moment they lay beyond the range of X-ray wavelengths commonly used for therapy, at

[6] For these papers, which were never actually read to the group but were published together, seeArbeiten und Verhandlungen der Sonderkommission für Dosimetervergleich der Deutschen Röntgengesellschaft. II Gruppe, Fortschr Röntgenstr. 1915;23:213–300, abgeschlossen im Juli 1915; Arbeiten und Verhandlungen des Sonderausschusses für Röntgenstrahlenmessung der Deutschen Röntgengesellschaft, III. Gruppe.:509–32, abgeschlossen am 22 XI. 1915; IV. Gruppe, Fortschr Röntgenstr. 1916;24:373–423, abgeschlossen am 15. VI. 1916; V. Gruppe, Fortschr. Röntgenstr. 25 (1917–18) 55–71; und Fortschr. Röntgenstr. 26. 1918;38–41.

[7] The British "Measurement" or "Dosimetry" Committee was formed late in 1913, see the Annual Report. Journal of the Röntgen Society. 1914;10:88–97 and reported inconclusively in 1915, see the "Interim Report on the Standardisation of X-ray Dosage," Interim Report on the Standardisation of X-ray Dosage. Journal of the Röntgen Society. 11:102–10, authorized to be printed in full by the Council at its meeting held on 1 June 1915. The Committee had ten members when it reported, of whom seven were nonphysicians, two were practicing physicians and one was a retired physician. For the French conclusion, see Ledoux-Lebard R, Dauvillier A. Principes rationnels de dosimétrie radiologique. Considération théoriques et pratiques. Journal of Radiology and Electrology. 1916;2:153–62, at 153: "...il est impossible d'arriver à une solution satisfaisante du problème du dosage des rayons X parce qu'il se présente sous une forme beaucoup trop complexe pour que soient réalisables des appareil s de mesure donnant des indications précises et toujours comparables à elles-mêmes."

voltages above 50,000. Outside areas of selective absorption, absorption changed with hardness in similar ways, so Grossmann suggested that the ideal dosimeter was one that had an atomic weight less than aluminum, the lightest element in which selective absorption had been observed. The obvious choice for the "test body" was air, and the obvious method to a physicist was the familiar technique of measuring the saturation current due to ionization.[8]

The medical radiological community was not won over immediately. Grossmann's work seemed "theoretical," and the question of the so-called "silver error" was regarded as unsolved.[9] At the same time, the Freiburg gynecologists who had been reporting high doses on the basis of their measurements with Kienböck's strips could not afford to ignore Grossmann's suggestions about the selective absorption of silver. One of them, Bernhard Krönig, brought Walter Friedrich, the Munich physicist mentioned in Chapter 4 who had demonstrated X-ray diffraction with Laue and Knipping, to Freiburg to work on the dosimetry problem as well as on determination of the biological effectiveness of X-rays of different quality. In 1918, Krönig and Friedrich published an extensive series of experiments undertaken in 1915 and 1916 at the Women's Hospital using Coolidge's high-vacuum, hot-cathode tube.[10] These experiments confirmed Grossmann's suspicions concerning the importance of selective absorption. The percentage absorption of X-rays of different wavelengths, and of gamma rays, in silver and in platinum was not parallel to the absorption in water, which Krönig and Friedrich demonstrated was equivalent to soft tissue. The absorption of X-rays and gamma rays in air was,

[8] Grossmann G (Charlottenburg). Grundprinzipien der Dosimetrie. Fortschr Röntgenstr. 1914;22:101–42.

[9] For experiments that indicated that the Kienböck strips and the Sabouraud-Noiré pastilles gave parallel results over a wide range of hardnesses, thus demonstrating that Grossmann's "theoretical" considerations were incorrect, see Meyer H. Fortschr Röntgenstr. 1915;23:75–6. It was later recognized that these experiments merely demonstrated that the strips and the pastilles were equally insensitive to changes in X-ray dosage.

[10] Krönig B (o. ö. Prof. der Geburtshilfe und Gynäkologie an der Universität Freiburg i. Br., Direktor der Univ.-Frauenklinik), Friedrich W (Privatdozent für Physik an der Universität Freiburg i. Br., wissenschaftlicher Assistent an der Univ. Frauenklinik). Physikalische und Biologische Grundlagen der Strahlentherapie, III. Sonderband zur Strahlentherapie. Berlin: Urban and Schwarzenberg; 1918. There is a clumsy but readable translation by Schmitz H. The Principles of Physics and Biology of Radiation Therapy. Rebman; 1922). For the sponsors (who included industry, government, private patrons and a local scientific society), see the Forward to the German edition.

however, closely parallel to their absorption in water and thus in tissue. As a practical matter, then, Krönig and Friedrich concluded that ionization measurements in air would give doses that were comparable over a wide range of wavelengths. They explicitly aimed to measure dose (the energy absorbed in a given volume) rather than X-ray quantity or intensity (the energy passing through a surface).

In order to make ionization measurements comparable among clinics, Krönig and Friedrich defined an absolute unit of radiation dosage as "that amount of radiation which by ionization in one cubic centimeter of air transfers one electrostatic unit of charge in a saturation current." This unit is similar to a unit that had been used by a French physicist a decade earlier as well as to the "Röntgen," the unit of X-ray dosage that a decade later would be adopted on the international level.[11] The recurrence of this proposal is not surprising. To the physicist, saturation current was the usual method of measuring X-ray intensity, and it was a short step to measure dosage in terms of the charge transported by the saturation current. There were, however, other possibilities for an ionization unit of radiation dosage. One possibility was the "megamegaion" (the number of ions, in million millions, produced in air). This unit required the same sorts of measurements as Krönig and Friedrich's but it also required an additional calculation after the amount of charge transported had been determined, or the calibration of the electrometer in number of ions rather than in electrostatic units. The "megamegaion" never came into general use.[12] Another possibility was to use the ionization produced by a given amount of radium as a unit of X-ray dosage, a proposal made even before the War in Britain. This procedure did not gain favor in Germany, where radium was however used to verify the constancy of measuring instruments. The French in the post-war period would, naturally, favor using radium as the basis of a unit of X-ray dosage.

More important than the definition of Krönig and Friedrich's unit were their procedures for measuring ionization. For the first time in the medical X-ray literature, they presented an extensive discussion of the physical

[11] Villard P. Instruments de mesure à lecture directe pour les rayons X. Arch Elec Med. 1908;16:692–9.

[12] For the "megamegaion," see Szilard B. Appareil pour la mesure de la quantité de rayons X. Radium. 1910;7:223–4 and on the Absolute Measurement of the Biological Action of the X-rays and Gamma Rays. Arch Rönt Ray. 12:3–20.

sources of error in ionization measurements, including inadequate insulation, the dielectric polarization, and depolarization of the insulating material, protection of the ionization chamber from electrostatic forces and from radiation other than the radiation in the primary beam, and the nature of the materials of which the ionization chamber was constructed. This last point concerning materials was especially important. Ionization chambers for clinical use had been introduced in Germany just before the War. They were small, usually one cubic centimeter in volume, so that they could be easily handled and even introduced into the patient's body. Rectal insertion during irradiation of the ovaries was one method of measuring the dose actually delivered near the target. The commercially available ionization chambers had metal walls. As Krönig and Friedrich pointed out, metal walls would give off secondary radiation when X-rays were absorbed in them. The ionization measured would then not be entirely from the air in the chamber but would include ionization by both characteristic X-rays and secondary cathode rays from the walls. To avoid the characteristic wall radiation, Krönig and Friedrich used an ionization chamber made of low atomic weight material, which did not emit secondary X-rays (they used cow's horn, whose walls were made conducting by a coating of graphite). Using this small chamber, Krönig and Friedrich calibrated their small unit using an ionization chamber that they believed sufficiently large to measure the total ionization due to the secondary cathode rays arising from the absorption of X-rays in air.

Krönig and Friedrich went on to answer two important questions for deep therapy in the human body: how did calculated deep doses compare with experimentally determined deep doses? and how did the biological effect of X-rays vary with quality? The former question was not one that others in the medical radiological community had asked, and it seems likely that Friedrich expected that the calculated doses and the measured doses would not agree. The exponential law of absorption, on which the calculations depended, did not consider scattered X-rays, which would add to the ionization a dose that came to be called the "*Streuzusatzdosis*." This "added scattering dose" would increase with the hardness of the primary beam, and because of scattering the dose delivered at the center of the "field" of the primary beam would be greater the larger the size of the field. Krönig and Friedrich readily confirmed these phenomena with experiments conducted in a basin of water. The practical problem of delivering a specified dose to deep-lying tissue thus became more complex than before. Numerous experimenters over the next decade would work on determining doses in water "phantoms" with different combinations of filters, focal distance, field size, and other parameters.[13]

Krönig and Friedrich also answered the question of whether X-rays of different quality had the same effects. With their answer came a simplification of therapeutic practice. Using frog larvae (*Rana temporaria* or *Rana esculenta*) that were known to suffer readily visible malformations as a result of exposure to radiation, they showed that biological effects were independent of the quality of the rays. The effects depended only on the absorbed dose measured by their ionization chamber, a quantity that they assumed to be identical to, or at least proportional to, the energy of the absorbed radiation. These experiments with frog larvae were confirmed by less extensive experiments on garden peas (*Vicea fava*) and on human ovaries.[14] The dependence of biological effects on absorbed doses alone suggested it might be possible to measure the doses required to bring about specific effects, regardless of the quality of the radiation used. Krönig and Friedrich defined, and made some preliminary attempts to measure, an "ovarian" dose (the dose required to produce cessation of ovulation and menstruation), an "erythema" dose (the dose required to produce a distinctly visible reaction on the skin), and a "carcinoma" dose (the dose required to produce a palpable decrease in the size of a carcinoma).

Ludwig Seitz, director of the Erlangen University Women's Hospital, and Hermann Wintz, the young physician who obtained a doctorate in physics, applied these concepts in extensive clinical trials.[15] Seitz and Wintz worked initially with pre-war X-ray tubes designed for deep therapy, but they turned eventually to Coolidge tubes excited with up to 200,000 volts. From 1914 on, they treated dozens of cases of carcinoma and sarcoma that came into the military clinic housed in the Erlangen

[13] For references to this literature, see Fricke H, Glasser O. Studies on the Physical Foundations of Röntgen-Ray Therapy I. American Journal of Roentgenology. 1924;11:435–42.

[14] If there were limits on human experimentation, they were not mentioned in the professional journals. Certainly nothing like current constraints on human experimentation existed.

[15] The full report of this work is Unsere Methode der Röntgen-Tiefentherapie und ihre Erfolge, V. Sonderband zu Strahlentherapie. Berlin: Urban and Schwarzenberg; 1920. For a summary account, see Wintz H (Erlangen). Die Grundlagen einer erfolgreichen Röntgentiefentherapie. Verh Deut Rönt Ges. 1920;11:64–8, auf Einladung der D. R.-G., with discussion at 92–98.

Women's Hospital during the War. They also treated five hundred cases of uterine fibroma and functional uterine bleeding. The Erlangen gynecologists measured their doses with an "iontoquantimeter" (an ionization measuring meter) produced by Reiniger, Gebbert and Schall, and with similar instruments designed in cooperation with an electrical engineer.

More than 20 years after the discovery of X-rays, reliable measuring instruments based on ionization, the usual method in scientific laboratories, were just starting to be used in medical clinics, especially in Germany. Up until then, medical radiologists had exposed themselves and many thousands of patients to highly uncertain radiation doses that varied widely from clinic to clinic. The trial-and-error methods were still not based on laboratory science or even comparable and accurate measurements. Radiation exposure of laboratory scientists was also common. It would however be another two decades before radiation protection on a quantitative basis would take root in medical radiology. Scientists had discovered X-rays and radium in laboratories, but their applications still proceeded without much help from contemporary science.

Biological Units Remain Preferred

In accordance with Krönig and Friedrich's suggestions, Seitz and Wintz tried to avoid radiation from the walls of the ionization chamber, but they did not use a physical unit for X-ray dosage. They had no large ionization chamber and thus lacked a way to standardize their ionization chambers in absolute units. Instead, Seitz and Wintz turned to what they called a "biological system of measurements" to ensure compatibility among different clinics. The basis of this system was Krönig and Friedrich's "erythema" dose, which Seitz and Wintz recast as the "unit skin dose" (*Hauteinheitdosis*). The unit skin dose was the dose of filtered X-rays required to produce a reddening of the skin within a specified time period. For healthy, previously unirradiated skin, Seitz and Wintz determined experimentally that the variations in skin sensitivity were relatively small, on the order of 10 or 15 percent, and they therefore thought themselves justified in expressing dosage in terms of the unit skin dose.

In their clinical trials, the Erlangen gynecologists found that the doses required to cause permanent cessation of ovulation, or to cure carcinoma or sarcoma, were also remarkably constant, as Krönig and Friedrich had suggested. The "castration" dose was 34 percent of the unit skin dose, the "carcinoma" dose was 110 percent of the unit skin dose, and the "sarcoma" dose was 60–70 percent of the unit skin dose. Seitz and Wintz delivered these doses, as far as possible, in a single sitting. They avoided burns by increasing the focal distance, by irradiating from several different directions, and by using fields that were as large as possible without overlap. They thus avoided what they termed, again following Krönig and Friedrich, the "dissipation" (*Verzettelung*) of the dose by the usual procedure of delivering it over the course of several sittings spread out over days or weeks. The objective in this intensive deep therapy was to kill the cancer cells, or in the case of ovarian treatments to kill the oogonia and ova. The success rates were extremely high, with 100 percent success reported in 500 cases of at least temporary female sterilization produced in one or more sittings. Of 170 cases in which sterilization had been produced in a single sitting, they reported that 77 percent had remained sterile for at least one year. Exposure of the intestines during treatment sometimes caused "Röntgen hangover" (*Röntgenkater*), they observed several instances of "late" effects (dermatitis developing long after irradiation), and there were often changes in the patient's blood. On the whole, however, Seitz and Wintz regarded serious harm as rare, without doing any epidemiological follow-up or obtaining informed consent. Experimentation on human beings was still very much part of clinical research, not only in Germany. Formal restrictions beyond the Hippocratic oath to do no harm as well as requirements for informed consent date from after World War II.[16]

The intensive deep therapy of Seitz and Wintz would rapidly become known abroad as the "German" style of therapy. Within Germany, however, the Erlangen technique faced a good deal of opposition. To many practitioners, the technique had the same disadvantages as the single-sitting technique that Kienböck had introduced for more superficial therapy twenty years earlier: it was overly schematic and did not permit adjusting the treatment to the progress of individual cases. The margins of safety seemed exceedingly small to professionals who were now convinced that protection was essential. In the many-sittings approach, the skin and blood of the patient were given an opportunity to recover between irradiations, the Röntgen hangover was less frequent, and in treatment of

[16] Bazzano LA, Durant J, Brantley PR. A Modern History of Informed Consent and the Role of Key Information. Ochsner Journal. 2021 Spring;21(1):81–85. https://doi.org/10.31486/toj.19.0105, accessed December 20, 2023. PMID: 33828429; PMCID: PMC7993430.

uterine fibromas the artificially induced menopause came about more slowly, and the fibromas disintegrated more gradually.[17] Opposition also came from practitioners who disagreed with the basic objective of the Erlangen technique, which was to kill cells. It was possible that radiation cured by stimulating the body's natural defense mechanisms. This notion, which is still sometimes debated, had been discussed earlier, and by 1920 it was a mainstream view in England.[18] In Germany, the introduction of intensive deep therapy raised the issue anew, since the stimulative effect of radiation was believed to exist at lower doses rather than at the higher doses Seitz and Wintz were using.[19] Repeated applications of the "stimulation" dose (*Reizdosis*) posed a sharp contrast to the application of large doses in a single setting.

The Erlangen technique also ran into opposition because it relied on ionization measurements. Opposition among practitioners was to be expected, but more important at the time was opposition among researchers to ionization as the basic mechanism of radiation effects. On the biological side, investigations of the precipitation of colloids by radiation had shown that breakdown of protein (denaturation) preceded precipitation. The primary effect of the radiation was then probably a chemical change, not a physical discharge of the colloidal particles by ionization.[20] Physicists were also starting to question the assumption that ionization in air measured the absorbed energy, an assumption implicit in most pre-war laboratory work with radiation. Ionization was not, however, the only effect observed when radiation was absorbed. Heating

[17] See the comments of Albers-Schönberg in the discussion following Wintz, ibid.

[18] See, for example, Mikhailov, VF, Zasukhina, G.D. A New Approach to the Stimulation of the Body's Defense Systems with Low Radiation Doses. Biology Bulletin Reviews 10, 475–482 (2020). https://doi.org/10.1134/S2079086420060031, accessed October 23, 2023.

[19] See, for example, Frankel M (Charlottenburg). Die Reizdosenanwendung, ihre Bedeutung für die Röntgentherapie. Verh Deut Rönt Ges. 1920;11:89–92, or the full text Die Bedeutung der Röntgen-Reizstrahlen in der Medizin mit besonderer Einwirkung auf das endokrine System und seiner Beeinflussung des Karzinoms. Strahlentherapie. 1921;12:603–38 and 850–99.

[20] Fernau A, Pauli W (aus der k. k. Radiumstation im allgemeinen Krankenhause und dem Laboratorium für physikalisch-chemische Biologie der k. k. Universität Wien, mit Unterstützung der Fürst Liechtenstein-Spende). Über die Einwirkung der durchdringenden Radiumstrahlung auf anorganische und Biokollide. I, Biochemische Zeitschrift. 1915;70:426–41, eingegangen am 4 Juni 1915. This W. Pauli was the father of the well-known physicist of the same name.

and chemical changes might also occur, and there was no guarantee that the proportion of these different physical effects would remain the same over a wide range of wavelengths. Theophil Christen, from his post at the Radiation Research Unit of Reiniger, Gebbert, and Schall, raised this question of the relationship between ionization and absorbed energy in 1916. Richard Glocker, in the first review of medical radiological dosage techniques published in a physical journal, reiterated the underlying assumption and emphasized its importance: "All ionization measurements of the energy of radiation rest on the assumption that the number of ions produced per unit volume of gas is, independent of the hardness of the rays, directly proportional to the radiation energy absorbed in the unit volume."[21] In other words, physicists assumed the electrical charge X-rays produced in a measuring device was proportional to the energy absorbed in the device.

Beginning in 1919, Hermann Holthusen, the physician who had worked with physicist Philipp Lenard and habilitated at Heidelberg, denied this vulnerable assumption of proportionality between ionization and absorbed energy, attacked the idea that ionization caused the biological effects of radiation, and put forward an alternative view of the underlying mechanism.[22] Krönig and Friedrich had ostensibly chosen ionization as the basis for their X-ray measurements on practical grounds. Their finding that biological effects were proportional to ionization independent of X-ray quality nevertheless strengthened the notion that ionization was the fundamental mechanism. Holthusen, by contrast, was

[21] Christen T (aus der Strahlenforschungsstelle der Reiniger, Gebbert und Schall-A.-G., München). Energiemessung von ionisierenden Strahlen insbesondere von Röntgenstrahlen. Physikalische Zeitschrift. 1916;17:23–5, eingegangen 17 Januar 1916, at 25: "...ein Zweifel auftaucht ob denn auch wirklich der Sättigungsstrom der in der Luft absorbierten Energie streng proportional sei oder ob nicht am Ende das als Proportionalitätskonstante aufzufassende Umsetzungsverhältnis zwischen der absorbierten Energie und der Ionisation eine Funktion der Wellenlänge sei, etwa auf Kosten von gleichzeitig entstehender Erwärmung der Luft"; Glocker R. Die Messmethoden der Röntgenstrahlen. Physikalische Zeitschrift. 1917;18:302–15 and 330–8, eingegangen 14 Mai 1917, at 306: "Alle Ionisations messungen von Strahlungsenergien beruhen auf der Voraussetzung, dass die pro Volumeneinheit des Gases erzeugte Ionenzahl, unabhängig von der Härte der Strahlen, direkt proportional der in der Volumeneinheit absorbierten Strahlungsenergie ist."

[22] Holthusen H (aus der Medizinischen Klinik Heidelberg). Über die Bedingungen der Röntgestrahlenenergiemessung bei verschiedenen Impulsbreiten auf luftelektrischem Wege. Fortschr Röntgenstr. 1918;26:211–31.

convinced that excitation of biologically important molecules (without ionization) could cause chemical reactions and thereby the observed radiation effects. To decide the issue, Holthusen proposed measuring biological effects resulting from exposures to X-rays of different qualities while maintaining, in one series, equal doses measured by ionization and, in another series, equal doses measured by absorbed energy. If the biological effects were the same when ionization was the same even though the quality of the X-rays had changed, Holthusen would conclude that ionization was the underlying mechanism. If the biological effects were the same when the absorbed energy was the same even though the quality of the X-rays had changed, Holthusen believed he would have *prima facie* evidence against ionization as the underlying mechanism and in favor of his own "chemical" view.

There ensued a complicated experimental and theoretical duel between Holthusen and his Erlangen colleagues.[23] Following up his attack on ionization as the fundamental mechanism of radiation effects, Holthusen put forward an ultimately fruitless proposal concerning dosage measurements and units. Instead of an ionization unit *e*, Holthusen preferred a biological system for measuring dosage and a biological unit, in part because he believed that variation in biological effect with changes in radiation quality would be parallel for all biological objects and that therefore a biological method would eliminate the need for considering X-ray quality separately.[24] The notion of a biological unit had considerable appeal. Two physicians who had proposed a "mouse" dose, which they defined as the quantity of radiation required to cause death in mice by damage to lymphoid tissue, argued in favor of biological measurements:

> ...because in therapy it is always a matter of producing an effect on a biological process, be it of normal or pathological character, so it would naturally be the best if one could undertake the graduation of the effect,

[23] This controversy is recounted in more detail in Serwer DP. The Rise of Radiation Protection: Science, Medicine and Technology in Society, 1896–1935. Brookhaven National Laboratory; Dec 1976. 161–9.

[24] Holthusen (Hamburg). Über die Beziehungen zwischen physikalischer und biologischer Dosierung. Verh Deut Rönt Ges. 1924;15. or Fortschr Röntgenstr. 32 (1. Kongressheft 1924):73–9.

> that is the measurement of the dose, by means of a biological measurement method.[25]

A unit based on the effect of radiation on the roots of pea plants was proposed in 1920.[26] In England, a physicist who was unaware of the controversy in Germany had proposed in 1918 a unit called the "rad," which he defined as the quantity of radiation which, when absorbed by sarcoma cells, caused their eventual destruction on implantation into rats.[27] Holthusen cited this suggestion and also proposed that Krönig and Friedrich's frog larvae, his own horse saliva worms, or the fruit flies used in the United States for genetics experiments (later to prove important not only to genetics but also to radiation protection) might serve as the basis for a biological unit of dosage.

This may all seem a bit comical or even macabre in retrospect, but as we shall see, biological units continued to have considerable appeal to those concerned with biological radiation effects. In practice, however, the only biological unit that was used extensively was Seitz and Wintz's unit skin dose. It became common throughout Germany in the early 1920s. The shift to the unit skin dose from earlier units was an easy one, since most of them, like Holzknecht's H, were fractions of the dose that caused a skin reaction. The use of biological units did not, however, bring use of biological measurements. Clinical measurement did not turn to mice or pea plants but rather to ionization chambers. Reiniger, Gebbert, and Schall, which was the only firm manufacturing the Kienböck strips, by 1923 was explicitly denying responsibility for any harm to patients caused when using the strips, and it was by then clear that in

[25] Meyer H (Privatdozent), Ritter H. Experimentelle Studien zur Feststellung eines biologischen Normalmasses für Röntgenstrahlen. Strahlentherapie. 1912;1:183–8, aus dem Institut für Strahlenbehandlung der Königl. Dermatol. Klinik zu Kiel (Direktor: Prof. Klingmüller), at 183:"...da es sich in der Therapie stets darum handelt, eine Wirkung auf biologische Prozesse hervorzurufen, seien sie nun normaler oder pathologischer Natur, so wäre es natürlich das beste, wenn man die Abstufung der Wirkung, d. h. also die Dosierung an der Hand eines biologischen Messverfahrens vornehmen könnte."

[26] Jüngling O (Priv.-Dozent, Assistenzarzt der Chirurgischen Universitätsklinik Tübingen, Vorstand: Prof. Dr. Perthes). Die praktische Verwendbarkeit der Wurzelreaktion von Vicia faba equina zur Bestimmung der biologischen Wertigkeit der Röntgenstrahlung. Münchener Medizinische Wochenschrift. 1920;672:1141–4.

[27] Russ S. A Suggestion for a New X-Ray Unit in Radiotherapy. Archives of Radiology and Electrotherapy. 1918 Dec;23(7):226–32. A different "rad" would come into common use after World War II.

a lawsuit their use would not be considered adequate to avoid a penalty for negligence.[28] Using whatever ionization chamber it chose, each clinic determined for itself the amount of ionization required to produce a skin reaction and then reported its dosages as percentages of this unit skin dose. The method was, above all, convenient: several companies had begun marketing ionization chambers to physicians, no standardization with a large ionization chamber was required, and each clinic could work independently. Many medical radiologists were prepared to do without standardization of ionization measurements among clinics, which scientific laboratories had done for years. They believed the unit skin dose would suffice for comparability. Physicians aggressively pursued clinical results on that flimsy basis for comparing or reproducing results.

To the German and other physicists who had entered medical radiology in the previous decade, the reliance among the medical practitioners on the unit skin dose was intolerable. In the first place, the unit skin dose did not meet the physicists' standard of precision. There were variations in the skin reaction used to define the dose in different clinics, and the small, commercially available chambers gave readings that depended on the hardness of the X-rays used. In 1922, a comparative study of the unit skin doses in different clinics yielded variations of around 50 percent.[29] In 1924, a more extensive study of fourteen clinics using twenty-seven different ionization chambers was undertaken by Leonard Grebe and Heinrich Martius, Bonn physicists.[30] They found that unit skin doses within Germany varied by as much as a factor of four. The physicists also found the combination of a physical method of measurement with a

[28] Küstner H (Göttingen). Vorarbeitung zur Schaffung eines Standardgeräts zur Dosierung der Röntgenstrahlen," from the report of the "Sitzung der von der Deutschen Röntgengesellschaft eingesetzten Kommission zwecks Schaffung eines Standardinstrumentes für die Röntgenstrahlenmessung," am 21 Oktober 1923 in Göttingen. Fortschr Röntgenstr. 1923;31:483–7, at 485: "Seine Anwendung kann den Arzt keinesfalls vor Schadenersatzansprüchen des Patienten schützen. Die Firma Reiniger, Gebbert und Schall, Erlangen, von der alle Streifen, Entwickeln und Geräte bezogen waren, lehnt diese Verantwortung auf Entschädigungsansprüche in ihrer Gebrauchsanweisung ebenfalls ab."

[29] Bachem A (Priv.-Doz., aus dem Institut für physikalische Grundlagen der Medizin in Frankfurt a. M., zurzeit Chicago). Zur praktischen Dosierung der Röntgenstrahlen verschiedener Härte. Strahlentherapie. 1922;13:605–10.

[30] Grebe L (Röntgen-Forschungs u. Unterrichtsinstitut der Universität Bonn), Martius H (Universitäts-Frauenklinik in Bonn). Vergleichende Messungen über der Grosse der zur Erreichung der Hauterythems gebrauchlichen Röntgenstrahlenmenge. Strahlentherapie. 1924;18:395–409.

biological unit anomalous. Ionization, in their view, belonged to physics and should be measured in physical units.

Friedrich, working with his student Otto Glasser, strengthened the physicists' hand by demonstrating in 1922 that the discrepancy between the results he had obtained with Krönig at Erlangen and Holthusen's Heidelberg results on the question of the variation of biological effects with hardness (penetrating power) was the result of a difference in their experimental arrangements.[31] While admitting Holthusen's claim that the chamber used in Friedrich's earlier work with Krönig was not sufficiently large relative to the range of the secondary cathode rays, Friedrich and Glasser believed that the discrepancy came from another source. Holthusen had irradiated his worms in a thin layer, but Krönig and Friedrich had irradiated their frog larvae submerged in a tank of water. Holthusen, then, had avoided significant scattering, but Krönig and Friedrich had measured a dose that included scattering from the water. The added scattering dose in their small chamber increased with increasing hardness in such a way that the ionization Krönig and Friedrich actually measured was proportional to the energy of the secondary cathode rays. The Krönig and Friedrich results, correctly interpreted, therefore agreed with Holthusen's and confirmed the notion that biological effect was proportional not to ionization but to absorbed energy.

With this fundamental question resolved, Friedrich and Glasser attacked Holthusen on another front. Holthusen had wanted to decide the dosimetry question by determining the mechanism of the radiation effects, which he thought were chemical rather than electrical. Friedrich and Glasser proposed separating these issues. Admitting that not enough was known of the mechanism of radiation effects to be sure that the processes that occurred in an ionization chamber were the same as those that occurred in biological materials, it was still possible to design sufficiently sensitive and reliable instruments, and units, to give reproducible results. From this point of view, ionization measurements and the *e* unit, measured in a large chamber and avoiding radiation from the walls, were still the best methods from the physicists' point of view, regardless of the mechanism of radiation effects. The physicists pressed this point of view in a new Commission for the Creation of a Standard Instrument for X-ray Measurement, created by the German Röntgen Society in

[31] Friedrich W, Glasser OA. Untersuchungen und Betrachtungen über das Problem der Dosimetrie. Strahlentherapie. 1922;14:362–88.

1923.[32] Moreover, physicist Hermann Behnken, who had moved from Friedrich's laboratory to the Physical-Technical Institute, went ahead without agreement from the medical radiologist and biologists.[33] Before the Commission had reached agreement, Behnken had already begun standardizing small ionization chambers using an "air-pressure" chamber that he had designed and that the firm of Siemens and Halske had produced.[34] It was Behnken who relabelled the *e* unit R, for Röntgen, following an earlier French proposal. The practical dosage problem, so far as the German physicists were concerned, appeared to be solved by 1924.

Scientific Theory Starts to Catch Up, but Protection Still Lags

Just as the physicists were separating the practical issues in X-ray dosimetry from the problem of understanding the mechanism of radiation effects, a physicist was proposing a theory of radiation effects that would provide an account of how ionization, as observed in Wilson's cloud-chamber photographs, caused biological effects. Friedrich Dessauer, the German X-ray tube manufacturer who obtained a doctorate in physics during the War, proposed in 1922 the "point heat" or, as it later became known, "hit" theory.[35] Noting that the total amount of energy transferred in the absorption of X-rays was no more than the energy transferred

[32] Sitzung der von der Deutschen Röntgengesellschaft eingesetzten Kommission zwecks Schaffung eines Standard-instrumentes für die Röntgenstrahlenmessung, am 21 Oktober 1923 in Göttingen. Fortschr Röntgenstr. 1923;31:483–7.

[33] Bekanntmachung betreffend die Eichung von Röntgenstrahlen Dosismessern in der Physikalisch-Technischen Reichsanstalt. Fortschr Röntgenstr. 1923;31:565–6. and Behnken (Berlin). Die Eichung von Dosismessern in absolutem Masse in der Physikalisch-technischen Reichsanstalt. Verh Deut Rönt Ges. 1924;15:92–4.

[34] Behnken H. Die Vereinheitlichung der Röntgenstrahlen-Dosismessung und die Eichung von Dosismessern. Zeitschrift fur technische Physik. 1924;5:3–16, eingegangen 4 September 1923.

[35] Dessauer F. Über einige Wirkungen von Strahlen. I. Zeitschrift für Physik. 1922;12:38–47, Mitteilung aus dem Universitäts institut für physikalische Grundlagen der Medizin in Frankfurt a. Main, eingegangen am 30 September 1922; and Blau M, Altenburger K. Über einige Wirkungen von Strahlen. II. Zeitschrift für Physik. 1922;12:315–29, Mitteilung aus dem Universitäts institut für physikalische Grundlagen der Medizin, eingegangen am 2 November 1922. See also Dessauer F (Direktor des Instituts für physikalische Grundlagen der Medizin an der Universität Frankfurt a. M.).

in a couple of swallows of warm water, Dessauer accounted for the difference in the biological effects caused by the way in which the energy was delivered. The hit theory treated the biological effects of radiation as the result of hits by one or more secondary cathode rays on especially sensitive structures or targets in the cell. A hit caused rapid motion of the molecules within a target, an event Dessauer thought of as "point heat." The nature of the targets was a matter of continuing debate, but the mathematical part of the theory did not require their specification. It was well known to physicists that hitting a target of a given size with randomly thrown projectiles was a process governed by a well-known probability law. At low doses, this law yielded a linear relationship between dose and effect. If more than one hit were required to bring about a given effect, the relationship between dose and effect would in general be sigmoid (S-shaped).

The hit theory would later in the 1920s and in the 1930s prove fruitful for radiation biology and provide, as Dessauer had hoped it would, a physical basis for radiation therapy and radiation genetics, but in the early 1920s it was a controversial theory that did not attract much immediate support in the medical radiological community. The mathematics used was beyond most medical practitioners, and in addition the evidence was not persuasive to biologists. The primary support came from experiments showing a sigmoid relationship between dose and effect, and such a relationship could derive from random variability in the biological materials as well as from random hits on cellular targets.[36] Holthusen summarized the initial attitude of physicians and biologists when he said, "The many ways in which the rays can affect the body do not allow themselves to be reduced to a formula."[37] Holthusen was more than Dessauer's equal

Dosierung und Wesen der Röntgenstrahlenwirkung in der Tiefen therapie vom physikalischen Standpunkt, Strahlentherapeutische Monographien Band II. Dresden and Leipzig: Theodor Steinkopff; 1923. especially Teil II. Apparently independent of Dessauer, an English physicist also proposed the hit theory and used it to calculate the size of the targets, see Crowther JA. Some considerations relative to the action of X-rays on tissue cells. Proceedings of the Royal Society. 1924 Apr 1;96B(674):207–11.

[36] See, for example, Packard C (Columbia University, Institute of Cancer Research, F. C. Wood, Director). The Measurement of Quantitative Biological Effects of X-Rays. The Journal of Cancer Research. 1926 Oct 1;10(3):319–39, and Mottram JC. The Survival Curves of Cells Under Radiation. Journal of Cancer Research. 1927;11:130–4.

[37] Holthusen H (Hamburg). Die Wirkung der Röntgenstrahlen in biologischer Hinsicht. Verh Deut Rönt Ges. 1924;15 (2. Teil 1924):3–4, from the Zwischentagung der

in physics and mathematics, so this statement should not be read as hostility arising from incomprehension. Holthusen and others believed that the physical hit theory did not consider the complexity of biological phenomena, so it did not provide significant support for the shift to ionization units and measurements. The creator of the theory, Dessauer, was in fact a diehard advocate of the Kienböck strips rather than ionization chambers for clinical use, provided that the practitioner followed his recommendation to use X-rays of a single wavelength.[38] Thus, even in Germany, where the gap between laboratory and clinic was narrowing, significant gaps between scientific theory and medical practice remained in the mid-1920s: ionization measurements were accepted in the clinic but without a firm theoretical basis and with continuing use of biological units.

Outside Germany, intensive deep therapy and ionization measurements were still novelties in the early 1920s. While the Germans were settling the problems of X-ray dosimetry among themselves, professional organizations in other countries (where radium was more readily available) had become concerned with protection against effects on the blood that resulted from exposure to radium as well as X-rays. By 1924, professional committees in Britain, France, and the United States would make recommendations on radium protection, and other countries also took action. These developments outside Germany again confirm the role of public concern in forcing medical radiological communities to put radium protection on par with X-ray protection.

The effects of radiation on blood and on blood-forming organs had been known since 1903. In addition to clinical trials in curing diseases like pseudoleukemia and leukemia, extensive experiments undertaken over the next decade aimed at determining whether the clinical manifestations were the result of effects on the white and red blood cells during circulation, or whether it was the lymphoid and myeloid tissues responsible for forming these blood cells that were affected. The issue was a complex one that was not satisfactorily settled until the mid-1920s, but in the

Deutschen Röntgen-Gesellschaft als Abteilung 22 der 88. Versammlung der Gesellschaft Deutscher Naturforscher und Ärzte in Innsbruck, 24–26 September 1924, at 4: "Die vielfältigen Wege, auf denen sich die Strahlen im Körper auswirken können, lassen sich nicht auf eine Formel bringen."

See also the other papers and the discussion, ibid., 4–13.

[38] Dessauer, *Dosierung und Wesen* …, note 32.

meanwhile it became clear that there were substantial dangers to both X-ray operators and radium workers.[39] In 1911, several Viennese physicians had reported the deaths of four X-ray operators and one radium worker from what they termed leukemia. In blood samples from ten healthy X-ray workers, they found reduced numbers of polynuclear leukocytes and increased numbers of lymphocytes.[40] In 1914, the death of an Italian physician who had worked with X-rays for fourteen years was reported prominently in Archives of the Röntgen Ray.[41] The diagnosis was pernicious anemia, a condition that was thought then to be secondary to destruction of other tissues, especially in the testicles, bone marrow, and spleen.

Professional alarm bells still did not sound. These blood-related incidents were regarded as isolated cases that did not alarm most practitioners. The weight of clinical evidence was again on the side of no effect, or an idiosyncratic effect physicians ignored in most instances. When an English physicist tried in 1916 to interest the Röntgen Society in further efforts in the area of radiation protection because of cumulative effects on blood, the reception from his physician colleagues was cool:

> If the effects of X-rays are steady and cumulative, workers like Sir MacKenzie Davidson [who in 1912 had been. knighted for his contributions to· radiology] and myself would have withered away long since.[42]

[39] As it turned out, the site of the primary lesion was the bone marrow, not the components of the blood in circulation, which are relatively resistant to radiation damage, see Jolly J, Laccasagne A. De la résistance des leucocytes du sang vis-a-vis rayons X. C R Soc Biol (Paris). 1923;89:379. and Laccasagne A, Lavedan J. Les modifications histologiques du sang consécutives aux irradiations expérimentales. Paris Med. 1924 Feb 2;21:97–103.

[40] V. Jagié N, Schwarz G, Van Siebenrock L (aus der I. Medizinischen Universitätsklinik in Wien, Vorstand: Prof. C. v. Noorden). Blutbefunde bei Röntgenologen. Berlin Klin Wschr. 1911;482:1220–2.

[41] The Autopsy of a Radiologist. Arch Rönt Ray. 1914 Apr 1;18(11):393–4. The radiologist was Emilio Tiraboschi, who worked at the Ospidale Maggiore in Bergamo. The original report was published in Gavazzeni S, Minelli S. L'Autopsie d'un radiologo. Radiologia Medica. 1914 Feb;1:66–71.

[42] The Injurious Effects Produced by X-rays; a Discussion at the Röntgen Society on 1 February 1916. Journal of the Röntgen Society. 1916;12:38–56. Sidney Russ (D. Sc.) opened the discussion. The comment quoted here was by Reginald Morton, at 40.

> Less than a pastille dose, especially if spread over a long period, is not going to do anyone any harm. Therefore, if the operator adopts the precaution of merely standing three yards from his apparatus, he is going to be pretty safe in any X-ray treatment.[43]

At the same meeting at which these comments were made, there was considerable concern with dermatitis reported among newly trained operators in the field. The lack of concern was limited to effects supposedly caused over a long period by repeated exposures when no acute symptoms were apparent. Though they themselves were the people most exposed over long periods, practitioners in Britain and France were convinced that such effects either did not occur or were so rare that they did not merit the attention of the profession. Another discussion of protection at the British Röntgen Society in 1919 that was concerned primarily with the harder X-rays available from Coolidge tubes led to "a hopeless divergence of opinion on the degree of screening required for the protection of the operator."[44] In retrospect, radiation experts were remarkably resistant to acknowledging the long-term effects that posed risks to themselves.

Public Concern Changes the Picture, Except in Germany

This situation changed rapidly in late 1920 and in 1921. J. C. Mottram, a physician who had been appointed head of the Research Department at the London Radium Institute, reported in August 1920 five cases of "aplastic pernicious anemia" occurring among clinical and laboratory workers at the Institute during the preceding several years. Three of the workers had died.[45] Mottram had been working for several years on effects on the blood, and one of his collaborators had been the physicist

[43] The comment was by N. S. Finzi, ibid., at 44.

[44] Editorial Notes. Journal of the Röntgen Society. 1919 Jul;15:66.

[45] Mottram JC. The Red Cell Blood Content of Those Handling Radium for Therapeutic Purposes. Archives of Radiology and Electrotherapy. 1920 Dec 1;25(7):194–7, read before the Pathological Society of Great Britain and Ireland, 3 August 1920. Mottram had already reported abnormalities in the blood of these workers, see Mottram JC (M. B.), Clarke JR. The Leucocytic Blood-Content of Those Handling Radium for Therapeutic Purposes. Proc Roy Soc Med. 1920;13(11):25–30, reprinted in Archives of Radiology and Electrotherapy. 1919;24:345–50. It turned out later that the immediate cause of death in two of these three cases was not pernicious anemia, but Mottram thought that the

who raised the question of protection from these effects at the Röntgen Society during the War.[46] By aplastic pernicious anemia, Mottram meant a severe decrease in the red blood cell count that was secondary to damage to the hematopoietic tissue in the bone marrow (not the B12 vitamin deficiency it entails today). He readily confirmed the effects on the bone marrow under laboratory conditions, and he also showed that with the introduction of simple protection measures in the clinic the red blood cell counts of the radium workers returned to normal.[47] The protection measures included better ventilation (to remove radium emanation); the use of forceps, of lead-lined boxes carried close to the floor in slings, and of lead rubber gloves in handling radium applicators; placement of filters on these applicators by temporary workers changed every three months; and the use of five-centimeter thick lead screens and similarly lined tables during manipulation of the applicators.

Mottram's reports from the London Radium Institute were already having an impact in the winter of 1921 on the French medical radiological community, but in Britain it was the death in March 1921 of a leading X-ray physician, Ironside Bruce, from acute aplastic anemia that galvanized public reaction and thereby generated a professional response.[48] The moment was an especially delicate one. A public fund-raising campaign to establish an Institute of Radiology had been launched in 1920.[49] The

anemia had weakened the resistance of the workers, see Foreign Letters. Journal of the American Medical Association. 1921 May 21;762:1412–3.

[46] For one product of this collaboration, see Russ S (D. Sc.), Chambers H (M. D. Lond.), Scott G, Mottram JC (M. B. Lond.). Experimental Studies with Small Doses of X-Rays. The Lancet. 1919 Apr 1;193(4991):692–5, undertaken at the request of the Medical Research Council and funded by the Cancer Investigation Fund of Middlesex Hospital.

[47] Mottram JC. Histological Changes in the Bone Marrow of Rats Exposed to the γ Radiations from Radium. Archives of Radiology and Electrotherapy. 25:197–9. and Mottram JC. The Effect of Increased Protection from Radiation upon the Blood Condition of Radium Workers. Archives of Radiology and Electrotherapy. 1921;25:368–72.

[48] For Bruce's obituary, which did not mention the cause of death but identified him as a "martyr," see Archives of Radiology and Electrotherapy. 1920;25:338. The case was later described, without identifying the victim, in Larkin FE. A Case of Acute Aplastic Anemia. Archives of Radiology and Electrotherapy. 25:380–2. Such were the sensitivities of a profession that had chosen to ignore this particular risk, but the lay press had already identified the victim and his disease.

[49] The MacKenzie Davidson Memorial Fund. Archives of Radiology and Electrotherapy. 24:306–7, where the original appeal and list of sponsoring luminaries (including A. Bonar

British Association for the Advancement of Radiology and Physiotherapy (BARP), which had been founded in 1917, was trying to sustain the war-time increase in the importance of radiology and raise the status of radiology within medicine. BARP had in 1919 convinced the University of Cambridge to offer the first postgraduate examination and diploma in medical radiology (and electrology, which was still an associated field in Britain).[50] The need for protection had been used as a justification for specialty status.[51] It would hardly do to have the practitioners of a field that was asking for public support and specialty status dying of injuries caused by the tools of their trade. A series of newspaper reports on Bruce's death and the dangers of X-rays led Robert Knox, a physician who had worked with physicist G. W. C. Kaye on the examination of aircraft timbers for faults using X-rays during the War, to propose in a letter to the London Times the establishment of a committee of physicists, physiologists, and radiologists to report on X-ray effects, especially effects on the blood, and on protective measures.[52] The intense pressures

Law, Stanley Baldwin, J. J. Thomson, Coolidge, and leading lights of the British medical radiological community) is reproduced. Failing an institute, plans called for a university chair.

[50] Report of the Special Board of Medicine upon a proposal to establish a Diploma in Medical Radiology and Electrology in the University [of Cambridge], dated 20 May 1919 and reprinted under the heading British Association of Radiology and Physiotherapy. Archives of Radiology and Electrotherapy. 24:31–4. This report to the Vice-Chancellor was communicated to the Senate, which on 17 June 1919 promulgated detailed plans for the syllabus of subjects to be covered by the examination, see the account in The Work of the British Association of Radiology and Physiotherapy. Archives of Radiology and Electrotherapy. 24:209–16. In the first of these reports, it is noted that a physician had contributed £1000 to cover the University's initial expenses in setting the examination, which would eventually become self-supporting from fees charged the candidates. The examination was given for the first time in July 1920, and the physicians were relieved that "no question on higher mathematics was asked, and a knowledge of only simple calculations would be required...," see The Diploma in Medical Radiology and Electrology. Archives of Radiology and Electrotherapy. 25:164–8, where the entire examination is reproduced.

[51] "Report of the Special Board," ibid., at 32: "...only medical men who have received special training in Physics and Practical Radiology, Electrotherapy and Electrology generally, are in a position to understand and foresee not only the development of their application to diagnosis and treatment, but also their limitations and dangers."

[52] Knox's letter to the Times was printed on March 29, 1921. It has been reprinted in Nauman JD. Pioneer Descriptions in the Story of X-ray Protection. In: Classic Descriptions in Diagnostic Röntgenology. Springfield Illinois: Charles C. Thomas; 1964:311–39. For Knox's war-time work with Kaye, see Captain Knox R, Kaye GWC. The Examination

that members of the medical radiological community were feeling as a result of newspaper reports in the spring of 1921 are reflected in a statement by a British X-ray equipment manufacturer at the Röntgen Society in April:

> I would remind those present that almost the only publicity we get is when someone dies, or swallows the radium.... Listen to these headings from the papers of the past two days. '[X-ray Dangers, a peril to people in rooms above the operating chamber'; 'Perilous X-rays, leaden screens to protect next door neighbors.' Not a word about the tens of thousands of people whose lives have been saved by X-rays, or whose sufferings have been relieved. I have reason to think that certain papers are deliberately putting forward the danger side of X-rays and radium, and that they will not publish re-assuring matter. Such a position would be scarcely possible if there were a Röntgen Society propaganda committee.[53]

Pressure from newspapers led to professional action, as is also clear from retrospective accounts.[54] Professional "self-regulation" was not automatic. It required an external stimulus.

of Aircraft Timber by X Rays, a contribution to a "General Discussion on the Examination of Materials by X Rays" held jointly by the Faraday Society and the Röntgen Society. Archives of Radiology and Electrotherapy. 1919 Apr 29;24.; G. W. C. Kaye, (0. B. E., M. A., D. Sc., R. A. F.), "The Examination of Aircraft Timber by X Rays," a contribution to a "General Discussion on the Examination of Materials by X Rays," held jointly by the Faraday Society and the Röntgen Society, 29 April 1919 and abstracted in Archives of Radiology and Electrotherapy. 24 (1919–20) 295–97.

[53] Andrews C. X-rays and Propaganda. Journal of the Röntgen Society. 1921;17:129–32, read 21 April 1921, at 131–2.

[54] The most detailed of these retrospective accounts is by Melville S. A Discussion on the International Protection Recommendations. The British Journal of Radiology. 1932 Jan 14 and 1931 Nov 19;2:215–233, at 218: "In the spring of 1921 radiology was very near to what might have been a terrific onslaught by the Press. On my way home from a Memorial Service for our old friend Ironside Bruce, whose untimely death caused much concern, I discussed with the Secretary to the Medical Society of London the many references that had been made in the public Press to his death. To my amazement, he informed me that he had been discussing the matter with a member of one of our most powerful papers, and that they had every intention of launching into a warning to the public against the dangers of X rays. I found on enquiry at the office of the paper that my information was correct." See also, Kaye GWC. Röntgenology: Its Early History, Some Basic Physical Principles and the Protective Measures. London: William Heinemann; 1928:69.

A committee established under the chairmanship of the President of the Royal Society of Medicine, Sir Humphrey Rolleston, was far from merely a propaganda committee, but it was nevertheless an attempt to defend medical radiology from what the profession regarded as undue public criticism. It issued its first report in June 1921 and did not dissolve until the 1950s. Mottram's concern for radium protection was incorporated along with X-ray protection. An informal cooperative venture of the leading medical radiological organizations in Britain, this British X-ray and Radium Protection Committee became an important forum for discussion among physicians and nonphysicians of protection measures and a model that other countries would imitate. The organizations involved included BARP, the Röntgen Society, and the Electrotherapeutic Section of the Royal Society of Medicine. As we shall see in the next chapter, these organizations had not been on good terms. Their cooperation in the Protection Committee should be viewed as a temporary show of unity in response to a common threat. They were forming what we now recognize as an interdisciplinary "epistemic community" of experts concerned with setting norms aimed to protect both patients and medical radiology.

In France, as in Britain, practitioners had largely discounted the effects of radiation on the blood as a serious source of concern. French biologists had done extensive experimental work on these effects before the War.[55] When, however, a French physician in 1918 reminded his colleagues of the death of the Italian radiologist of pernicious anemia, a leading radiologist replied that the case was an isolated one and may not have been caused by X-rays.[56] In late March 1921, Henri Bordier, a physician and professor of medicine at Lyons who had done research with both X-rays and radium, reported on Mottram's work to the French Academy of Medicine, claiming that radium was more dangerous so far as effects on

[55] For one of many articles, see Aubertin C, Beaujard E. Actions des rayons X sur le sang et la moelle osseuse. I. Action d'une dose unique d'intensité moyenne en irradiation totale. Arch Med Exp. 1908;20:273–88.

[56] Mignon (M. le Docteur). La Protection en radiologie. Journal of Radiology and Electrology. 1918;3:165–72, communication faite à la Réunion des radiologistes de la XIIIe Région, with discussion. It was Belot who emphasized that this was an isolated case.

the blood were concerned than X-rays.[57] The Paris Radium Institute had only recently opened its new buildings, the completion of which had been delayed by the War. There was a good deal of talk about curing cancer with radium. Marie Curie had only recently succeeded in convincing the American public to buy her a gram of radium partly with the promise of progress in the fight against cancer.[58]

The report on Mottram's work in Britain brought public concern, and in response the appointment of a special commission of the French Academy of Medicine in 1921 to advise on the need for protection measures. The rapporteur of the commission was clear about the importance of public pressure in its creation: "The well known dangers of radioactive materials and X-rays have for some time drawn the attention of the public at large in a remarkable way, and have provoked unjustified fears."[59] After the death of Ironside Bruce, Bordier made an attempt to interest the French Society for Medical Radiology, a group that excluded nonphysicians, in undertaking blood examinations of X-ray workers. The reply was negative: This observation [that the protection being used is insufficient] is perhaps true for his service, but it cannot be generalized without supporting evidence, under penalty of discouraging young radiologists.[60]

[57] Bordier H (Professeur à la Faculté de Médecine de Lyon). Les dangers du radium. Utilité des mesures de protection. Bulletin of the Academy of Medicine (Paris). 1921;85:416–7, séance du 29 mars.

[58] Reid R. Marie Curie. New York: New American Library; 1974. gives an extensive account of this post-war period in France and Curie's trip to the United States in Chapter 20 and 21. Reid is, however, wrong in saying (at p. 240) that there was no committee concerned with radium protection in France as late as 1922.

[59] Broca. Sur les dangers des radiations pénétrantes et les moyens de les éviter, au nom de la Commission du Radium. British Academy of Medicine (Paris). 1921;85:651–60, séance du 7 juin, at 651: "Les dangers bien connus des corps radioactifs et des rayons X ont attiré depuis quelque temps d'une manière spéciale l'attention du grand public, et ont provoqué des craintes injustifiées." See also the retrospective account of the 1921 events in Bouchacourt and Morel-Kahn (les docteurs), De quelques point fondamentaux concernant la protection des personnes utilisant les R. X. Bulletin of the Society of Radiology and Medicine (Paris). 1928 Feb 14;16:59–65.

[60] Haret, in the discussion, ibid., at 160: "cette observation est peut-être vraie pour son service, mais elle ne peut-être généralisée, sans preuve à l'appui, sous peine de décourager les jeunes radiologistes." Béclère added: "Nous pouvons tous un jour ou l'autre être atteints d'une affection grave sans qu'il soit absolument besoin de mettre en cause les rayons de Röntgen. Il ne s'ensuit pas, d'ailleurs, que nous ne devions pas nous entourer du maximum de tous les moyens de protection."

For physicians, the weight of the evidence and the interests of the profession still weighed against even collecting data, never mind acting.[61]

In addition to the direct public pressure, there were other mechanisms at work in encouraging the French medical community to take radium protection measures: insurance companies and the laws governing industrial health and workmen's compensation. At least one French company that insured X-ray and radium clinics for liability for harm to their own personnel and to visitors was concerned with the reports of effects on blood. A physician hastened to reassure the insurers that there was no risk to patients and little risk to the personnel.[62] At the same time, inquiries from insurance companies made it clear that it would be desirable if the medical radiological community could agree on appropriate protection measures and thereby avoid the imposition of even more burdensome procedures.[63] So far as existing laws were concerned, France had in 1919 extended the protection of its industrial accident law to most occupational diseases. The medical radiological community was concerned that radium institutes not be classified among the "dirty industries" that were excluded from the workmen's compensation scheme.[64]

The British and French recommendations for radium protection were in many respects similar.[65] As the Röntgen Society noted, "The attitude of the [French] Commission towards these dangers is identical with that

[61] Bordier H (le docteur, professeur agrégé à la Faculté de Médecine de Lyon). Sur un cas d'anémie mortelle due aux rayons X. Bulletin of the Society of Radiology and Medicine (Paris). 1921 Nov 8;9:158–60, with discussion.

[62] Laquerrière, note 2.

[63] See Regaud C. Sur les dangers du radium. Bulletin of the Academy of Medicine (Paris). 1921;85:608–12, séance du 24 mai, where Regaud argued against the lead protection surrounding patients undergoing radium treatments suggested by Bordier H (Professeur à la Faculté de médecine de Lyon). Dangers du radium et mesures à prendre pour les éviter. ibid. 512–13, séance du 26 avril.

[64] For mention of the extension of the French law on workmen's compensation to occupational diseases, see Flaskamp W (Dr. med., aus der Universitäts-Frauenklinik Erlangen). Röntgenschädigungen als Unfälle und Gewerbekrankheiten. Fortschr Röntgenstr. 1924;32:641–7. For the concern with being classified among the "industries insalubres," see A. Broca, note 59, at 654.

[65] For the first recommendations of the British X-ray and Radium Protection Committee, dated June 1921, see Journal of the Röntgen Society. 1921 Jul;17:100–3. For the report of the French commission, see Broca, note 59. The British committee had ten members, including the chairman and honorary secretaries, of whom only three appear to have been nonphysicians (two physicists and one X-ray tube manufacturer). The

of the British Committee; it is held that the dangers may be avoided by the adoption of well-recognized precautions."[66] These precautions included those that Mottram had suggested. The Paris Radium Institute, even before the discussion at the Academy of Medicine, had indicated its willingness to adopt similar measures, except that the French preferred lead screens two centimeters (rather than five centimeters) thick for the tables at which manipulations were carried out on the radium applicators.[67] The British and French recommendations also included blood examinations for the personnel, and limitations on working hours or provisions for additional vacation time. The philosophy underlying the British recommendations was not explicitly stated, but it was implied that with proper precautions no harm would occur.[68] The French were more explicit:

> ...there is, as always, a threshold. We are sure of the existence of this threshold because there is often, perhaps always, some emanation in the air that we breathe, especially near certain mineral springs, and these areas are inhabited by thriving populations; many sick people even go there for their health.[69]
>
> There is surely a threshold for the effect of penetrating radiation, as for all kinds of energy, and this notion is confirmed by the fact that we live continuously in a very weak penetrating radiation.[70]

French committee had five members, all presumably physicians since it was appointed by the Academy of Medicine.

[66] Journal of the Röntgen Society. 1921;17:99.

[67] Felix A (Institut de Radium de l'Université de Paris). Dispositifs de protection contre les rayons du radium, à l'usage des radiumologistes-manipulateurs. Journal of Radiology and Electrology. 1921 Feb;6:61–6.

[68] See the report, note 65, at 100: "The danger of over exposure to X-rays and radium can be avoided by the provision of efficient protection and suitable working conditions..."

[69] Broca, note 59, at 654: "...il y a, comme partout, un seuil. Nous sommes certains de l'existence de ce seuil, car il y a souvent, peut-être toujours, de l'émanation dans l'air que nous respirons, en particulier au voisinage de certaines sources minérales, et ces contrées sont habitées par des populations florissantes; beaucoup de malades même y vont rétablir leur santé."

[70] Ibid., at 657: "Il y a certainement un seuil d'action pour les radiations pénétrantes, comme pour toutes les formes d'énergie, et cette vue de l'esprit est confirmée par le fait que nous vivons constamment dans une radiation pénétrante très faible..."

> We cannot in fact effect a complete suppression of penetrating radiation in order to ensure protection; it suffices to reduce it below the threshold for the harmful effect, and that is easily done.[71]

Neither British nor French physicians tried to verify experimentally that no effect occurred below a quantitatively determined threshold or to design protection measures that would assure that it was not exceeded. Physicists, as we shall see, took these steps, not physicians. The issue of whether a threshold exists for some biological effects due to radiation, especially genetic mutation, remains debated until today.

The British and French initiatives for radium protection had counterparts in other countries as well. The deaths at the London Radium Institute raised concern about the insurability of workers in radiology and inspired a survey of 1500 radiologists in the United States by the President of the American Radium Society, who also proposed that the Society appoint a protection committee to cooperate with the Safety Committee of the American Röntgen Ray Society and the Bureau of Standards.[72] This particular proposal was not acted on, but the survey of radiologists produced results showing few effects on the blood of radium and X-ray workers, an outcome that the organizer regarded as helpful to radiologists in obtaining insurance at reasonable rates.[73] The Safety Committee of the American Röntgen Ray Society, which had been established in 1920 to recommend electrical safety precautions following the electrocution of a French physician during an X-ray examination, refocused its attention on X-ray protection.[74] In the meanwhile, an investigation of

[71] Ibid., at 659: "Il n'y a pas lieu, en effet, pour assurer la protection, de réaliser la suppression complète des radiations pénétrantes; il suffit de les amener au-dessous du seuil d'action nocive, et cela est aisé."

[72] Pfahler GE. Protection in Radiology, Presidential Address, read at the 7th Annual Meeting of the American Radium Society, St. Louis Missouri. American Journal of Roentgenology. 1922 May 22;9:803–8.

[73] Pfahler GE. The Effects of the X-rays and Radium on the Blood and General Health of Radiologists, read at the 23rd Annual Meeting of the American Röntgen Ray Society, American Journal of Roentgenology. 1922 Sep 12;9:647–56, discussion at 771–74.

[74] For reports on the electrocution of Dr. Auguste Jaugeas at Beclere's X-ray clinic, see Electrocution of a Radiologist. Archives of Radiology and Electrotherapy. 1919;24:267–9, and American Journal of Roentgenology. 1921;7:167–8. For the creation of the Safety Committee,

see American Journal of Roentgenology, 8 (1921) 204, and for its report on electrical dangers, delayed by the death of its chairman, see "Report of the Safety Committee,"

workers engaged in measuring samples against the radium standard at the Bureau of Standards was undertaken by the United States Public Health Service.[75] In Norway, the "alarming news" from Britain and the death of a Norwegian radiologist in 1923 from pernicious anemia led to X-ray and radium protection measures at the Royal Hospital.[76] In Holland, the Ministry of Health set up a committee concerned with radium as well as with X-ray protection, and in the Soviet Union the Radiological Congress established a protection committee.[77]

Germany is conspicuously absent from this list of countries in which action was taken on radium protection. X-ray protection however continued to receive the attention of the German Röntgen Society, which in 1922 began an extensive survey of injuries.[78] In 1924, the Society adopted several "guidelines" for work with X-rays that reiterated the physician's obligation to provide for protection, suggested the use of a 0.5 mm aluminum filter in radiography, and emphasized that dose measurements were indispensable.[79] The British Röntgen Society had explicitly extended its purview to medical uses of radioactive substances, which in any case had long appeared as a subject at its annual congresses. Radium

presented at the Los Angeles meeting of the American Röntgen Ray Society, American Journal of Roentgenology, 10 (1923) 246–47. I have been unable to find the Safety Committee's first report (1923) on X-ray protection, but for a follow-up report see Report of the Safety Committee of the American Röntgen Ray Society presented at the 25th Annual Meeting of the American Röntgen Ray Society, Swampscott, Massachusetts. American Journal of Roentgenology. 1924 Sep 3;12:566–71. All of the members are mistakenly identified there as M. D.'s, but at least two (William D. Coolidge and William Duane) were physicists and not physicians.

[75] Williams RC. Preliminary Note on Observation Made on Physical Condition of Persons Engaged in Measuring Radium Preparations. Public Health Reports. 1923 Sep 21;38:3007–28.

[76] Amundsen P. Blood Anomalies in Radiologists and in Persons Employed in Radiological Service. Acta Radiologica. 1924;3:1–7.

[77] Kaye, note 53.

[78] Groede (Frankfurt a. M.-Bad Nauheim). Einleitung. Sammelreferat über Röntgenschädigungen. Verh Deut Ront Ges. 1922;13:75. The survey was to be conducted by the Sonderausschuss für die Beurteilung von Röntgenschädigungen und zurn Studium ihrer Verhütung.

[79] Levy-Dorn M (Prof. Dr., Vorsitzendem des Sonderausschusses für die Beurteilungen von Röntgenschädigungen und zum Studium ihrer Verhütung). Leitsätze für das Arbeiten mit Röntgenstrahlen gemäss Beschluss der Deutschen Röntgengesellschaft vom 28 April 1924. Deut Zeit Ges Gericht Med. 1924;4:288–9.

did not, however, have the public visibility in Germany that it had in other countries, and its prospects as a therapeutic agent do not appear to have excited medical or popular interest. The deaths at the London Radium Institute did not excite interest either. Without pressure from outside the profession, Germany thus lagged in professional activities concerned with radium protection.

CHAPTER 6

Establishment of International Norms, 1922–40

> The race is to the swift and the Hun will take the hindmost.
>
> —G. W. C. Kaye (D. Sc.), in his Presidential Address to the Röntgen Society, November 1917[1]

> This Congress was not only a congress of scientists, no, it was an assembly of nations.
>
> —Gosta Forsell (M. D.), at the closing of the First (post-War) International Congress of Radiology, London, July 1925[2]

The seven International Conferences of Medical Radiology and Electrology held between 1900 and 1914 were meetings at which individual speakers delivered papers to audiences organized in sections according to their scientific and medical interests. Such conferences unquestionably

[1] Kaye GWC. "X-rays and the War," Presidential Address delivered 6 November 1917. Journal of the Röntgen Society. 1918;4:2–17, at 16. Kaye had served as a Captain in the London Electrical Engineers (Territorials), see Griffiths E. G. W. C. Kaye. ICRP Archives, Archive Files. Archive File 66 (Stockholm 1928.pdf, 74–89):66–75.

[2] Gosta Forsell, as quoted in Erster Internationaler Radiologen Kongress. Fortschr Röntgenstr. 1925;33:797–800, at 800: "Dieser Kongress war nicht nur ein Kongress von Wissenschaftlern, nein, er war eine Versammlung der Nationen.".

D. Serwer, *Strengthening International Regimes*,
Palgrave Studies in International Relations,
https://doi.org/10.1007/978-3-031-53724-0_6

influence professional standards and behavior, but they do so through the give and take among individuals. There is another kind of professional conference at which collective decisions in addition to scholarly meetings of the sections are a major activity. At these conferences, committees are appointed to study particular problems, plenary sessions pass resolutions, and an executive committee is often required to manage the flow of deliberations and decisions. Norms of professional behavior result. This is the work of an interdisciplinary epistemic community of global experts committed to policy outcomes in its area of expertise. Before the War, this latter sort of professional activity had been limited to the national medical radiological organizations. Previous chapters have mentioned some of the normative decisions taken, especially in the German and British Röntgen Societies.

Formal decision-making of this type on the international level might be viewed as an entirely natural development growing from the inherently international character of science and medicine and belief in the objective character of knowledge. In this view, science and medicine are, except for minor aberrations, immune to nationalist appeals. Scholarship suggests, however, that the internationalist ethic of science often does not account for the actual behavior of scientists vis-a-vis their colleagues in other countries.[3] Instead, it has been suggested that cooperative efforts grow from competitive, and often nationalist, motives. The function of international cooperation in this view is to provide a basis for further competition. In the case of international cooperation on radium and X-ray units and standards, we shall see that, as Forman has put it in another context, "in many cases 'cooperation' and 'competition' are not behaviorally antithetic, and therefore need not be...motivationally antithetic."[4] The point can also be

[3] For a general statement of this view, see Salomon JJ. Science and Politics. tr. Noel Lindsay. MIT Press; 1973. For specialized studies, see Schroeder-Gudehus B. Deutsche Wissenschaft und international Zusammenarbeit, 1914–28: Ein Beitrag zum Studium kultureller Beziehungen in politischen Krisenzeiten. Genève: Thèse présentée à l'université de Genève, Dumaret et Golay; 1966.; Kevles DJ. Into Hostile Political Camps: The Reorganization of International Science in World War I. Isis. 1970;62:47–60.; and Forman P. Scientific Internationalism and the Weimar Physicists: The Ideology and Its Manipulation in Germany after World War I. Isis. 1973;64:151–80.

[4] Forman P. The Environment and Practice of Atomic Physics in Weimar Germany: A Study in the History of Science. University of California, Berkeley, Ph.D., Ann Arbor, Michigan: University Microfilms; 1968, at 139.

stated positively, as Forman has also suggested: cooperation can depend on competition, and competition can in turn depend on cooperation.[5]

In addition to illustrating the causal relationship between nationalist competition and international cooperation, the development of international norms in medical radiology will reveal a causal relationship between competition *within* national communities and international cooperation. Even when inspired by nationalist goals, a professional community does not necessarily find itself unified in all respects. In medical radiology, differences between physicians and nonphysicians had long been evident. These groups split further once physician-specialists and physicists started emerging as small but aggressive subgroups. As minorities, such subgroups face difficulties in having their claims to special status recognized. Superior academic credentials may hinder more than help. The majority in a professional community may resent efforts to establish specialist subgroups with higher status and interest in imposing norms that generalist members find it difficult or expensive to meet. Appealing to international cooperation is one of the strategies the more highly qualified subgroups use in outflanking domestic opposition. Better represented at international meetings and more aggressive in pursuing agreement with their colleagues in other countries, the physicists and physician-specialists in medical radiology could achieve influence on the international level that was not so readily available to them within national medical radiological organizations, where less qualified generalists outnumbered them and were more likely to prevail.

Nationalist Sentiments Stimulate Competition

By the end of the War, nationalist feelings were much higher than they had been at the time of radium standardization to meet the needs of commerce, described in Chapter 5. Nationalism would play a major role in achieving X-ray standardization. In addition to the material disruptions to professional activities, the War brought intense anti-German feelings to the radiological communities in Allied countries. Both physicians and physicists shared in the popular resentment of Germany. Any restraint they may have felt because of the internationalist ethic of science and medicine was short-lived. The organizers of the seventh International

[5] Ibid.

Congress of Medical Radiology and Electrology, which had taken place in Lyons on the eve of the pre-war mobilization in July 1914, delayed distribution of the Proceedings for nationalist reasons:

> ...inspired by a thought which each of us will find echoed in himself, the Minister of War has asked...that the distribution of the volume be postponed until the end of the hostilities in order to avoid the ill-timed publication of several German papers contributed to the Congress, which are in any case of little consequence.[6]

Allied scientists and physicians often justified anti-German comments and acts by reference to German nationalism. Physicians in Allied countries strongly resented the Prussian Ministry of War order prohibiting distribution of medical journals beyond Germany, even though it was not strictly enforced. In France, a war-time review of the German medical radiological literature based on materials obtained from neutral countries referred to the Germans as "*boches*," denounced the mathematician-physician Theophil Christen as a "despicable renegade" for leaving Switzerland to work in Germany, and concluded—after quoting anti-French comments from a German journal—that "the German mentality is furthermore something very extraordinary and remains incomprehensible for us in the baseness and crudeness of its processes and its conceptions."[7]

In Britain, the physician-controlled Archives of the Röntgen Ray changed its name in 1915 to the Archives of Radiology and Electrotherapy. That was done to rid it of the taint of the German professor who had signed a nationalist Proclamation in 1914 and who had donated his gold Rumford Medal, which the Royal Society had given him in 1896,

[6] VIIe Congrès International d'Électrologie et de la Radiologie Médicale (Lyon, 27–31 juillet 1914). Journal of Radiology and Electrology. 1916;2:659–61, at 659: "...s'inspirant d'une pensée dont chacun trouvera l'écho en lui-même, le Ministre de la guerre a, au mois de novembre dernier, demandé qu'il fût sursis à la distribution du volume jusqu'à la cessation des hostilités, afin d'éviter la publication déplacée pour le moment, des quelques mémoires allemands, d'ailleurs peu considérables, communiqués au Congrès.".

[7] Ledoux-Lebard R. Causeries sur les livres. III–La Radiologie chez les austro-allemands depuis la guerre. Journal of Radiology and Electrology. 1916;2:520–30, at 528.: "La·mentalité germanique est d'ailleurs quelque chose de bien particulier qui reste incompréhensible pour nous dans la bassesse et la primitivité de ses moyens d'action et de ses conceptions.".

to what the Allies considered a nationalist cause, the German Red Cross.[8] The Röntgen Society removed Röntgen, and two other Germans, from its list of honorary members and considered a change in name in order to remove "all taint of Germanism from the Society," as physicist G. W. C. Kaye put it. Even the arguments against the proposed change were couched in anti-German terms. Röntgen, it was noted, was "of Dutch origin" (his mother was Dutch) and changing the name of the Society was "rather too closely characteristic of learned German professors…to imitate."[9] The change was not made. In Italy, France, and England, committees were organized during the War to fight against post-war domination of the scientific and medical instruments industry by German manufacturers.[10]

Boycotts of German manufacturers were generally unsuccessful after the Armistice. The few small British X-ray equipment manufacturers failed to amalgamate so that they could compete with the larger German firms. German products once again began to dominate the British market, despite a one-third tax imposed by the Safeguarding of Industries Act

[8] The change of name was attributed in an editorial to the need for broader cooperation among all those concerned with medical electricity, and the words "Archives of the Röntgen Ray" were preserved in parentheses on the masthead, see Archives of Radiology and Electrotherapy. 1915 Jun;20:1–2. However, as early as the previous December there had apparently been pressure to change the name of the journal, for W. Deane Butcher, the editor, wrote "It may be noticed that we have not erased from our list of collaborators the names of the German and Austrian radiologists who have done so much to promote the success of this journal, an expression of our lasting belief that the brief frenzy of war should not cause any lasting breach between radiologists of different tongues.…We have no intention of retaliating [against Röntgen] by altering the title of our paper, a discourtesy which would rather savour of the religious rancour of two hundred years ago than of the cool, scientific culture of the twentieth century," Archives of Radiology and Electrotherapy. 1914 Dec;19:239–40. Butcher left the editorship in January 1915 because of illness, the Germans and Austrians were dropped from the list of collaborators in February 1915, and by June 1916 Röntgen's name was not to be found on the journal. As late as 1923, the *New York Tribune* of November 2 reminded its readers on the occasion of Röntgen's death that "because of his hatred for England," he had donated his Rumford medal to the German Red Cross, see BARP Clippings File V (Volume 5 of the BARP Clippings File in the library of the British Institute of Radiology).

[9] Discussion of the Proposed New Rules of the Society, 7 May 1918. Journal of the Röntgen Society. 1918 Oct;14:107–18, at 109. The members present at this meeting voted in favor of a change to "The Society of Radiology (Röntgen Society)," but the general membership turned down the proposal in a postal vote, ibid., at 115.

[10] Comité médical et scientifique d'expansion économique. Arch Elec Med. 1916;24:23 (feuilles de garde).

in 1921.[11] In the privacy of their order forms, and with the quality of their equipment important to the success of their practices and the safety of their own bodies, British radiologists apparently failed to heed the demands of nationalism.

These demands, however, continued to influence the public activities of the medical radiological community. Germans were excluded from many scientific and medical meetings in Allied countries in the early 1920s.[12] Medical radiologists participated in this so-called "boycott," which has been described elsewhere.[13] In 1920 and in 1922, "bilingual" radiology conferences, conducted in English and French, were held in Antwerp and in London. Exclusion of the Germans was not justified by denial of the international character of science and medicine, but rather on personal grounds:

> We frequently hear the remark that science is international in its aims and objects, and there are few who would dissent from this view, but we never interpreted this as meaning that scientists are devoid of personal feeling. We can read any scientific publications, including those of German authors, without memories of the war being thereby evoked, but a Congress is essentially a personal and friendly matter; we think the time will come for international greetings, but that it has not yet arrived.[14]

The post-war exclusion of the Germans from professional meetings did not require government action, and insofar as government rules did affect these meetings the Allies were not exempt. The 1922 bilingual conference in London had originally been scheduled for 1921, but "the adverse exchange, and the absurd regulations as to passports and costly visas"

[11] For amalgamation proposals, see Pearce G. The Future of the British X-ray Industry. Journal of the Röntgen Society. 1917;13:60–87 and 91–106., with discussion, and Kaye, note 1. For reference to the Safeguarding of Industries Act, see the Yorkshire Observer. 1921 Nov 5;in BARP Clippings File II:at 58. note 8. For one objection to the post-War resurgence of German equipment in Britain, see the letter from an unidentified British manufacturer, German-Made X-ray Apparatus. Journal of the Röntgen Society. 1922;18:95.

[12] In 1923, Germans were excluded from 70 percent of the 50 international congresses and other events, and in 1924 from 50 percent, see His W. Mitteilungen der Gesellschaft Deutscher Naturforscher und Ärtze. 2. 1925 Feb;1–4, published with Naturwissenschaften. 13 (1925).

[13] Schroeder-Gudehus, note 3.

[14] Editorial. Archives of Radiology and Electrotherapy. 1920;25:321–5, at 321.

made it difficult for the French and Belgians to attend and caused a postponement.[15]

Despite the disavowal of prejudice in evaluating the technical literature, reception of German innovations in Britain and in France was cool, and in the case of the Erlangen deep therapy technique Allied scientists were often hostile and nationalist. News of the technique reached the British public in mid-1921 through newspaper reports inspired by the West London Hospital, which had purchased German apparatus for deep therapy. Provoked by a favorable editorial in The Lancet (Britain's leading medical weekly), the British Association for the Advancement of Radiology and Physiotherapy (BARP) issued a warning against the Erlangen technique and its exaggerated claims.[16] "Public disappointment" from "unfulfilled promises" would, BARP thought, discredit radiotherapy. In France, the Erlangen technique was quickly identified as the "German" method and contrasted with the superior, "French" method of less intense exposures and more sittings.[17] Some British and French objections were similar to those German critics had put forward: the Erlangen technique was more dangerous because it could not be discontinued when the first sign of an adverse reaction appeared, and it was overly schematic. As Antoine Béclère, the leading French advocate of radiotherapy in gynecology, put it:

> The judicious employment of a pliable method which can be adapted to the exigencies of each particular case is preferable to the blind acceptance of a uniform formula; but after all, we must insist that the radiotherapist be not only an able technician, but also an excellent clinician.[18]

[15] Congress of Radiology and Physiotherapy 14–16 April 1921. Archives of Radiology and Electrotherapy. 1920;25:316. For mention of the postponement, see Journal of the Röntgen Society. 1922;18:55. For a report of the meeting finally held in 1922, see Congress of Radiology and Physiotherapy. British Medical Journal. 1922 Jun 17;1:958–60.

[16] The X Rays in Malignant Disease. Lancet. 1921 Jul 2;2:25. and for the BARP reply, X-ray Treatment-of Cancer. Med Press. 1921 Aug 24;2:15–55. See also X-Ray Treatment of Cancer–Erlangen Claims–Radiologists' Warning. The Times. 1921 Aug 22.

[17] Gunsett A (Strasbourg). Considérations sur les doses en radiothérapie profonde. Méthodes françaises—méthodes allemandes. Journal of Radiology and Electrology. 1921;5:543–51.

[18] Béclère (M. D., Academy of Medicine, Paris). What is the Best Method for the Treatment of Uterine Fibromyomata by Means of the Röntgen Rays? American Journal

For physicians, the clinic still had its own requirements, distinct from scientific measurements.

In addition to their objections to the Erlangen technique as excessively dangerous and schematic, the British thought that the Germans misunderstood the mechanism of the therapeutic action of radiation against cancer. The Germans aimed to kill the cancer cells. The British thought this goal unattainable and perhaps even counter-productive, as well as dangerous because it required such high doses. A British physician had suggested in 1907 that X-rays and radium could stimulate the body's natural defenses against cancer.[19] This notion had gained support with the discovery in 1911 in the United States of a transmissible sarcoma of fowls.[20] Cancer appeared to be a transmissible disease. X-rays did not have any marked effect on known disease microorganisms, but most British radiologists by the end of the War probably believed that the purpose of radiation therapy was not to kill the cancer cells or microorganisms directly, but rather to stimulate immunity with short, repeated doses.[21] The intensive therapy used at Erlangen was, from this point of view, entirely misconceived.

British radiologists could be openly hostile toward the Erlangen technique, but the German claims were difficult to ignore once brought to

of Roentgenology. 1922;9:797–802. read at the 23rd Annual Meeting of the American Röntgen Ray Society, Los Angeles, 12–16 September 1922, at 802.

[19] Butcher WD. The Future of Electricity in Medicine. Proceedings of the Royal Society of Medicine. Electrotherapeutical Sect. 1907;1(delivered 25 October 1907):1–14.

[20] Rous P. Transmission of a Malignant New Growth by Means of a Cell-Free Filtrate. Journal of the American Medical Association. 1911;56:198, from the Laboratories of the Rockefeller Institute for Medical Research.

[21] See, for example, Morrell (M. R. C. S. (Eng.), L. R. C. P. (Lond.), Honorary Radiologist to the Sheffield Royal Hospital, Hon. Radiologist and Medical Officer-in-Charge of the Electrical Department, the Chesterfield and North Derbyshire Royal Hospital) RA. The Present Position of Radio-Therapy in the Treatment of Malignant Disease: a Critical Note with Special Reference to the Erlangen Technique. Med Press. 1922 Aug 30;2:177–9. See also.

Hernamen-Johnson F. X Rays in Malignant Disease. Lancet. 1921 Jul 16;2:153. For a discussion of both suppression and excitation of immunity, see Russ (D. Sc.) S, Chambers (M. D. Lond.) H, Scott (M. B. Lond.) G, Mottram (M. B. Lond.) JC. Experimental Studies with Small Doses of X Rays. Lancet. 1919 Apr 26;196:692–5, undertaken at the request of the Medical Research Council and funded by the Cancer Investigation Fund of Middlesex Hospital. There are still advocates of "hormesis": Calabrese EJ. LNT and Cancer Risk assessment: Its Flawed Foundations Part 1: Radiation and leukemia: Where LNT Began. Environmental Research. 2021 Jun;197:111025. accessed May 14, 2022.

public attention. At stake appeared to be no less than a cure for cancer. There was public dissatisfaction in Britain with the twenty-year-old Cancer Research Fund, and a more activist Anti-Cancer League had been established to promote early diagnosis and treatment.[22] Hospitals found it relatively easy to raise funds for the sort of high-voltage X-ray equipment that the Erlangen technique required. The Bradford Royal Infirmary received a 1000-pound donation from a "yam and stuff" merchant in the summer of 1921 for its equipment, and BARP itself received an anonymous donation of 4000 pounds, intended in part to send someone to Erlangen.[23] By the end of 1921, Wintz found that the large number of foreign visitors was hampering the work of his clinic.[24] Many of the visitors returned from Erlangen with favorable reports. Especially impressive, and unknown in clinics outside Germany, were the precise ionization measurements. One British physician lauded the "scientific method," and another reported that "the whole process is mathematical and accurate."[25]

The earlier hostility toward the Erlangen technique and the continuing enmity toward the Germans heightened the impact of favorable reports and excited competitive efforts. The French adopted small, graphite-lined ionization chambers like those Krönig and Friedrich had used, but instead of standardizing against a larger ionization chamber the French adopted a simpler procedure. Iser Solomon, a physician with a degree in physics, proposed in 1921 using the radiation from one gram of radium filtered

[22] See the 17 July 1922 letter to the *Daily Telegraph*, in BARP Clippings File IV, note 8.

[23] For the donation by W. H. Shaw to the Bradford Royal Infirmary, see the article from the 23 August 1921 *Yorkshire Observer*, in BARP Clippings File I, note 8. For the donation to BARP, see Archives of Radiology and Electrotherapy. 1921 Aug;26:38–9.

[24] The Study of Deep X Ray Therapy. Lancet. 1921 Dec 31;2:1381.

[25] The former was Ward HK (M. C., M. B. Sydney, D. P. H. Oxford, Department of Pathology, University of Oxford). Deep X Ray Treatment of Cancer: A Personal Impression of the Erlangen Frauenklinik. Lancet. 1921 Feb 25;1:366–8, at 368; the latter was Webb JC (Hon. Radiologist, Gloucester Royal Infirmary). The Erlangen Technique in X Ray Therapy. Lancet. 1921 Oct 1;2:729–30, at 729. For favorable American reports, see Case JT (M. D., F. A. C. S., from the Surgical Department of the Battle Creek Sanitarium). Technical and Clinical Aspects of the New Deep Therapy. American Journal of Roentgenology. 1922;9:530–7, read at the Midwinter Meeting of the Eastern Section of the American Röntgen Ray Society, Atlantic City, 28 January 1922; and Stewart WH (M. D., New York City). The Present Status of Deep Röntgen Therapy in Europe. American Journal of Roentgenology. 1922;9:315–8.

through one-half millimeter of platinum and placed at a distance of two centimeters from the ionization chamber. Ignoring the details of the German research on ionization methods, French physicians regarded the amount of ionization produced under these standard conditions as a unit of dosage, which Solomon dubbed the "Röntgen," an early indication that some nationalist sentiments were fading. The French assumed that this unit could be used to compare X-rays of different quality.[26] In Britain, the image of foreigners moving ahead was used to goad the profession to compete more effectively, and even to justify buying German apparatus:

> Our friends and rivals are wide enough awake to the necessities of the work and are working strenuously with more powerful apparatus than we employ—such a state of things cannot be allowed to continue—we must have the apparatus wherever it is made.[27]

The campaign for a British Institute of Radiology was directly linked to the effort to catch up with the Germans in deep therapy, but there was an even more effective goad available:

> Let us take an example from Russia…two new Institutes have been inaugurated at Petrograd. One of these is an Institute of Röntgenology and Radiology…. In the midst of the upheaval—the like of which the world has never seen—Bolshevik Russia can erect an Institute of Radiology. Are we in Britain going to be outdone in a matter of scientific research by Russia?[28]

Competition with the Germans and the Russians constituted strong stimulus.

[26] Solomon I (Chef du laboratoire de M. le Dr Béclère, à l'hôpital Saint-Antoine). Ionomètre radiologique. J Radiol Electrol. 1921;5:509–12. Solomon, born in Romania, was *licencié es sciences physiques* as well as a physician, see the obituary by Béclère in Paris Med. 1939;471:498.

[27] Knox R. Presidential Address. Journal of the Röntgen Society. 1921;17:5–22, at 19.

[28] Ibid., at 20.

The Competition Between Specialists and Generalists Heats Up

In addition to this international competition with foreigners, there was an internal conflict among British medical radiological organizations that eventually came to bear on the question of international cooperation. The setting of the Cambridge radiology examination in 1920, and the organization in the same year of a Society of Radiographers that pledged its membership to practice only under the supervision of physicians, fulfilled BARP's initial goals of physician control and specialty status. BARP's leadership feared that the organization might drift into competition with the Electrotherapeutic Section of the Royal Society of Medicine (an organization under the exclusive control of physicians) and with the Röntgen Society (where physicians and nonphysicians participated on an equal footing). Amalgamation with the Electrotherapeutic Section was out of the question because the Royal Society of Medicine could not permit "activities of a medico-political nature," which were BARP's primary interest. The Council of BARP, which was dominated by physicians interested in radiology as a specialty, therefore decided that, provided an independent medical section could be maintained, amalgamation with the British Röntgen Society would be desirable. The rank-and-file membership of BARP, which included many physician general practitioners opposed to joining with a society composed in large part of "laymen," defeated the Council's proposal. Discredited, its Council was enlarged, and BARP was incorporated as a legal entity for the first time in 1921.[29]

The British Röntgen Society, in the meanwhile, was undergoing important changes and began as a result to bid for a stronger role in medical radiology. As in Germany, the War had brought more academically trained physicists into what came to be called "applied" research, and into the Röntgen Society. Though their numbers were still small relative to the total membership, which increased dramatically as the X-ray operators trained for military service joined, the physicists were well-represented on the Council of the Röntgen Society. After 1916 the post of President alternated between physicians and academically trained physicists.[30] Some

[29] The B. A. R. P. Archives of Radiology and Electrotherapy. 1920;25:30–2.

[30] Of the six nonphysicians on the Council in 1920, four were physicists or engineers (B. Sc., D. Sc. or F. R. S. E.), see Journal of the Röntgen Society. 16 (1920) 91. For a list of the Presidents of the Röntgen Society, see the Handbook of the British Institute of

of the physicists had only tenuous connections with medical radiology and participated in the Röntgen Society sporadically, but there was a small group whose professional interests focused increasingly on the medical applications of X-rays and radium. Physicist G. W. C. Kaye, who had been trained under J. J. Thompson, became head of the radiological unit at the National Physical Laboratory, where activities had been expanded beyond custodianship of a British radium standard to include testing of X-ray protection materials and standardization of X-ray measurements. Sidney Russ, another physicist trained under J. J. Thomson, occupied a newly endowed position at the Middlesex Cancer Hospital. J. A. Crowther, University Lecturer in Physics Applied to Medical Radiology at Cambridge, taught the physics section of the course for the Diploma in Medical Radiology and Electrology. These academically trained physicists did not make their living practicing medical radiology, and they were therefore not in direct competition with physicians, as some less academically trained lay practitioners were.

On the whole, the academic physicists supported the physicians in their efforts to gain supervisory control over radiological practice and in their campaign for specialty status. The physicist J. W. Nicholson, who as a student in 1901 and 1902 had worked as a lay medical radiologist at the Cancer Hospital in Manchester, in his Presidential Address to the Röntgen Society in 1922 referred to

> ...the anxiety we share with the medical profession that operators entrusted with such work must have a medical qualification...I can only say that, as a physicist, I am in the most complete sympathy with my medical colleagues in this matter...[31]

While supporting physician control of radiological practice, the physicists were also acutely aware of the shortcomings of their physician colleagues in maintaining adequate X-ray and radium protection. Kaye had become aware of the difficulties in protection during the War, when his unit at the National Physical Laboratory checked lead glass and other materials

Radiology, 3rd edition, 1966, at 42. The physicist Presidents after 1916 were G. W. C. Kaye (1917–1918), Sidney Russ (1919–1920), J. W. Nicholson (1921–1922), Sir Oliver Lodge (1923–1924) and F. W. Aston (1925–1926).

[31] Nicholson JW (M. A., D. Sc., F. R. S.). Presidential Address. Journal of the Röntgen Society. 1922;18:5–14, at 10.

and found them variable in quality. In its second memorandum, issued in December 1921, the British X-ray and Radium Protection Committee, of which Kaye was a member, recommended that the National Physical Laboratory check the physical layout of X-ray clinics, their protection devices, and their electrical measuring instruments.[32] Nicholson reported the disappointing results to the Röntgen Society:

> The NPL...has examined a large number of X-ray departments in various hospitals, and almost invariably found their equipment as regards protective appliances is by no means satisfactory...the question is essentially an international one...I cannot say too strongly that though the investigation of X-ray phenomena from the point of view of the patient is of necessity the fundamental activity of our medical members, it is vital, in view of the new dangers which arise from radiations now in use, that operators should have some concern for their own welfare.[33]

Nicholson, Kaye, Russ, and other physicists in the Röntgen Society saw the solution to protection problems, and also the solution to the problem of competing with the Germans, in closer cooperation between the scientific and medical sides of the radiological community. The Journal of the Röntgen Society had deplored the founding of the (nonphysician) Society of Radiographers in 1920 as a step in the wrong direction, and it had pleaded for amalgamation of all the radiological organizations into a single national entity:

> If unreasoning prejudice could be swept away, a powerful British Society of Radiology (with a truly representative journal) could well look after the combined interests of the Röntgen Society, the Electrotherapeutic Section of the Royal Society of Medicine, the B. A. R. P., and this new Society of Radiographers.[34]

This amalgamation would eventually be achieved, but only after a complex series of negotiations that culminated in 1927.

[32] X-ray and Radium Protection Committee. Memorandum No. 2. Journal of the Röntgen Society. 1922;18:3–4.

[33] Nicholson, note 31, at 6.

[34] Society of Radiographers. Journal of the Röntgen Society. 1920;16:82–3, at 83. The *Journal* later softened its position on the Society of Radiographers, but it continued to favor amalgamation in principle.

The major issue in this conflict over amalgamation was physician control over radiological practice. Discussions on amalgamation began in 1924 between the Röntgen Society and BARP, which in that year changed its name to the British Institute of Radiology, but the negotiations stalled repeatedly on this issue. The conflict was not however a simple two-part conflict between physicians and nonphysicians. There were actually four groups involved. Among the physicians, one group included those who were practicing radiology as a specialty as well as those who were engaged in research; a second group consisted of general practitioners who did not want, or could not afford, to practice only radiology, and who contributed little to research. Among the nonphysicians, there were the so-called "lay" radiographers who actually operated X-ray machines as well as tube and other equipment manufacturers and interested amateurs; and there were also the academic physicists, who did not practice radiology.

Initially, the major conflict occurred between the physician general practitioners and the nonphysician radiographers, especially those lay practitioners of the older generation who had refused to join the Society of Radiographers. The physicists supported this older generation of lay practitioners more strongly than might be supposed, partly out of respect for elder colleagues who formed an important part of the membership of the Röntgen Society and partly because some of the proposals put forward for amalgamation would have lumped all the nonphysicians together in a lower category of membership. Similarly, the physician-specialists supported the general practitioners more strongly than might be supposed, partly because the general practitioners formed an important part of the membership of BARP/British Institute of Radiology and partly because as physicians the specialists shared with generalists an interest in maintaining strict provisions for physician control.[35]

[35] See the notes of the Joint Committee of Röntgen (sic) Society and British Institute of Radiology in a box of Röntgen Society documents in the Library of the British Institute of Radiology referred to below as RS (BIR) and also Amalgamation. British Journal of Radiology. 1927 Jan;23:1–2. For a sample of the conflict between physicians and nonphysicians, see Hernamen-Johnson F (M. D., Radiologist to the French Hospital, Physician to the X-ray Department, the Margaret Street Hospital for Consumption, etc.; late Consulting Radiologist, Aldershot Command). The Place of the Radiologist and his Kindred in the World of Medicine. Archives of Radiology and Electrotherapy. 1919;24:181–7. and Oddie CF (Radiographer to North Stafford Infirmary) Letter to the Editor. Archives of Radiology and Electrotherapy. 1920;25:149–51. The Röntgen Society already had a provision in its rules that gave physicians veto power over nonphysician memberships and prohibited therapeutic work by nonphysicians, see Journal of the

Despite this four-part conflict, there were substantial areas of common interest to the physicists and the physician-specialists. Research was one such common interest. In 1923, the Electrotherapeutic Section of the Royal Society of Medicine and the Röntgen Society began to hold annual meetings together at which a joint prize was awarded, alternately to a physician and a nonphysician.[36] In 1924, the Journal of the Röntgen Society and the Archives of Radiology and Electrotherapy, which had become the official organ of the British Institute of Radiology, joined forces as separate but equal "sections" of a newly founded British Journal of Radiology. Deep therapy and the ionization measurements of X-ray doses associated with it were some of the areas of research that attracted the interest of both the specialists and the physicists. Another important common interest was X-ray and radium protection. Despite some grumbling about its excessive requirements among general practitioners, the X-ray and Radium Protection Committee continued its work. The press campaign on the dangers of X-rays proved less threatening than anticipated, and the Committee in 1924 convinced the Home Secretary to include X-ray and radium work in the Schedule of Dangerous Occupations covered under the Workmen's Compensation Act.[37]

The physician-specialists were pleased that the emphasis on protection confirmed their view that specialized knowledge was required to practice radiology. In addition, the specialists found the strictness of the requirements beneficial in terms of professional advancement as well as in terms of health. They could afford the costly shielding and elaborate protection procedures because a greater proportion of their incomes came from

Röntgen Society. 1918 Oct;14:116.: "No person engaged in the practice of medical or surgical radiography shall be eligible for membership unless he or she is proposed and seconded by a medical practitioner, who must have personal knowledge of the candidate, the final decision to rest with the Council. No person engaged in therapeutic work shall be eligible for membership unless duly qualified in medicine." These provisions were not, however, retroactive and several nonphysician diagnostic practitioners remained in the Röntgen Society.

36 The Mackenzie-Davidson Memorial Lecture and Medal. Journal of the Röntgen Society. 1923;19(151).

37 Rolleston H (Bart., K. C. B., M. D., Hon. D. Sc., D. C. L., LL. D., President of the British Institute of Radiology, Regius Professor of Physic in the University of Cambridge). On the Effects of Radiations on Patients and Radiologists, and on Protection Eighth Mackenzie-Davidson Memorial Lecture. British Journal of Radiology (Röntgen Society Sect. 1927;23:266–91. with discussion.

radiological work. The general practitioner who did only a few diagnostic exposures per week was much less ready to accept such encumbrances, and he may well have thought it unfair that the Protection Committee required the same precautions to protect X-ray operators regardless of the extent of their exposure.[38] Protection requirements thus increased the competitive edge of the specialist over the general practitioner, and interest in protection brought the specialist into closer alignment with the physicist. Competition, or more precisely the desire for competitive advantage, can sometimes favor norms.

Competition Produces International Cooperation

While the British Institute of Radiology and the Röntgen Society continued at odds over the precise wording of a clause on physician control over radiological practice, the common interests of the specialists and the physicists developed into an effort at international cooperation. BARP had acquired a building at 32 Welbeck Street, not far from the Royal Society of Medicine. The British Institute of Radiology, as BARP became shortly thereafter, planned to open this permanent headquarters in 1924 and invited non-German foreign radiological societies to send representatives to the event. Economic conditions on the Continent had improved greatly since the postponement of the bilingual conference in 1921, and the response to this invitation was much greater than expected.[39] As a result, the Röntgen Society in the summer of 1924 joined the Electrotherapeutic Section of the Royal Society of Medicine and the British Institute of Radiology in nominating representatives to a Provisional Committee, which polled radiological societies, journals, and individuals, including some German radiologists, on the question

[38] For explicit criticism of the British recommendations on this score, see Altschul W. Internationale Strahlenschutzbestimmungen. Strahlentherapie. 1926;24:766–8, Vortrag gehalten auf der V. wissenschaftlichen Tagung der Vereinigung Deutscher Röntgenologen und Radiologen in der tschecholslovakischen Republik in Prag am 23 und 24 Oktober 1926. For traces of general opposition to the Protection Committee, see the discussion following Finzi NS. Research in Radiology, British Journal of Radiology. 1927 Jan;23:4–18, Presidential Paper read 2 November 1926.

[39] For the limitation to non-German radiological societies, see Jaches L. Sir Archibald Douglas Reid, K. B. E., C. M. G., D. M. R. E., American Journal of Roentgenology 1924;11:288–9. and for a retrospective account see the report on the Third International Congress of Radiology (Paris, 1931). British Journal of Radiology. 1931 May;4:365–8.

of calling an international conference for July 1925 in London.[40] The response was sufficiently positive for the Provisional Committee to be converted to an Organizing Committee that sent out announcements early in 1925 of what was still cautiously regarded as a "preliminary" meeting.[41]

Not all of the German medical radiological community was keen on the notion of participating in the conference. The Germans had suffered little tangible harm by exclusion from the two post-war bilingual conferences, which did not equal in either quality or quantity the research presented at the annual German Röntgen Society Congresses that had resumed in 1920. The boycott had been galling to the Germans. When word of the projected London conference reached them in late 1924, probably by means of the Provisional Committee's poll, the question of participation was brought before the Council of the German Röntgen Society and discussed during the annual meeting of the German Society of Scientists and Physicians at Innsbruck. The discussion has not been preserved, and no decision was recorded in the proceedings of the meeting. But after the official announcement emphasized that all nations would be invited, the Council recommended that members of the German Röntgen Society participate.[42] About forty Germans attended out of a total of 500 participants. This percentage was much smaller than might have been expected from the relative sizes of the radiological communities and also much

[40] The minute book of the Provisional Committee, Organizing Committee and Grand Committee, in RS (BIR), note 35.

[41] For the official British announcement, see International Congress of Radiology. Acta Radiologica. 1925 Mar 20;4:81–2.

[42] Some Germans may even have received invitations to the conference in late 1924, see Internationaler Radiologenkongress 1925. Fortschr Röntgenstr. 1924;32:725.: "Seitens eines vorbereitenden Komitees englischer Röntgenologen ist an eine Reihe von Mitgliedern der Deutschen Röntgen-Gesellschaft die Aufforderung ergangen, sich an einem im Sommer 1925 stattfindenden internationalen Kongress zu beteiligen. Anlässlich der Tagung der Deutschen Röntgen-Gesellschaft während der Naturforscherversammlung in Innsbruck wurde beschlossen, an dem Kongress teilzunehmen." There appears to be no report on this question in the proceedings of the Innsbruck meeting in Fortschr Röntgenstr. 32:2. Kongressheft 1924., but after printing the official announcement in Internationaler Kongress für Radiologie, Vorbereitende Tagung, London, 1. bis 4. Juli 1925. Fortschr Röntgenstr. 1925;33:333–4., Haenisch (Hamburg) reported, "Der Ausschuss der Deutschen Röntgen-Gesellschaft hat beschlossen, den Mitgliedern die Beteiligung an dem Kongress zu empfehlen.".

smaller than the percentage of German participation in the subsequent international conferences held before World War II.

In both Britain and Germany, it is likely that it was the physicists, perhaps supported by the physician-specialists, who advocated German participation in the 1925 London conference. More than anyone else associated with the medical radiological community, the physicists appreciated the importance of an internationally agreed unit of X-ray dosage. Once the work of Krönig and Friedrich, Holthusen, and Seitz and Wintz had become known it was difficult to consider the dosage problem without the Germans. At a joint meeting of the Physical Society and the Röntgen Society in 1923, the Middlesex Hospital physicist Russ had called for international standardization, and the two Societies soon thereafter appointed a joint committee to consider the dosage problem.[43] In Germany, the initiation of standardization activities at the Physical-Technical Institute in 1924 seemed to the physicists to be a preliminary step toward international standardization. As the Charlottenburg physicist Behnken put it, "international standardization is then the next goal to keep an eye on."[44] With the official adoption of the Röntgen unit by the German Röntgen Society in April 1925, the stage was set for the London conference, where physicists would press for ionization measurements, international standardization of X-ray units, and radiation protection.

The London conference was successful in re-establishing formal communication among the German, British, and French radiological communities. The participants declared it the first International Congress of Radiology and decided that the second would meet in Stockholm in 1928. An International Commission on X-ray Units was formed, and the groundwork was laid for international cooperation on radiation protection. The Germans returned home praising British hospitality, boasting that radiology was the first medical discipline to return to true international cooperation, and pleased that Röntgen had been given his due in

[43] Russ S. The Measurement of X-ray Intensity, and the Necessity for an International Method, in the Report on the Joint Meeting with the Physical Society. Journal of the Röntgen Society. 1923 Feb 23;19 (and "Annual Report of the Council–Session 1922–1923," ibid., 191–94):163–71 at 166.

[44] "Als nächstes Ziel ist dann die internationale Standardisierung der Dosismessung ins Auge zu fassen," at 94 in Behnken (Berlin). Die Eichung von Dosismessern in absolutem Masse in der Physikalisch-technischen Reichsanstalt. Verh Deut Rönt Ges. 1924;15:92–4.

the speeches at the conference dinner.[45] The British were delighted with the decision to make the conference the first of a series, and the French, anxious to have pictures of the Curies and of Becquerel on the dinner program at the next Congress, were snarkily relieved that the Germans behaved themselves in a civilized manner.[46]

The sudden emergence of cooperation from conflict should not be surprising. If the British physician-specialists and their Allied colleagues were to compete with the Germans in doing intensive deep therapy, or if they were to deny the Erlangen claims and put forward their own, their results would have to be comparable with the results of the German clinics. Making the results comparable required cooperation in standardizing doses. The physicists pushed this necessary cooperation on standardizing doses a step further to a less necessary, but highly significant, cooperation on radiation protection. In doing so, they again found supporters among the physician-specialists.

Physicists and Physician-Specialists Take Charge

The pre-1925 nationalism nevertheless continued at the Conference and fueled its most important decision: to establish an International Commission on X-ray Units. After opening speeches emphasizing common interests and international friendship, a joint meeting of the sections on physics and radiology under the chairmanship of William Bragg, who had become Britain's leading X-ray physicist, debated the problem of X-ray dosage measurements.[47] French gynecologist Béclère presented the case for the French, radium-based "Röntgen."[48] German physicist Behnken presented the case for the German "Röntgen" defined in terms of the

[45] See the report on the Congress, note 2.

[46] The First International Congress Radiologists from Twentyone Countries Meet in London. British Journal of Radiology. (B I R Section). 1925 Aug 25;30:284–94, at 92.

[47] Discussion on International Units and Standards for X-Ray Work, in the Proceedings of the Section of Physics, the First International Congress of Radiology (London, 30 June–4 July 1925, Central Hall, Westminster). British Journal of Radiology (Röntgen Society Section). 1927 Apr;23:64–101.

[48] Béclère A. (Membre de l'Académie de Médecine à Paris), On International Standardisation of Measures in Röntgentherapy. British Journal of Radiology (Röntgen Society Section). 1927 Apr;23:66–72.

charge produced by the ionization of air.[49] German physicists Grebe and Martius presented the case against the unit skin dose by showing that it varied, even within Germany, by as much as a factor of four.[50] No one defended the unit skin dose openly, but the medical practitioners had certainly not abandoned it. Using the unit skin dose in the clinic and defending it to an audience that included physicists were two quite different activities. The unit skin dose remained in clinical use until the 1930s, when it only gradually lost its hold.

There were other proposals as well, including a last-ditch effort by Dessauer to defend photographic measurements, a proposal by a French physicist to measure dose in energy (ergs) absorbed per gram of tissue (this unit later became known as the "rad" and came temporarily into common use), and also a proposal to adopt the common clinical procedure of specifying the voltage across the tube and the current through it. The discussion brought the major conflict, between the French and German Röntgens, into the open.[51] TheBritish X-ray Unit Committee that had been formed by the Röntgen Society and the Physical Society in late 1923 refrained from offering its own proposal. The Congress rewarded this restraint by giving the British the task of calling together an International X-ray Unit Commission to decide the issue at the second International Congress three years hence.[52]

The physicists were less successful in pressing the issue of protection. G. W. C. Kaye took the lead, proposing "...international agreement on, at any rate, the main questions of protective measures." He claimed that "such a step would have obvious advantages."[53] In making this proposal, Kaye reviewed the history of the British X-ray and Radium Protection Committee and mentioned its counterparts in other countries, but the

[49] Behnken H (Physikalisch-Technische-Reichsanstalt, Charlottenburg). The German Unit of X-Radiation. British Journal of Radiology (Röntgen Society Section). 1927 Apr;23:72–7.

[50] Grebe L, Martius H. Röntgen-Ray Measurements in Absolute Units and Ray-Doses Necessary for Skin-Erythema. British Journal of Radiology (Röntgen Society Section). 1927 Apr;23:78–81.

[51] Ibid.

[52] Discussion on International Units and Standards. British Journal of Radiology (Röntgen Society Section). 1927 Apr;23:101.

[53] Kaye GWC (O.B.E., M.A., D.Sc., Physics Department, the National Physical Laboratory. British Journal of Radiology (Röntgen Society Section). 1927 Apr;23:152–63, at 162.

tangible advantages of his proposal were by no means obvious to clinicians. Comparability of therapeutic results depended on international agreement on an X-ray unit, but not on international agreement on protection requirements. One might be tempted to assign to Kaye idealistic motives, but they would hardly account for the success of his proposal within the Physics Section of the conference, which adopted a resolution placing "on record the desirability of adopting a standard scheme of X-ray and Radium protection throughout the world."[54] There were still strong nationalist feelings in this group, and Kaye himself had expressed vehement anti-German sentiments only a few years before. Kaye was appealing for agreement on the international level to strengthen the hand of the physicists, and their physician-specialist supporters, on the national level. Had there been a significant number of non-specialist physicians in the Physics Section (which naturally there were not) or had the Kaye proposal been submitted to the Congress as a whole, the outcome would have been different.

Within the Physics Section, however, Kaye found a good deal of sympathy. The receptivity of the physicists to strengthening radiation protection was not entirely disinterested. Their role in medical radiology was still being defined, and they stood to gain status and security if they could demonstrate their usefulness in designing and monitoring protection measures. There was in addition ample evidence to support the physicists' view that physicians, left to themselves, would not adopt and maintain adequate protection measures, even though it was the physicians themselves who often suffered most from laxity. The National Physical Laboratory inspections had revealed many shortcomings. By 1925 similar investigations undertaken at the four largest X-ray clinics in Stockholm and at the Saint Antoine Hospital in Paris had shown significant quantities of so-called "stray" radiation arising from inadequate shielding and from scattering in the body of the patient and in the walls, ceiling and floor.[55] Many physicians appear to have been unaware of the increasing

[54] H. Pilon (Paris). Protection in Radiotherapy. British Journal of Radiology (Röntgen Society Section). 1927 Apr;23:164–70 at 170.

[55] Sievert RM. Einige Untersuchtungen über Vorrichtungen zum Schutz gegen Röntgenstrahlen. Acta Radiologica. 1925;4:61–75. and Solomon I. Recherches sur la valeur des moyens de protection contre l'action à distance de rayons de Röntgen. Journal of Radiology and Electrology. 1924;8:62–3, communication présentée à l'Académie de

proportion of scattered relative to absorbed radiation with increasing X-ray hardness. In Germany, the Röntgen Society survey of X-ray injuries to patients was not yet published, but it was already known that the survey included a significant proportion of injuries due to negligence or ignorance on the part of X-ray operators, including physicians and technicians under physician supervision.[56]

Kaye's proposal for international protection recommendations was not formally discussed among the physicians at the 1925 Congress, an omission that confirms the leading role of the physicists in pressing for international protection standards. The position of the physicians can, however, be inferred from later developments. Among physicians, radiation protection became part of a dual strategy for promoting specialization: on the one hand, there was a need for higher educational standards; on the other hand, there was a need for improving the apparatus used in radiology, including protection devices. Raising educational standards and improving apparatus would help to place radiology in the hands of those who practiced it full time. The general practitioner, who might rely on nothing more than a short course offered by an X-ray tube salesman for his knowledge of radiology and who at best had a few weeks of instruction during medical school, would be the eventual victim of this dual strategy. The physician-specialists had much to gain from the physicists' initiative in favor of radiation protection.

The London Congress had a broad impact, and it set the agenda for international cooperation in the medical radiological community in a number of important respects. The common interests of the physicists and the physician-specialists would become increasingly evident in the decade

Médecine le 16 octobre 1923. Sievert, a Swedish physicist, would later play a central role in international radiation protection cooperation.

[56] This conclusion was already cited in Groedel, Liniger, Lassen (Frankfurt a. M.). Schädigungen aus unserer Gutachtersammlung der Röntgenschäden. Fortschr Röntgenstr. 32((1. Kongressheft 1924)):160–3. The full survey was published in two parts, Materialiensammlung der Unfälle und Schäden in Röntgenbetrieben. Fortschr Röntgenstr, Ergänzungsband. 1925;36. and Ergänzungsband. 1927;38. For a summary, see Lassen H (Dr. med., Facharzt für die gesamte Röntgenkunde). Über Ergebnisse unserer Materialiensammlung der Unfälle und Schäden in Reichsdeutschen Röntgenbetrieben (Groedel-Liniger und Lossen). Acta Radiologica. 1927;8:45–62, vorgetragen auf der XIV. ordentlichen Hauptversammlung der Schweizerischen Röntgen Gesellschaft am 28. Mai 1927 in Luzern.

after 1925. The physicists would have their way, achieving both international standardization of X-ray dosage and international recommendations for X-ray and radium protection. Measuring dosage posed technical difficulties that were solved largely within the physicists' part of the medical radiological community. Protection posed difficulties of a different sort involving the relationship of the physicists to physicians, and of both to the issue of specialization. Taking protection seriously was not automatic, even for the physicians most likely to suffer harm.

Physicists Solve the International X-ray Measurement Problem, At Last

When the Physical-Technical Institute began its standardization program in 1924, Behnken and other physicists were convinced that the technical difficulties had been overcome with the introduction of the air-pressure chamber. German physicians, however, found maintaining the standardization in Röntgens under clinical conditions difficult, and even physician-specialists who used ionization chambers often continued to express doses in terms of the unit skin dose rather than in terms of Röntgens.[57] This practice seemed eminently sensible after the physicists discovered in 1926 and 1927 that the dose in Röntgens required to produce an erythema was different in Germany and the United States. The Bonn physicists Grebe and Martius, using ionization chambers standardized by Behnken's air-pressure chamber, had found an average "erythema" dose (the dose required to produce mild irritation of the skin) of 600 Röntgens in their survey of German clinics.[58] Glasser, the student of Friedrich who

[57] See Holthusen H (Hamburg). Über die Standardisierung der Röntgendosismessung, Referat III to the 17th Röntgenkongress, 11–13 April 1926. Verh Deut Rönt Ges. 1926;17:156–7. and also the succeeding papers and discussion, pp. 158–74. G. Gabriel summed up the practitioners' view in replying to a paper by Fried (Worms) on the use of a Siemens ionization dosimeter: "Es liegen heute in den physikalischen Dosierungsmethoden noch so viel unbekannte Komponenten, dass wir für die Praxis durchaus an den alten Dosierungsmethoden festhalten.

müssen.Wenn Herr Fried in seinem Vortrage die HED [Hauteinheitdosis] feierlichst zu Grabe getragen hat, so wollen wir sie schleunigst von ihrem Scheintode erwecken, da wir sie als Grundlage für unser weiteres Arbeiten notwendig brauchen.".

[58] Grebe L (Röntgen-Forschungs und Unterrichtsinstitut der Universität Bonn), Martius H (Universitäts-Frauenklinik in Bonn). Vergleichende Messungen über der Grösse der zur Erreichung der Hauterythems gebräuchlichen Röngenstrahlermenge. Strahlentherapie. 1924;18:395–409.

had emigrated to the United States, found an erythema dose of 1400 Röntgens using clinical ionization chambers standardized against a large chamber at atmospheric pressure.[59] Part of the problem arose because Glasser placed his ionization chambers directly on the skin, thus including in his measurements the dose due to back scattering from the body; Grebe and Martius positioned their ionization chambers in the air at the same distance from the tube as the exposed skin. Even after this difference was recognized, however, there remained a significant discrepancy that was traced to a difference in the size of the Röntgen unit measured in Germany and in the United States.

Glasser found that his own Röntgen unit agreed with those of two other United States-based investigators (one of whom, like Glasser, was a recent immigrant from Germany) to within 4 percent. The Röntgen units measured by Behnken, by Grebe and Martius, and by Friedrich also agreed well, but they were 50 percent larger than the "American" Röntgen.[60] The fact that two of the three "American" investigators were German-born and German-trained physicists was irrelevant: the competition was cast in terms of a rivalry between the United States and Germany. The French, gleeful at the discrepancy, leapt into the fray and tried to reassert the claims of the French, radium-based Röntgen. Béclère put it this way:

> It is necessary that an impartial arbitrator intervene between the physicists of Germany and of the United States....I hope that a French physicist has this ambition and that the honor will come to him to settle [the question].[61]

Béclère had in mind his own laboratory chief, Solomon, who had proposed the French, radium-based Röntgen in 1921. Solomon was

[59] Glasser O. Erythemdosen in Röntgeneinheiten. Strahlentherapie. 1925;20:141–3.

[60] Glasser O (Ph. D., Cleveland Clinic Foundation), Portmann UV (M. D., Cleveland Clinic Foundation). The Standardization of the Röntgen-Ray Dose read at the 28th Annual Meeting of the American Röntgen Ray Society, Montreal, Canada, 20–23 September 1927. American Journal of Roentgenology. 1928;19:47–61, at 54

[61] Béclère A. La discordance des mesures pour l'évaluation de l'unité de dose radiothérapique en Allemagne et aux États-Unis. Journal of Radiology and Electrology. 1927;112:535–9, at 539: "Entre les physiciens de l'Allemagne et des États Unis, il est nécessaire qu'intervienne un arbitre impartial. Pour terminer par un vœu, je souhaite qu'un physicien français ait cette ambition et que l'honneur lui advienne de la justifier.".

aware of the arbitrary character of his unit and suggested that the distance at which the radium was placed might be altered to make the unit agree with the German Röntgen.[62] Glasser welcomed this suggestion by showing in 1927 that the French Röntgen bore a constant relationship to the American Röntgen (with a variation of less than ±5 percent).[63]

At the same time, Glasser found that seven German laboratory ionization chambers calibrated in German Röntgens varied by ±13.5 percent among themselves. Such a variation might at the time have been tolerable in X-ray clinics, but it reflected badly on the laboratory skills of the German physicists. Behnken replied with a detailed description of the German equipment and procedures.[64] With the second International Congress of Radiology only a few months away, a major battle among the physicists over X-ray units appeared to be brewing. Conflict was averted at the last minute, when Behnken traveled to the United States and checked the German ionization chambers that Glasser was using in Cleveland. The sources of error and Behnken's means of correcting them are not clear. Glasser merely cited in general terms "faulty construction and lack of proper control of the instruments used in the transportation of the German R unit."[65] After Behnken's repairs, the German and American instruments agreed.

The British, in the meanwhile, had carried out their mandate from the 1925 Congress and had invited national physical and radiological societies to send representatives to the International Commission on X-ray Units, which met for the first time in Stockholm during the second International Congress of Radiology in July 1928. This group adopted the German definition of the Röntgen, which both the Americans and the Germans had used, and the Congress as a whole endorsed this decision. The French were given their due in a recommendation that the constancy of ionization chambers standardized in (German) Röntgens be checked

[62] Solomon I. Sur la nécessité de la standardisation des chambres d'ionisation utilisées en dosimétrie radiologique. Journal of Radiology and Electrology. 1927;111:286–90.

[63] Glasser and Portmann, note 60.

[64] Behnken H. Die Absolutbestimmung der Dosiseinheit'1' Röntgen in der Physikalisch-Technischen-Reichsanstalt. Strahlentherapie. 1927;26:78–100.

[65] Glasser and Portmann, note 60, in a footnote added after the reading of the paper, at 54.

using radium.[66] At the third International Congress (Paris, 1931), the "international Röntgen" was declared satisfactory.[67] With the physicists at last agreeing among themselves, this unit gradually entered clinical practice, becoming well-established by the mid-1930s.

There would be a variety of new difficulties before World War II arising from the increasing voltages used in generating X-rays and from the suggestion that the dosage of gamma rays from radium be measured in Röntgens, but by 1934 doses of X-rays from tubes excited with several hundred thousand volts were comparable to within ±1 percent.[68] The problem of measuring X-ray exposure seemed at long last solved, though as we shall see new units would eventually be required to measure absorbed doses not only of X-rays but also of other ionizing radiation. This triumph came close to 40 years after the discovery of X-rays, decades during which countless claims were made to the "scientific" character of X-rays and radium and their application in medicine. No doubt clinicians had applied many doses to patients without accurate measurement, not to mention the doses they themselves had absorbed.

Protection Comes into Its Own

As for radiation protection, the resolution passed at the 1925 Congress by its Physics Section had called for an international scheme but failed to specify a procedure for reaching an agreement, and the Congress took no action on the suggestion. In 1928 at the Stockholm Conference, Kaye proposed to the physicists that the recommendations of the British X-ray and Radium Protection Committee be adopted as international recommendations.[69] The British recommendations included specific thicknesses

[66] A Report of the Second International Congress of Radiology (Stockholm, 23–27 July 1928) and the Proceedings of the Joint Scientific Meetings of the Congress. Acta Radiologica, Supplementum III, Pars I. 1929;60.

[67] British Journal of Radiology. 1931;4:484.

[68] General Recommendations of the National Laboratories for the Standardisation of the X-Ray Dosimeters. British Journal of Radiology. 1934;7:304–8.These recommendations included the use of a large standardization chamber of the sort Glasser had advocated rather than the Behnken air-pressure chamber.

[69] Proposals from the British X-Ray and Radium Protection Committee to Be Submitted for International Approval by the IInd International Congress of Radiology, Designed to Unify Protection Measures and to Improve the Working Conditions of X-ray and Radium Operators in All Countries. ICRP Archives, Archive Files 66–75, Archive File

of lead shielding for X-ray tubes to be used in diagnostic work, in superficial therapy, and in deep therapy. These shielding requirements were to prove a major item of contention. The British Committee had aimed to reduce the dose to the operator as much as possible without interfering with radiological practice.[70] This goal was a reasonable one that would remain a basic tenet of radiation protection, but the specification of shielding requirements failed to allow for the variety of tube designs, for the increasing voltages becoming available, or for the possibility of adequate shielding but inadequate protection because of scattering in the patient's body and in the room.

The way around these difficulties in the physicists' view was to specify a dose limit to the operator of the X-ray tube, or to the manipulator of radium applicators, and to calculate the shielding required from this dose limit. Equipped with their ionization chambers, the physicists could then check whether the dose limit was exceeded. The question that neither the physicists nor the physicians could answer was how high the dose limit should be. If it were too high, then the operators would suffer harm, but if it were too low the shielding required would hinder radiological practice. One way to decide the size of the dose limit would have been to weigh the risk to the operators against the benefits of radiological practice, a procedure that at least in principle is today often advocated for controlling other sorts of technological risks. Even before World War I, it had been common in replying to public fears concerning the risks of radiation exposure for members of the radiological community to emphasize the benefits of X-rays and radium in medicine, but explicit efforts to determine a dose limit by risk-benefit analysis were still decades in the future.

The strategy used was based, instead, on the assumption that there was a threshold for the biological effects of radiation. The assumption did not have, and did not seem to require, experimental confirmation. To both physicists and physicians, clinical experience suggested that many people had been exposed to radiation, some for many years, without suffering harm. By the 1920s, obvious harm to patients was rare. Though the threshold assumption had been common previously, it was only

68. 1928;Stockholm, July 23–27:1–30. The approved "International Recommendations for X-Ray and Radium Protection" are at 32–44.

70 X-ray and Radium Protection Committee. Preliminary Report. Journal of the Röntgen Society. 1921;17:100–3.

in the mid-1920s that anyone made a serious effort to determine the threshold quantitatively. Late in 1924, an American physicist, Arthur Mutscheller, initiated these efforts by attempting to measure the "tolerance dose," which he defined as "the dose which an operator can, for a prolonged period of time, tolerate, without ultimately suffering injury."[71] Mutscheller's procedure was to measure the dose actually delivered to the X-ray operators in "several typical good installations" and on the basis of these figures and "fair averages" to calculate the dose to the operators over the period of a month.[72] Mutsheller in this way arrived at 1/100 unit skin dose (which he termed the erythema dose) received over a period of a month as the tolerance dose. He put forward the figure tentatively and called for "close cooperation between physicists and biologists and a systematic cooperation of Röntgenologists, and careful examination of the blood and other organs of Röntgen-ray operators [to] decide the point."[73]

In the wake of the 1925 Congress, Mutscheller's proposal received an enthusiastic response among physicists. The German physicist Glocker, commenting in 1926 on the recommendations of the British X-ray and Radium Protection Committee, concluded by pointing toward the importance of the tolerance dose for future decisions on radiation protection:

> To get an exact basis for the drafting of radiation protection measures it is indispensable that, through as many statistical contributions as possible from the membership of the German Röntgen Society, a more precise value of the tolerance dose be obtained. Cooperation to this end thus lies in the Röntgenologists' very own interest![74]

[71] Mutscheller A. Physical Standards of Protection Against Röntgen-Ray Danger. American Journal of Roentgenology. 1925;13:65–70, at 67.

[72] Ibid.

[73] Ibid.

[74] Glocker R (Prof. Dr., Suttgart). Internationale Strahlenschutzbestimmungen. Strahlentherapie. 1926;22:193–204, Referat IV erstattet auf dem Röntgenkongress 1926, at 204: "Um eine exakte Grundlage für die Ausarbeitung von Strahlenschutzbestimmungen zu gewinnen, ist es unerlässlich, dass durch möglichst zahlreiche statistische Beiträge aus dem Kreise der Mitglieder der Deutschen Röntgengesellschaft ein genauerer Wert für die Toleranzdosis gewonnen wird. Eine Mitarbeit an dieser Aufgabe liegt also im eigensten Interesse jede Röntgenlogen!"See also Glocker R, Kaupp E (aus dem Röntgenlaboratorium an der Technischen Hochschule Stuttgart). Über den Strahlenschutz und die Toleranzdosis. Strahlentherapie. 1925;20:144–52.

Glocker preferred to express the tolerance dose on an hourly basis rather than on Mutscheller's monthly basis, but he accepted Mutscheller's figure of 1/100 unit skin dose per month in calculating his own tolerance dose of 1/20,000 unit skin dose per/hour. Behnken also accepted Mutscheller's figure, and the Swedish physicist Rolf Sievert (who would play an important role in radiation protection for decades to come), in the study of protection in Stockholm's four largest X-ray clinics referred to above, assumed a tolerance dose of 1/10 unit skin dose per year, which with one month vacation would be approximately the same as Mutscheller's tolerance dose.[75] In Britain, a physician and a physicist working together confirmed Mutscheller's figure with data on two workers at the Manchester Royal Infirmary and showed that this tolerance dose could be readily achieved in diagnostic work.[76] Kaye showed that the shielding thicknesses recommended by the British X-ray and Radium Protection Committee were consistent with a tolerance dose about 40 percent lower than Mutscheller's.[77]

Thus the time duration for which the tolerance dose was specified varied (and would remain a subject of discussion for decades to come, because the biological effects depended on the duration of exposure), but physicists generally agreed on the approach. They were also prepared to compromise with the physicians in their continued adherence to the unit skin dose, which seemed to be appropriate for protection in clinics. Kaye in late 1927 outlined the ideal procedure for determining protection measures from the physicists' point of view as follows:

> ...a scheme of X-ray protection which rests on a sound physical and biological basis involves:

[75] Behnken, in the discussion following the oral presentation of Glocker, ibid., as reproduced in Verh. Deut. Rönt. Ges. 17 (1926) 177–87, at 183; Sievert, note 55.

[76] Barclay AE (M. D.), Cox S (B. Sc.) (Manchester). The Radiation Risks of the Röntgenologist: An Attempt to Measure the Quantity of Röntgen Rays Used in Diagnosis and to Assess the Dangers. American Journal of Roentgenology. 1928;12:551–61.

[77] Kaye GWC (0. B. E., M. A., D. Sc., Superintendent of the Physics Department, the National Physical Laboratory. Protection and Working Conditions in X-Ray Departments. British Journal of Radiology. 1928;1:295–312, read 18 November 1927 and revised in proof August 1928.

a) Measuring under specified conditions the intensity of X-rays in terms of a specifiable and reproducible physical standard expressed, if possible, in absolute units.

b)Establishing a maximum tolerance dose in terms of a specifiable and reproducible biological standard, and if possible, expressing this biological standard in physical units.

c) Establishing reliable figures for the transmission of X-rays of specified quality by lead and other absorbents.

d) Calculating the thickness of the absorbent necessary to reduce the intensity of a given beam of X-rays to that corresponding to the tolerance dose at some specified point.[78]

In carrying out this dose-limiting procedure, it was more important to have a single agreed number for the tolerance dose, a rule of thumb or "heuristic," rather than the precisely correct number. That would remain the approach for decades into the future. The physicists argued little over variations as great as 50 percent in estimates of the tolerance dose. Just before the 1928 Stockholm Conference, Mutscheller let it be known that, with the approval of Kaye and Glocker, he intended to propose international adoption of a tolerance dose of 1/100 erythema dose per month.[79] The proposal was well-received by the physicists present, who included Glasser and Lauriston Taylor, an American physicist who had begun to play a major role in radiological work at the National Bureau of Standards and would remain involved for decades more.

The tolerance dose was more than an additional requirement for radiation protection. It added a new dimension to "command-and-control" regulation, which specified the best way to operate and shield an X-ray tube, and moved toward what is now termed "performance-based" regulation.[80] The former is more readily verified but can be expensive and less

[78] Ibid.

[79] Mutscheller A (Ph. D., New York). Safety Standards and Protection Against X-Ray Dangers. Radiology. 1928;10:468–76, with discussion.

[80] Pritchett W. Types of Regulation | the Regulatory Review [Internet]. www.theregreview.org. 2016. Available from: https://www.theregreview.org/2016/04/05/pritchett-types-of-regulation/, accessed June 23, 2023.

than optimal, especially in practices that are changing rapidly with innovation. The latter sets a norm that is more difficult to verify but can be met in any way the operator sees fit, thus encouraging innovation and allowing minimization of costs. In radiation protection, performance norms would in the future be termed "basic radiation protection" norms. These would become the main focus of international cooperation, as they would be independent of equipment employed. Command-and-control norms were not abandoned, and in principle they would be derived from the basic radiation protection norms—often labeled generically "dose limits" or "permissible doses."

While the physicists were occupied with the tolerance dose in the aftermath of the 1925 Congress, physician-specialists welcomed Kaye's proposal for international protection recommendations and began ratcheting up the related requirements. They focused initially on training and command-and-control protection measures. In Austria, Holzknecht began to press the government, through a report written for the Technical Testing Bureau, to issue rules governing both the equipment used in X-ray clinics for protection and the training required of radiologists and X-ray operators.[81] Holzknecht claimed that the worst injuries to patients were caused by forgetting to place a filter in the primary beam to remove the softest X-rays. An automatic device that prevented operation of the X-ray tube if the filter was not in place cost 0.1 percent of the 12,000 marks required to buy an X-ray installation, and yet he believed as many as 90 percent of the X-ray tubes lacked the device. In Germany, the Röntgen Society in 1926 decided to revise its 1913 Instruction Sheet to consider the higher voltage X-ray tubes that had come into use.[82]

At the same time, the German Röntgen Society Special Committee for the Judgment of Röntgen Injuries and the Study of their Prevention reported on "Foreign Legal Prescriptions for the Exercise of the

[81] Holzknecht G (Professor für Röntgenkunde an der Wiener Universität). Zur Frage gesetzlicher Sicherheitsbestimmungen für die Anwendung der Röntgenstrahlen. Wien Klin Wschr. 1928;41:202–5., which is a 1926 or 1927 report to the medizinische Prüf- und Beratungsstelle (Vorsitzender Prof. Durig) am Technischen Versuchsamt in Wien (Leiter Präsident Ing. Dr. Exner). The report was brought before the Bundesministerium für soziale Verwaltung in November 1927.

[82] See Glocker, note 74, for the proposal to revise the 1913 Instruction Sheet and for the finished product see Merkblatt der D. R.-G. über den Gebrauch von Schutzmassnahmen gegen Röntgenstrahlen vom Jahre 1926. Fortschr Röntgenstr. 1926 May;34:848.

Röntgen Procedure."[83] This report cited approvingly a French requirement of two- or three-years study, plus a year of practical experience, before being examined for recognition as a "specialist." It also advocated licensing of X-ray installations by the government, a procedure that had been adopted in Denmark and in New York City. In France, the educational requirements for recognition as an X-ray specialist had, as the German report noted, been greatly expanded, and in addition consideration was again being given to rules for X-ray and radium protection.[84] In Sweden, an X-ray and Radium Protection Committee modeled after the British Committee adopted similar recommendations.[85] At the same time, the Swedes chose "Instruction and Training in Medical Radiology" as a theme for the 1928 Congress of Radiology in Stockholm, a theme that necessarily raised questions about specialization, including the need for radiation protection. In the Soviet Union, the People's Commissariat for Work issued rules for X-ray protection in the fall of 1925 that required upgrading or closing down X-ray installations that could not comply within three months, a requirement that at least in principle would eliminate the smaller, less busy X-ray installations run by non-specialists.[86]

Notably lacking from these efforts by physicians to promote, in tandem, protection, and specialization was much explicit consideration of the tolerance dose. Some medical objections to the tolerance dose arose from the necessary variations in clinical conditions and practices:

[83] "Gesetzliche Bestimmungen zur Ausübung des Röntgenverfahrens im Auslande," Referat aus dem Sonderausschuss für die Beurteilung von Röntgenschädigungen und zum Studium ihrer Verhütung, 27.

April 1927 (Referent: Herr Levy-Dorn, Berlin), Fortschr Röntgenstr. 1927;36:410–1.

[84] Jaulin (Orléans). Rapports sur les dangers des rayons X et des substances radioaktives pour les professionnels–moyens de s'en préserver. Journal of Radiology and Electrology. 1927 Apr;111:193–8. and Bouchacourt, Morel-Kahn (les docteurs). De quelques points fondamentaux, concernant la protection des personnes utilisant les R. X. Bull Soc Radiol Med (Paris). 1928;16:59–65.

[85] See the reference in Wintz H (M. D., Ph. D., Director of the University Gynecological Clinic and Röntgen Institute, Erlangen), Rump W (Privatdozent, Ph. D.). Protective Measures against Dangers Resulting from the Use of Radium, Röntgen and Ultraviolet Rays, Prepared for the Health Organization of the League of Nations (Geneva: League of Nations, III. HEALTH. 1931. III. 9). at 73.

[86] Verfügung des "Volkskommissariats der Arbeit" der Räterepublik vom 9, September 1925, Nr. 233/389 betreffs des Arbeitsschutzes der in Röntgenkabinetten tätigen Arbeiter. Fortschr Röntgenstr. 1926;35:781–3.

idiosyncratic reactions of individuals, though recognized as less frequent than had been thought before the use of ionization chambers to measure doses, were still regarded as possible. In addition, reaction to radiation varied with the time in which a given dose was delivered, so that four exposures over a period of a month would not have the same effect as the same dose delivered in a single sitting. Though from a physical point of view it made no difference for what time period the tolerance dose was specified, from the biological point of view the time factor was critical. Dose rate would remain an issue for decades to come.

In addition to these medical arguments and probably more important in accounting for lack of physician interest in the tolerance dose, the calculation of shielding thicknesses was still a mysterious mathematical procedure to most physicians, however routine it had become for the physicist in medical radiology. Behnken, in proposing in 1926 that the first protection rule always be "the tolerance dose should, in the places protected, nowhere and never be exceeded," tried to allay the physicians' fears:

> A Röntgenologist need hardly get the creeps from 'higher' mathematics that enter..., especially since the practitioner needs to use only the condensed table corresponding to average [voltage] requirements.

The physicians' reply was that protection measures had to be phrased "so that everyone will be able to understand them."[87]

Physicians did not confront the physicists on the issue of the tolerance dose, and they were content to let it be used to calculate recommended shielding thicknesses. At the same time, however, the tolerance dose went unspecified in the protection recommendations, which then read like a compendium of good clinical practice based on the collective experience of physicians. If the notion that protection lay within the prerogatives of the physician were to be maintained, it would hardly do to have the

[87] Behnken, note 75, at 183: "Durch die am Anfang vorkommende 'höhere' Mathematik braucht sich wohl kaum ein Röntgenologe gruselig machen zu lassen, zumal da ja der Praktiker nur die dem Durchschnittbedürfnis entsprechend gekürzten Tabellen zu benutzen braucht." The reply was by the physicist Grossmann (Berlin), ibid., who may have been more sensitive to the practitioner's requirements because he worked in the X-ray industry: "Auch müssen die Vorschriften–worauf ich besonders hinweisen möchte–populär gefasst sein, so dass sie von jedermann verstanden werden konnen.".

tolerance dose cited as the basis for the rest of the protection recommendations. Thus, when the British X-ray and Radium Protection Committee extended its recommendations to higher voltages in 1927 in a way that was consistent with a tolerance dose of 1/100 unit skin dose per month, this figure was not mentioned in the recommendations.[88] The second International Congress of Radiology, meeting in Stockholm in 1928, adopted at the behest of the Physics Section simplified and abridged international protection recommendations that for most practical purposes followed the British recommendations, but Mutscheller's effort to have the tolerance dose formally adopted failed.[89]

International Protection Takes Institutional Form and Endorses the Tolerance Dose

In addition to adopting international protection recommendations, the Stockholm Congress created the International X-ray and Radium Protection Commission, with five of the initial seven members physicists (including Solomon, who was also a physician).[90] The creation of this Commission raised the issue of protection to a new level of international visibility, gave focus to the growing epistemic community concerned

[88] Recommendations of the X-ray and Radium Protection Committee Third Revised Report, May 1927. British Journal of Radiology (Archives of Radiology and Electrotherapy). 1927;32:330–6.

[89] International Recommendations for X-Ray and Radium Protection: Stockholm 1929. Annals of the ICRP, Volume OS_1, Issue 1. 1929. Available from: https://doi.org/10.1016/S0074-27402880010-9, accessed September 1, 2023. For the adoption of the international protection recommendations, see A Report of the Second International Congress of Radiology (Stockholm, 23–27 July 1928) and the Proceedings of the Joint Scientific Meetings of the Congress. Acta Radiologica, Supplementum III, Pars I. 1929. Mutscheller announced his intention in 388. Safety Standards of Protection against X-ray Dangers (read before the Radiological Society of North America, at the Thirteenth Annual Meeting, at New Orleans, Dec. 2, 1927). Radiology. 1928 Jun;10(6):468–76.

[90] The original members of the International X-ray and Radium Protection Commission were the Chairman Rolf Sievert, the Swedish physicist; G. W. C. Kaye, the British physicist; Stanley Melville, a British physician; Guilio Ceresole, an Italian physician; Gustav Grossmann, a German physicist who worked for an X-ray tube manufacturer; Iser Solomon, the French physicist and physician; and Lauriston Taylor, the American Bureau of Standards physicist. The list is in ICRP Archives, Archive Files 66–75, Archive File 68, Stockholm 1928.pdf, 31. Sievert later gave an inaccurate description of the membership and also said Kaye was Chairman, see The International Commission on Radiological Protection. Inter Ass. 1957;9:589–93.

with radiation dosimetry and protection, and generated a wave of activities on the national level. The League of Nations Health Organization asked the German physician-physicist Wintz in 1931 to review national protection measures. He was able to cite detailed protection rules under consideration or adopted in Austria, Czechoslovakia, Denmark, Britain, Germany, Greece, Hungary, the Soviet Union, Sweden, and Switzerland.[91] In the United States, the creation of the international protection commission incentivized the formation of an Advisory Committee on X-ray and Radium Protection with representatives from the American Röntgen Ray Society, the less restrictive Radiological Society of North America, the American Medical Association, the National Bureau of Standards, and equipment manufacturers.[92] The British X-ray and Radium Protection Committee continued its work, and in Germany the Röntgen Society, which in 1927 had formed a Standards Bureau that affiliated with the German Standards Committee, promulgated radiation protection recommendations in 1930 after two years of discussion and redrafting.[93]

The American Advisory Committee would after World War II become an important pillar of both domestic and international efforts for radiation protection. But it started as a norm-taker, not a norm-maker. The committee initially undertook to study foreign recommendations on radiation protection, especially stemming from analogous German, Swedish, and British professional groups, as well as the International X-ray and Radium Protection Commission version. It also sought to use its influence to prevent the passage of what it regarded as harmful legislation or the issuance of harmful rules by the Underwriters Association. As Lauriston Taylor later wrote, the committee referred often to its own work as legislation or regulation, but it in fact had no force of law. Whom it was

[91] Wintz and Rump, note 85.

[92] Taylor, L. "Brief History of the National Committee on Radiation Protection and Measurements (NCRP) Covering the Period 1929–1946," Health Physics. 1958;1:3–10. See also Taylor, L. Organization for Radiation Protection: the Operations of the ICRP and NCRP, 1928–1974, published by the U.S. Department of Energy, DOE/TIC-10124, 1979, 4-001-8 and Whittemore, GF. The National Committee on Radiation Protection, 1928–1960: from professional guidelines to government regulation. Harvard University Ph.D. dissertation, 1986.

[93] For a brief history of the *Normenstelle* and its affiliation with the Deutsche Normenausschuss, see Graf H. Die Entwicklung der radiologischen Normung in Deutschland. DIN-Mitt. 1975;54:531–5.

advising was never specified. But the value added of the recommendations was nevertheless clear to Taylor:

> ...lack of legal standing will probably not in any way detract from their legal value. They are a recognized set of recommendations, drawn up by qualified representatives of the art and freely distributed to those interested. A court decision involving X-ray protection would in all probability, for lack of another source, be guided by these recommendations, and persons ignoring them may be held liable for negligence.[94]

They might also be "useful for regulatory or legislative purposes by some other appropriate body should such a trend and need develop."[95] Radiation protection norms aimed not only to protect people from the harmful effects of radiation, but also to protect the medical and other professionals using radiation from what they might regard as unwarranted interference. The concern with lawsuits would persist, as did the threat of insurance requirements and legislation.

The International X-Ray and Radium Protection Commission met in Paris in 1931 during the third International Congress of Radiology and made a number of changes in the international recommendations. Among the most important were the extension of the table of recommended shielding thicknesses for X-rays from 225,000 volts to 400,000 volts and the addition of a table of recommended shielding thicknesses for radium that replaced an earlier requirement of 5 cm of lead shielding for each 100 mg.[96] The first table was determined from a tolerance dose of 10^{-5} Röntgens per second, which was the equivalent (assuming 200 working hours per month and a unit skin dose of 600 Röntgens) of Mutscheller's original 1/100 unit skin dose per month. The recommended shielding thicknesses for radium were approximately those that would have been derived from

[94] Taylor, L. "The Work of the National and International Committees on X-ray and Radium Protection Radiology," Radiology. July 1932;19(1):1–4, Available from: https://doi.org/10.1148/19.1.1, accessed August 2, 2023.

[95] Taylor, note 92, Organization for Radiation Protection, 4-003.

[96] For the changes introduced in 1931, see Recommendations of the International X-ray and Radium Protection Commission. British Journal of Radiology. 1931;4:85–7, and for the recommendations as they stood after these changes were made see International Recommendations for X-ray and Radium Protection, Revised by the International X-ray and Radium Protection Commission and Adopted by the Third International Congress of Radiology, Paris, July 1931. British Journal of Radiology. 1932;5:82–5.

a tolerance dose one third the size of Mutscheller's, an added precaution taken because of the continuous emission of radiation from radium while X-ray tubes were assumed to be used only eight hours per day.[97] In neither case did the international recommendations specify the tolerance dose on which they were based.

National and international discussions of the protection recommendations could not, however, continue to ignore the tolerance dose, as controversy over protection measures revolved increasingly about this performance-based norm. In 1930, for example, two physicists working for the Dutch Philips Company, a major X-ray tube manufacturer since its introduction of a tube that had most of the required protection built inside rather than surrounding the glass bulb, challenged the draft German recommendations on the grounds that they did not follow the international recommendations and cited the tolerance dose as the basis for the latter.[98] In 1931, when a British physician attacked the international recommendations as too strict, the reply he received from both physicists and physicians present was that the international recommendations were consistent with the tolerance dose.[99] Wintz, in his 1931 report to the League of Nations outlined in detail the procedure for deriving shielding thicknesses from the tolerance dose and discussed checking the effectiveness of protection measures in terms of verifying that the tolerance dose had not been exceeded.[100] Mutscheller's own effort in the early 1930s to get the American Advisory Committee to lower the implicit tolerance dose also forced ever more explicit attention to it.[101]

The tolerance dose was gradually coming into open circulation and achieving acceptance among at least physician-specialists as well as physicists. When the International X-Ray and Radium Protection Commission

[97] Wintz and Rump, note 85, pp. 19–21.

[98] Van der Tuuk JH, Boldingh WH (Naturkundig Laboratorium der N. V. Philips' Gloeilampenfabrieken). Die Bleischutzdicken in den deutschen Strahlenschutzvorschriften. Fortschr Röntgenstr. 1920;412:965–7. and the reply by Glocker R, Zur Frage der 'Bleischutzdicken' in den internationalen und in den deutschen Strahlenschutzvorschriften, ibid., 967–71.

[99] A Discussion on the International Protection Recommendations, 19 November 1931 and 14 January 1932. British Journal of Radiology. 1932;5:215–33, especially the comments of G. E. Bell, W. Binks and the President, A. E. Barclay.

[100] Wintz and Rump, note 85.

[101] Whittemore, note 92, 75–85.

met at the fourth International Congress of Radiology in Zurich in 1934, five of its nine members were physicians (once again including Solomon, who was also a physicist). The X-ray protection recommendations the Commission approved cited the tolerance dose prominently and explicitly, though still cautiously: "The evidence at present available appears to suggest that under satisfactory working conditions a person in normal health can tolerate exposure to X-rays to an extent of about 0.2 international Röntgens (r) per day."[102] This figure was approximately equivalent to 10^{-5} Röntgens per second assuming a seven-hour working day, and its adoption should be viewed as the acknowledgment of a heuristic best practice rather than as an innovation. Clinical requirements, not laboratory science, were still the major factor in determining the tolerance dose, even if more scientific measurement methods and units had been adopted.

The American Advisory Committee on X-ray and Radium Protection had already adopted a lower tolerance dose of 0.1 r per day, rounded down, Taylor later said, from 0.24 per day "so as not to imply a degree of knowledge about the number that was clearly not borne out by established facts."[103] That was not the whole story. Concern about the deeply penetrating gamma rays of radium was also a motive. Gioacchino Failla, a physicist working at Memorial Hospital in New York City and a member of the Advisory Committee, had recommended in 1931 (on the basis of experience with technicians handling radium) 1/1000 of the 600 r erythema dose, which would have been 0.6 r per month or 0.024 r per day.[104] The number was moved up from Failla's recommendation, but down from the International Commission's. The tolerance dose was

[102] ICRP. International Recommendations for X-ray and Radium Protection Revised by the International X-ray and Radium Protection Commission at the Fourth International Congress of Radiology, Zürich, July 1934. British Journal of Radiology. 1934;7:695–9, at 695.

[103] Taylor, note 92, Organization for Radiation Protection, "Meetings of Advisory Committee on X-ray and Radium Protection," p. 4-011. The tolerance dose was not however mentioned in the 1931 National Bureau of Standards Handbook 15 on "X-ray Protection," Available from: https://www.orau.org/health-physics-museum/files/library/nbs/nbs-15.pdf, accessed April 10, 2023. Instead, it was published in the preface to a report on radium protection only published in 1934.

[104] Failla G. Radium Protection. Radiology. 1932 Jul;19(1): read before the Radiological Society of North America at the Seventeenth Annual Meeting, at St. Louis, Nov. 30–Dec. 4, 1931, 12–21, Available from: https://doi.org/10.1148/19.1.12, accessed August 2, 2023. Failla, as we shall see, would later change his view, based on the difficulty of meeting his recommendation in clinical practice.

intended to protect the use of radium in medicine as well as the physicians and technicians using it. Mutscheller himself reportedly proposed the equivalent of 0.1 r per day to Taylor.[105]

A General Electric representative (Coolidge, who had invented the high-voltage, hot-cathode "Coolidge tube") was on the committee that decided on the 0.1 r per day tolerance dose. He had forwarded a General Electric objection but lost the consensus.[106] No brouhaha ensued. The manufacturers wanted government inspections and lowered insurance rates to ensure compliance.[107] They did not resist a public statement on unsafe equipment but advocated "several years grace" to bring protection up to standards.[108] Protection requirements might even be welcome, as they would reduce the risks of liability as well as competition from less scrupulous manufacturers.[109]

The Americans likely advocated 0.1 r per day at the international level as well but failed until after World War II to convince their colleagues from other countries. Divergence between the American committee and its international counterpart would be common in the decades to come, with the Americans sometimes setting tighter standards and sometimes laxer ones. The international recommendations were not intended to bind national authorities, a feature that would make the international regime more resilient than it might otherwise have been. Eventual national convergence would become the rule rather than the exception.

Genetic Effects Get Little Traction

Hermann J. Muller had demonstrated in his laboratory at the University of Texas in Austin in 1927 that X-rays could produce genetic mutations. Despite Muller's repeated efforts, two decades would pass before that

[105] Lindell B. Bo Lindell's History of Radiation, Radioactivity, and Radiological Protection [Internet]. www.nks.org. 1996 [accessed 2023 April 10]. Available from: https://www.nks.org/en/news/bo-lindells-history-of-radiation-radioactivity-and-radiological-protection.htm.

[106] Whittemore, note 92, at 87.

[107] See Taylor, note 92, "Meetings of Advisory Committee on X-ray and Radium Protection, December 2, 1931," 4-008-9.

[108] Ibid.

[109] Whittemore, note 92, at 93 and 98–100.

knowledge emerged from the laboratory to arouse public and consequently professional concern. Before World War II, genetic effects had little influence on the norm-setting process either at the national or international level.[110]

An advocate of evolution and thechromosome theory of heredity, Muller believed that genes were the basis for all life. He was looking in the mid-1920s for a way of producing more frequent mutations in fruit flies (*Drosophila*), as these would facilitate research aimed at understanding how genes were distributed and redistributed on chromosomes. Captivated by the potential of radium, Muller was familiar with previous work showing its effects on embryos as well as prior claims to having demonstrated radiation-induced mutations, which he regarded as inconclusive and would later be forgotten in the wake of his own more dramatic success.[111] By the mid-1920s he had shifted to using X-rays, which he rightly regarded as similar to the gamma rays of radium, and his techniques for detecting mutations were far more advanced. He demonstrated a 15,000 percent rise in the frequency of mutations in fruit flies due to X-ray exposure and labeled the phenomenon "artificial transmutation of the gene," an obvious nod to the transmutations wrought by radioactivity.[112] Soon thereafter, American geneticist Lewis John Stadler independently confirmed that radium could cause mutations in corn.[113]

The spectacular success of Muller's experiments made him famous in scientific circles and generated a flush of laboratory experiments, but before World War II aroused little public concern. The gap between the medical clinic and the genetics laboratory was still wide. Medical radiologists rejected the notion that laboratory experiments on fruit flies could shed light on heredity in human beings. Clinicians even reacted angrily to

[110] Muller is dissected in Carlson EA. Genes, Radiation, and Society: The Life and Work of H. J. Muller. Ithaca and London: Cornell University Press; 1981. But note Campos, note 111.

[111] The prior claims and Muller's attitude towards them is discussed in Campos LA. Radium and the Secret of Life. Chicago: University Of Chicago Press; 2016. 101–239.

[112] Muller HJ. The Problem of Gene Modification, Verhandlungen des V. Internationalen Kongresses für Vererbungswissenschaft (Berlin, 1927). In: Z Induk Abst Vererb, Supplement Band 1. 1928. p. 234–60. This article is reprinted in Muller HJ. Studies in Genetics: the Selected Papers. Bloomington, Indiana: Indiana University Press; 1962. For a more popular version, see his Artificial Transmutation of the Gene. Science. 1928;66:84–7.

[113] Stadler LJ. Genetic Effects of X-rays in Maize. Proceedings of the National Academy of Sciences of the United States of America. 1928;14:69–75.

Muller's suggestions that they protect themselves from genetic effects.[114] Though interested in eugenics as a means for improving human offspring, Muller believed most mutations would be harmful. He tried to warn the public of potential harm not only to individuals but also to future generations, and therefore the human race, from mutations caused by radiation.

A leftist affiliated in the early 1930s with a student-run, Communist-front organization, Muller spent 1933–1937 at the Soviet Academy of Sciences in Moscow. While there, he attributed his discovery of X-ray-induced mutations to "a strong direct Marxian influence," though he had earlier (in 1921 at Cold Spring Harbor) emphasized the central importance to his thinking of Thomas Hunt Morgan, leader of the "Drosophila group" at Columbia University.[115] Muller had worked there even while an undergraduate, but his relationship with Morgan was fraught.[116] Neither Marx nor Morgan was likely the key influence, though the latter was certainly important to Muller's career. There was incentive to laud Morgan at Cold Spring Harbor. Muller, who spent much of his early career in Houston and Austin, liked to spend summers on Long Island or Cape Cod rather than in Texas, which he disliked for personal, climate, professional, and political reasons.[117] There was also incentive to

[114] Carlson, note 110, 160 and 255.

[115] H. J. Muller, An Episode in Science, a thirty-page typed manuscript with hand-written corrections and the notation "Title and subject chosen by Dr. C. B. Davenport. This lecture was given at the Biological Laboratory of the Brooklyn Institute, Cold Spring Harbor, L. I., the evening of July 25, 1921." The manuscript is on deposit at the Library of the American Philosophical Society (Philadelphia). The later account is available in Muller HJ. Lenin's Doctrines in Relation to Genetics," as reprinted in Appendix II of Loren R. Graham, Science and Philosophy in the Soviet Union. New York: Alfred A Knopf. 1972;453–69, at 462. Muller went on to avoid naming names, saying "this is not the place to go into personal details," but it is clear from his description of the influences within the Drosophila group that he meant to be including himself among the Marxists.

[116] Carlson EA. The Drosophila Group. Genetics. 1975;79:15–27. and The Drosophila Group: the Transition from the Mendelian Unit to the Individual Gene. Journal of the History of Biology. 1974;7:31–48. Carlson has mentioned the possible relevance of Muller's political views to the disputes with Morgan, but only in passing, see Elof Axel Carson, "An Unacknowledged Founding of Molecular Biology: H. J. Muller's Contributions to Gene Theory, 1910–1936," Journal of the History of Biology. 4 (1971) 149–70, at 158.

[117] Muller later wrote to L. C. Dunn, à propos of Texas, in a letter of 27 March 1928 (Dunn Collection, American Philosophical Society): "(a) they fired my wife for having a child (before it came and before they knew it was coming–except that she notified them)

laud Marx in Stalin's Moscow, especially as Trofim Lysenko, a favorite ofStalin's, opposed the chromosome theory of heredity that Muller advocated. But other leftist influences, not Marxist, more likely pointed Muller toward his experiments with radiation. Among those who had tried as early as 1911 to produce mutations with X-rays or radium was Jacques Loeb, a German biologist who had emigrated to the United States in the 1890s and who had become a close friend of Morgan. Muller admired Loeb, who is most remembered for his discovery of artificial parthenogenesis, a procedure in which embryological development of an egg is initiated by treatment with a salt solution or even by the prick of a pin rather than by fertilization.[118]

This experimental work was linked to theoretical preoccupations. Loeb was heir to a reductionist tradition in biology and medicine. He believed, as did Muller, that all of life was reducible to physical and chemical laws and emphasized that this assertion was a first principle rather than a limited methodological assumption. Like his predecessors, the "medical materialists," Loeb's reductionism was combined with leftist political views, the common root of both being an uncompromising materialism.[119] Muller's demonstration of radiation-induced mutation quickly attracted efforts to explain mutation in terms of physical and chemical events like ionization and chemical reactions. These efforts appeared to succeed in 1935, when three Göttingen scientists applied Dessauer's "point-heat" theory, mentioned in Chapter 5, to experimental studies of

and won't give her job back, tho she has a Ph. D. in math. from Illinois, had taught here 4 years and they acknowledged her 'loyal and efficient service,' and intended to go on indefinitely. (b) one can't do fly work here in the summer, (c) there is a dearth of suitable graduate material, even my colleagues are willing to take the work out of my hands for themselves before I can get around to it. (d) there are other objections, connected with its being in the South." Muller was a staunch anti-racist, and a good part of this letter is concerned with efforts to help a black geneticist who could find neither a suitable post nor research support.

118 Elof Axel Carlson, in a private communication, kindly informed me that Muller did not correspond with Loeb but that he admired Loeb's early materialist writings, that he had a photograph of Loeb in his office at Indiana University after World War II, and that he mentioned Loeb's influence in a biographical sketch for the National Academy of Sciences (on deposit at the Lilly Library of the University of Indiana).

119 Fleming D. Introduction. In: The Mechanistic Conception of Life. Cambridge, Massachusetts: Harvard University Press; 1964. Originally published in 1912.

radiation-induced mutation.[120] N. W. Timofeeff-Ressovsky (a geneticist who had worked with Muller), K. G. Zimmer (a radiation biologist), and M. Delbrück (a physicist, also known to Muller) demonstrated that mutation was a single-hit process, in which only a single ionization event was required to produce the observed linear dose/effect relationship. This work, though no longer considered valid in the form in which it was initially presented, played an important role in twentieth-century biology, inspiring Erwin Schrödinger's popular reductionist presentation "What is Life?" and leading thereby to James Watson's overweening (though correct) faith in the molecular character of the gene.[121]

The *Dreimännerwerk* of Timofeeff-Ressovsky, Zimmer, and Delbrück directly contradicted the idea of a tolerance dose, which by the 1930s was in common use. If the "point-heat" theory was correct and mutation was a single-hit process, there was no threshold even at low doses. The tolerance dose would not provide the protection that it appeared to promise. This possibility raised two questions: should mutation be considered in radiation protection, and did the linear relationship between dose and mutation found in the *Drosophila* laboratory exist as well in the real world? Both of these questions entailed, and to some degree continue to entail, profound difficulties for the professional radiological community and for the public. No one had ever demonstrated radiation-induced mutation in mammals outside the laboratory. Even inside the laboratory the demonstration for low doses, though apparently straightforward, would have involved numbers of test animals so large that the experiment lies beyond imaginable capabilities. Radiation-induced mutation at low

120 Timoféeff-Ressovsky NW, Zimmer RG, Delbrück M. Über die Natur der Genmutation und der Genstruktur. Nach Ges wissen (Göttingen). 1925;189–245.

121 Schrödinger E. What is Life? The Physical Aspect of the Living Cell, reprinted with "Mind and Matter." Cambridge: University Press; 1969. For the connection with Watson, see Fleming D. Emigré Physicists and the Biological Revolution. Pers Amer Hist. 1968;2:152–89. If the connection between Loeb and Muller suggested above is correct, and if Fleming's analysis of both the medical materialists and Watson is accepted, then the connections between what Paul Cranefield calls The Organic Physics of 1847 and the Biophysics of Today. Journal of the History of Medicine. 1957;12:407–23, are stronger than sometimes supposed: du Bois-Raymond, Helmholtz and Brücke; the leftist medical materialists; Loeb; Muller; Timofeef-Ressovsky, Zimmer and Delbrück; Schrodinger; Watson.

doses thus lay in the sphere of what Alvin Weinberg has called "trans-science," or questions that can reasonably be asked but which science could not answer.[122]

With radiation-induced mutation, the gap between the laboratory and the clinic again opened wide. Experiments can show, in a fruit fly laboratory, that mutation is apparently a one-hit process for which there is no threshold. In practice, however, we do not know the relevance of these experiments for mutation in human beings, and the surveys undertaken beginning in the late 1920s concerning genetic damage in human beings exposed to radiation did not show significant results. Given this uncertainty, it is not surprising that the views of both scientists and nonscientists on the importance of genetic effects have varied, often depending more on cultural and political values than on verifiable evidence. As early as 1933, a Joint Committee on the Question of Genetic Damage of the German Society for the Science of Heredity and of the German Röntgen Society, although recognizing that in individual cases it could never be proven whether radiation had caused genetic damage, urged the greatest caution in medical irradiation because of the possibility of damage to the "germinal heritage of our nation."[123] It appears the Nazi emphasis on genetic purity and eugenic progress had already had an impact on thinking in German professional circles.

Genetic risks did not arouse much public concern in the rest of Europe and the United States before World War II, despite Muller's pleas. In the United States, radiation-induced genetic effects did however generate debate within the Advisory Committee on X-ray and Radium Protection. It considered, adopted, and reversed in 1940 and 1941 a proposal to lower the tolerance dose.[124] After its adoption was mentioned at an

[122] Weinberg AM. Science and Transscience, in the Ciba Foundation Symposium Volume Civilization and Science: in Conflict or Collaboration? Amsterdam: Associated Scientific Publishers; 1972:105–22, with discussion.

[123] "...die Gefährdung des Keimgutes unseres Volkes," in Zur Erbschädigungsfrage, Verh Deut Ront Ges. 1933;26:111. In 1958 Holthusen told Sievert that the Germans had adopted in 1929 50 rems as the maximum permissible gonad dose, H. Holthusen to Sievert, "Recommendations of the ICRP," January 28, 1958 (translation), ICRP Archives, Box W-18, Archive file 23, Sect. Correspondence 1.8.57-31.12.58, 64–71, at 67.

[124] Taylor, note 92, Organization for Radiation Protection, Report of the Advisory Committee on X-ray and Radium Protection, December 3, 1940, 5-011-13 and Notes of the Meeting of Advisory Protection Committee, December 4, 1940, 5-013-4. This complicated back and forth is treated in detail in Whittemore, note 92, 135–72.

American Medical Association meeting, a more intense debate ensued within the Advisory Committee. Failla, the physicist who had suggested a stringent tolerance dose for gamma rays from radium, objected:

> I feel this is a mistake for the following reasons: .1 roentgen per day is certainly a safe dose so far as systemic changes are concerned. If we bring in the genetic criteria, then there is no limit at all and .02 roentgen per day is just as arbitrary as .1 roentgen per day. To be sure the smaller the dose the less the genetic damage but the possible damage from .1 roentgen per day is so slight that one can just as well stop at this point.[125]

Admitting that X-ray practitioners could readily meet the proposed new requirement, he noted however that those administering radon for therapeutic purposes could not. Failla would take a different position on genetic effects after World War II, but in 1941 he added:

> I do not think it wise to publish a statement at this time since it would probably be used by state authorities working on codes, and once the new tolerance dose gets into these codes it will be very difficult to get it out.[126]

Preventing medical radiology from government regulation was still a higher priority than protecting radiologists and others from uncertain genetic effects. A physician added:

> In the course of the last thirty years, we have had a very large number of technicians, doctors, nurses and workers here, who have been working with radium and x ray, and who have received very much greater dosage than that suggested by the new requirements. A large number are married, and healthy children have been born to the females as well as the males. There have been no observed malformations or gross changes in any of the children. Of course, I realize that the geneticists may say we should wait until the second or third generations.[127]

[125] Taylor, note 92, Organization for Radiation Protection, Remarks by Dr. Failla, 5-016.

[126] Ibid.

[127] Ibid., To members of the Advisory Committee on X-ray and Radium Protection, 5-016-7. The physician was Curtis F. Burnam, who was affiliated with the American Radium Society.

Without public pressure and no geneticist among its members, the pre-war committee felt little pressure to protect the profession, even at risk of not protecting the professionals.

The "medico-legal" factor militated against lowering the tolerance dose, "since almost any level that is likely to be used at present in diagnostic work is liable to exceed a tolerance dose."[128] Setting a separate tolerance dose for genetic effects might lead to "endless lawsuits."[129] While a survey of American users of X-rays and radium had shown that it was possible to keep doses down to one-fifth of the then current recommendation of 0.1 r per day, and Taylor anticipated such a tightening of the permissible dose, the Advisory Committee eventually reversed its decision to lower the tolerance dose and failed to come to agreement on anything but continuing the discussion of genetic effects, a discussion World War II interrupted.[130] The lower figure would only be reached in ICRP recommendations decided almost 50 years later, in 1990.

The pre-war consideration of genetic effects did however cause one small but significant change in terminology. Members of the U.S. Advisory Committee began to call what had previously been termed the "tolerance dose" a "maximum permissible dose."[131] "Tolerance" implied a threshold, which still made sense to medical doctors, many of whom continued to use the term. Physicists and geneticists knew no reason to assume there was a threshold. This change persisted after the war, at least among those associated with norm-setting in the United States, and

[128] Advisory Committee on X-Ray and Radium Protection, September 25, 1942, Taylor, note 92, Organization for Radiation Protection, 5-019.

[129] Ibid., 5-020.

[130] Cowie DB, Scheele LA. A Survey of Radiation Protection in Hospitals. JNCI: Journal of the National Cancer Institute. 1941 Jun;1(6):767–87, https://doi-org.proxy1.library.jhu.edu/10.1093/jnci/1.6.767, accessed September 2, 2023. Cowie and Scheele say that the tolerance dose had been reduced to .02 r per day by the Advisory Committee, attributing the information to Taylor, who had cited .02 r, based on a survey by G. W. C. Kaye in Taylor L, "X-Ray Protection," JAMA 1941;116(2):136–140, https://doi.org/10.1001/jama.1941.62820020006012, accessed September 4, 2023. But Taylor later reported that no action was taken on the recommendation to lower the tolerance dose to .02 r per day before World War II, and after the War the figure .1 r was accepted as the Advisory Committee recommendation, Taylor, Organization for Radiation Protection, note 92, 5-022.

[131] Taylor, Ibid., 5-018.

gradually spread beyond. It opens difficult issues that will be discussed in later chapters. Permissible to whom and why are questions without easy answers.

Radium Protection Lags Again

The international recommendations of 1934 noted that no tolerance dose for exposure to the gamma rays of radium was available, but without citing reasons.[132] The Americans had already determined that it would not be possible to work with radium at anything like a tolerance dose as low as 0.1 r per day. They instead adopted a tolerance dose of 5 r per day for the fingers of those handling small quantities of radium.[133] Only in 1938 did the NCRP use 0.1 r per day to calculate distances and shielding that they thought would be adequate to protect from the gamma rays of radium.[134] These recommendations were not based on a careful assessment of biological effects.

Those effects had, however, already become apparent in two newly discovered instances of injuries caused by radium and its decay product, radium emanation (now known as radon): to radium dial painters and to miners. Luminescent dials were in increasing demand after the Great War due to the rapid expansion of military and civilian aviation, including at night. The women had ingested radium while tipping their brushes to a fine point between their lips. Several people involved in running the companies they worked for knew that this practice was dangerous, and one even advised the women to stop. But nothing more serious was done. A physician reported a peculiar and sometimes fatal necrosis of the jaw among women working as dial painters to New Jersey health officials by the end of 1922, but an investigation produced no results.

[132] ICRP, note 102.

[133] Taylor, Organization for Radiation Protection, note 92, 4-015.

[134] "Radium Protection," Radiology, 1938 31:4, 481–490, https://doi.org/10.1148/31.4.481, accessed September 3, 2023.

Reports began to appear in the medical literature by 1924.[135] The incident first came to the attention of the public through the efforts of the New Jersey Consumers' League. Only after its campaign and the court case of the "five women doomed to death" did government authorities and the medical profession beyond the local community become actively interested.[136] An out-of-court settlement was reached in 1928, but shortly thereafter it was discovered that some of the radium dial painters were developing osteogenic sarcomas at the sites of previously observed irritations of their bones.[137]

[135] Theodore Blum in a footnote to "Osteomyelitis of the Mandible and Maxilla," an address to the American Dental Association, September 1924 was apparently the first report, see Hoffmann FL (Newark, N. J. O, Radium (Mesothorium). Necrosis. Journal of the American Medical Association. 1925;851:961–5), read before the Section on Preventive and Industrial Medicine and Public Health at the 76th Annual Session of the American Medical Association, Atlantic City, May 1925. The entire radium dial painters' story, including remarkable details about the individuals involved, is thoroughly and passionately recounted in Clark C. Radium Girls: Women and Industrial Health Reform, 1910–1935. Chicago: University of Chicago Press; 1997 and Moore K. The Radium Girls The Dark Story of America's Shining Women. Naperville, Illinois: Sourcebooks; 2017.

[136] Hoffmann, ibid., credited the New Jersey Consumer League with bringing the case to his attention, and he was the first to report in the medical literature on the dial painters. For one of many newspaper reports, see Radium and Gas as Death Cause Open New Issue. New York Times. 1925 May 19;14. Hoffmann noted that the New Jersey Bureau of Labor had investigated the situation but found nothing, investigators from the Harvard Medical School did not publish a report they had prepared, and the U. S. Public Health Service considered investigating but did not. Two local physicians and a dentist, however, had been working on the radium dial painters, and Hoffman's publication precipitated the early publication of their more detailed report, see Martland HS (M. D.), Conlon P (M. D.), Knef JP (D. D. S.). Some Unrecognized Dangers in the Use and Handling of Radioactive Substances: With a Special Reference to the Storage of Insoluble Products of Radium and Mesothorium in the Reticulo-endothelial System. Journal of the American Medical Association. 1925 Dec 5;85:1769–76, from the Medical Service of St. Mary's Hospital, Orange, N. J.; the Pathologic Department of the City Hospital, Newark; and the office of the County Physician of Essex County, N. J.

[137] For reference to the out-of-court settlement, see Maurice De Laet (Agrégé à l'Université de Bruxelles), "La pathologie professionnelle due aux corps radioactifs," Annales de Medecine Legale, Criminologie, Police Scientifique et Toxicologie. 8 (1928) 443–52 and also Harrison S. Martland (M. D., the Department of Pathology of ·the Newark City Hospital and the Office of the Chief Medical Examiner of Essex County, Newark, N. J.), "The Occurrence of Malignancies in Radioactive Persons. A General Review of Data Gathered in the Study of the Radium Dial Painters, With Special Reference to the Occurrence of Osteogenic Sarcoma and the Interrelationship of Certain Blood Diseases," American Journal of Cancer Research. 15 (1931) 2435–2516. Osteogenic sarcoma was first reported in H. S. Martland and R. E. Humphries, "Osteogenic Sarcoma

At about the same time as the initial discovery of "radium jaw," a lung disease characteristic of arsenic ore miners in the Schneeberg mountains of Germany was attracting the attention of research workers sponsored by the Saxon Regional Committee for the Investigation and Control of Cancer.[138] By the early 1930s, radium emanation (radon) in the Schneeberg mines and in the uranium mines at Joachimsthal (Czechoslovakia) had become a prime suspect as the causal agent of lung cancer manifested in some of the miners.[139] Neither the radium dial painters affair nor the Schneeberg and Joachimsthal miners incident had been caused directly by medical uses of radiation, as earlier radiation-induced injuries had been, but both raised questions about the long-term effects of using radium and radium emanation in therapy. Radium protection faced new and poorly understood challenges. Specifying a tolerance dose in the face of these uncertainties may well have seemed unwise, even though it was used to determine the relevant procedures for applying radium.

On the eve of World War II, professional groups of physicists and physician-specialists based in the United States and Europe had reached agreement on units for the measurement of X-rays and radium as well as pragmatic protection measures applicable in medical radiology ratified at the international level. But outside medical radiology the situation was less professionally disciplined, as illustrated by radium dial painters and uranium miners. The main radiation protection concerns of the remaining decades of the twentieth century would likewise arise outside medical radiology, even if medical diagnosis and therapy remain (until today) the main source of radiation exposure for most people. Radiation protection would instead become vital to two major new enterprises: the building and testing of nuclear weapons and the operation of nuclear power plants for electrical generation, in addition to far more extensive use of X-rays in industry and radioactive isotopes in medicine. Even as miners continued

in Dial Painters Using Luminous Paint," Archives of Pathology & Laboratory Medicine. 7 (1929) 406–17.

[138] Thiele, Rostoski, Saupe, Schmorl. Ueber den Schneeberger Lungenkrebs. Münchener Medizinische Wochenschrift. 1924;711:24–5, Sitzung vom 8 Oktober 1923 of the Gesellschaft für Natur und Heilkunde in Dresden. This work was sponsored by the Sächsischen Landesausschusses zur Erforschung und Bekämpfung der Krebskrankheit.

[139] Pirshan A (Head Physician, State Radium Institute, Jàchymov), Sikl H (Extraordinary Professor of Pathology at the Czech University, Prague). Cancer of the Lung in the Miners of Jàchymov (Joachimstal). Report of Cases Observed 1929–30. American Journal of Cancer. 1932;681–722.

to go largely unprotected for decades more, public pressure, imagined and real, would ensure that nuclear weapons testing and nuclear power plants got more attention from qualified professionals working both nationally and internationally in epistemic communities that set norms for the atomic age.

CHAPTER 7

War Generates Radioactive and Political Fallout, 1939–1965

The applications of radiation and radioactivity would vastly enlarge, unbeknownst to most of the world, during World War II. The United States mounted, starting in 1942, the Manhattan Project, a top-priority, secret, crash program to develop an atomic bomb. The Americans used both plutonium and enriched uranium, fissile materials that could generate a chain reaction, in addition to producing many previously unknown isotopes. The uncontrolled chain reactions generated by isotopes of uranium and plutonium manifested in August 1945 at Hiroshima and Nagasaki as the largest explosions human beings had ever created, killing between 100,000 and 200,000 people.[1] The handling of enriched uranium and especially plutonium in the building of atomic bombs posed dramatic risks not only to hundreds of scientists but also to tens of thousands of workers.[2]

[1] Wellerstein A. Counting the Dead at Hiroshima and Nagasaki [Internet]. Bulletin of the Atomic Scientists. 2020. Available from: https://thebulletin.org/2020/08/counting-the-dead-at-hiroshima-and-nagasaki/, accessed December 22, 2023.

[2] Hacker BC. The Dragon's Tail: Radiation Safety in the Manhattan Project, 1942–1946. Berkeley: University of California Press; 1987. Is the authoritative account of the role of radiation protection in the Manhattan Project.

D. Serwer, *Strengthening International Regimes*,
Palgrave Studies in International Relations,
https://doi.org/10.1007/978-3-031-53724-0_7

The Manhattan Project Worries About Lawsuits

The Manhattan Project chose to apply the pre-war tolerance dose, which the Americans increasingly termed the "maximum permissible dose," throughout the war as a yardstick for preventing harm to its workers, though at times it exposed workers to doses that exceeded the limit. Why did the builders of the atomic bomb not take the opportunity of working in secret and urgently on a top-priority weapon to cut corners and accelerate the work by ignoring norms designed for other (primarily medical) purposes? Why did the urgency of national security not take absolute precedence over radiation protection? Under what circumstances were the pre-war norms exceeded, and what were the consequences?

The short answer is that the leadership of the Manhattan Project decided to accept the established norms, both in their frequent observance and in the occasional breach, precisely because building atomic bombs was a top-priority, secret, crash program. There were no applicable legal requirements at the federal or state levels. The decision was not due to continuity in personnel. None of the radiation protection experts hired into the Manhattan Project during the war had had any direct role in the development of the pre-war tolerance dose and related norms.[3] The project's overall administrator, Army General Leslie Groves, and the scientific director of the Los Alamos laboratory where the bombs were designed and built, J. Robert Oppenheimer, could have decided to ignore the existing norms entirely and develop their own standards for radiation protection. They did not. The reasons boil down to three:

1. Protection of the Manhattan Project's workers was vital to ensuring the quickest possible manufacture, testing, and use of atomic weapons. Rapid recruitment and stable retention of staff were top priorities if the job was to get done before the Germans succeeded, the Americans thought.[4]

[3] Ibid., 27. Several of them did however work in the Manhattan Project, see Taylor L. Organization for Radiation Protection: the Operations of the ICRP and NCRP, 1928–74. Assistant Secretary for Environment, Office of Health and Environmental Research and Office of Technical Information, U.S. Department of Energy (DOE/TIC-10124), 1979, 7-001. This is an invaluable compilation of primary source documents with Taylor's commentary, on which this chapter will rely heavily.

[4] The Germans were, it was discovered at the end of the war, nowhere near producing an atomic weapon, as demonstrated in Bernstein J. Hitler's Uranium Club: the Secret

2. The secrecy required meant no one could be given any reason to sue the project or otherwise cause a public outcry. That risked revealing the project and its purpose as well as alarming thousands of vital workers, including scientists and physicians who knew about the pre-war tolerance dose as well as the radium dial painters' tragedy.
3. Resources seemed constrained to the scientists and military officers involved, but in practice the project was such a high priority that the funding required to protect employees, work quickly, and maintain secrecy was adequate. Time, not funding, was the main constraint.

Seeking to recruit a medical doctor to Los Alamos, Oppenheimer wrote early in the project: "I think it will be reassuring to people who come in that we have a doctor and a nurse or two available."[5] Radiation protection, which came to be known within the Manhattan Project and in America thereafter as "health physics" and in the U.S. military as "rad safe," grew much larger than Oppenheimer anticipated. It remained, however, focused on workers' health, not the environment, as the origin of health physics lay in industrial hygiene. That tradition strictly separated the human body and the environment, a distinction that would prove post-war an important limitation.[6]

There were crucial moments during the Manhattan Project when its leadership might have abandoned the existing norms for radiation protection entirely. Recounting them will enrich the picture of why they did not do so. The key junctures were these: (1) initiation starting in 1942 of the main project efforts in Chicago, Oak Ridge, Hanford, and Los Alamos; (2) testing of the first atomic bomb at Alamogordo, New Mexico in July 1945; (3) the post-war testing of nuclear weapons at Bikini Atoll in 1946. Throughout, the scientists and military officers who led the project were concerned primarily with demonstrating that an atomic bomb was feasible

Recordings at Farm Hall. Woodbury, New York: American Institute of Physics Press; 1996. Nor had the Japanese made significant progress.

[5] Quoted in Nolan, Jr. JL. Atomic Doctors: Conscience and Complicity at the Dawn of the Nuclear Age. Cambridge, MA: Harvard University Press; 2020:7. Nolan's book amply confirms the priority given to "medico-legal" issues in the Manhattan Project and American testing of nuclear weapons.

[6] Jessee EJ. Radiation Ecologies: Bombs, Bodies, and Environment During the Atmospheric Nuclear Weapons Testing Period, 1942–1965. Montana State University Ph.D. thesis, https://scholarworks.montana.edu/xmlui/handle/1/1561?show=full, accessed November 29, 2023.

and usable. Radiation protection was not their mission. But at each of these critical junctures they decided to devote resources and pay high-level attention to radiation protection. The main motive was to protect the enterprise from lawsuits and public outcry that might delay it. As before the war with regard to medical radiology, radiation protection served not only to protect radiation workers but also to protect an enterprise that otherwise might have slowed, faltered, or even failed.

In Chicago in December 1942, Enrico Fermi demonstrated in his "Met [allurgical] Lab" that natural uranium (which is mainly the isotope U235) could sustain a chain reaction as well as convert the scarcer isotope U238 to plutonium, which could then be separated chemically and also used to produce a chain reaction. Fermi's reactor "pile" lay on the campus of the University of Chicago, in a densely populated urban area. University of Chicago Professor Arthur Compton, who supervised the effort, needed to recruit top scientists quickly to his research group. Significant potential exposure to radiation could have resulted from the pile's radiation as well as the handling and separation of plutonium. Compton decided early that he required medical monitoring of the workers involved, because physicists knew that radiation could cause blood changes. Vigorous health monitoring was intended to enable recruitment, promote retention, and prevent public concern.[7] He and any potential recruits would have been aware of the plight of the radium dial painters. It was impossible by 1942 to avoid newspaper coverage of their diseases and deaths. Concerned about legal challenges, a group of health physicists from the Met Lab and Oak Ridge visited one of the dial-painting plants in 1944 to observe the procedures they were using and set up similar precautions at Los Alamos.[8] They would also have been aware that X-rays could cause genetic mutations. While not yet a subject of public alarm, H. J. Muller's work using X-rays to produce mutations in fruit flies—for which he won the Nobel Prize only later, in 1946—was well-known among scientists. Knowledgeable biologists thought that most mutations produce negative traits. The eugenics movement of the 1920s and 1930s had made a public issue of protecting the gene pool. In addition to these concerns, knowledge of biological effects was important to ensure the health of American troops, should an enemy acquire

[7] Hacker, note 2, 29.

[8] Nolan, note 5, 28.

and use atomic weapons or just a "dirty bomb," one that spreads radioactivity in the environment. Some Americans also contemplated this use of radioactivity as a weapon, without a nuclear explosion.[9]

Thus, it was reasonable for Compton to spend part of his budget on ensuring that workers on the Fermi pile in Chicago were not overexposed to radiation and to document the consequences for any that were. For want of better, the Met Lab adopted the 1934 tolerance dose as the yardstick.[10] The decision was a practical one. No new scientific information was produced to justify it. This yardstick prevailed also at Oak Ridge, Hanford, and Los Alamos. The enrichment work at Oak Ridge posed lesser risks, but Stafford Warren, the Manhattan Project's medical director, was headquartered there and Oak Ridge did extensive research on biological effects, which made it an important research and training center after the war.[11] Production of plutonium at Hanford and the design, fabrication, and testing of atomic weapons in New Mexico posed much greater risks to worker health, not least because plutonium was a newly discovered element first isolated in 1940. It was impossible to know what its biological effects might be. There was no applicable tolerance dose. Common sense dictated caution and the need for secrecy dictated precautions. Hanford monitored the health of its workers, but worried far less about environmental impacts beyond the confines of the secret site, except insofar as they might arouse the ire and lawsuits of ranchers and fishermen.[12] The experiments at Los Alamos required to determine how much fissile material—either enriched uranium or plutonium—was needed for (potentially explosive) "criticality" were also inherently dangerous, as they produced intense radiation. Any incident with either might have brought unwanted attention and likely delay.[13]

[9] Meyer S, Bidgood S, Potter WC. Death Dust: The Little-Known Story of U.S. and Soviet Pursuit of Radiological Weapons. International Security. 2020;45(2):51–94. https://doi.org/10.1162/isec_a_00391, accessed June 4, 2022.

[10] Hacker, note 2, 28.

[11] Morgan KZ. Education and Training [Internet]. Available from: https://www.osti.gov/opennet/servlets/purl/16108401.pdf, accessed April 20, 2022.

[12] Stacy I. Roads to Ruin on the Atomic Frontier: Environmental Decision Making at the Hanford Nuclear Reservation, 1942–1952. Environmental History. 2010 Jul 1;15(3):415–48. https://www.jstor.org/stable/25764461, accessed May 18, 2022.

[13] One such fatal incident did occur shortly after the bombing of Hiroshima and Nagasaki in August 1945 and another in May 1946. The account in Alex Wellerstein,

Legal concerns and public exposure were not the least of the Manhattan Project's worries. The overall director, General Groves, was contemptuous of his own medical officers but still no less than obsessed with the need to avoid health-related lawsuits that could compromise the project's secrecy and cause delay.[14] Oppenheimer likewise wanted "to safeguard the project against being sued by people claiming to have been damaged."[15] Concern about lawsuits and public outcry was a main motive for monitoring radiation levels in the air and soil surrounding the first atomic bomb test, Trinity, in July 1945 at Alamogordo, New Mexico. Groves' military lawyers thought extensive record-keeping would be vital to protecting the U.S. government from citizens suing for damages. The monitoring detected surprisingly high levels of radiation in a few places. To avoid a lawsuit, the U.S. government bought some cows that had visibly suffered harm, but it managed to avoid any liability for alleged harm to people by keeping the radiation levels under wraps. Only years later did the local population seek redress, without success. Some are still campaigning for recompense.

Planning for the Trinity test had raised alarm in advance among the Manhattan Project scientists concerned with health effects. Prior calculations led to warnings, in particular if it were to rain at the time of the test, which it did not. These calculations suggested significant possible radiation exposure well beyond the tolerance dose, even if one assumed that a one-time accidental dose could be many times higher than repeated exposure without causing harm. Under the veil of secrecy, the scientists' warnings were largely ignored.[16] The Army hoped that "...the measures keeping Trinity safe from prying eyes could help keep the public safe from the test and testers safe from lawsuits."[17] It also decided to permit significantly higher exposures than the tolerance dose for those gathering data immediately after the test, a precedent that the military would continue to follow. The Manhattan Project was under the presidential gun to produce

"The Demon Core and the Strange Death of Louis Slotin," *The New Yorker* (May 21, 2016) includes photographs of the (reconstructed) equipment involved in the second of these incidents. A prior criticality incident in June 1945 was not fatal.

[14] Nolan, note 5, 47.

[15] Quoted in Hacker, note 2, 106.

[16] Nolan, note 5, tells this story well, 43–7.

[17] Hacker, note 2, 84.

a successful test before the Allied Summit in Potsdam (July/August 1945) and in order to end the war in the Pacific. Under the veil of secrecy, urgency came into direct conflict with radiation protection for the Trinity test. Radiation protection lost.

The Manhattan Project's success became dramatically apparent worldwide with the bombing of Hiroshima and Nagasaki in August 1945. Unable to maintain secrecy any longer, the U.S. military moved quickly to minimize in the press the notion that radiation had caused the deaths of tens of thousands of people.[18] The military claimed the blast, not radiation or residual radioactivity, was responsible. Groves and others were anxious that the stigma of chemical and biological weapons, which had led to a ban in 1925, not be associated with atomic weapons.[19] In addition, they wanted to deploy U.S. troops to Hiroshima and Nagasaki as quickly as possible, which required minimizing the residual radiation risks. Groves ignored reports from scientists and physicians he had sent to Hiroshima and Nagasaki, lied to Congress about radiation effects and residual radiation there, and even claimed low levels of radiation might be a good way to die.[20] Five weeks after the Hiroshima bombing, he and Oppenheimer conducted a press briefing at the Trinity site denying the existence of residual radiation, but measurements showed it far higher than anticipated.[21] The public relations effort was initially but only briefly successful. The publication in August 1946 of John Hershey's New Yorker article and book *Hiroshima* gave Americans a clear description of the horrors, including radiation effects, apparent after the bombing.[22]

[18] Blume MM. Fallout: the Hiroshima Cover-Up and the Reporter Who Revealed It to the World. New York: Simon & Schuster; 2020.

[19] Brodie JF. Radiation Secrecy and Censorship after Hiroshima and Nagasaki. Journal of Social History. 2015 May 15;48(4):842–64, https://doi-org.proxy1.library.jhu.edu/10.1093/jsh/shu150 and Looking Back Helps Us Look Forward [Internet]. OPCW. Available from: https://www.opcw.org/about/history#:~:text=The%201925%20Protocol%20for%20the, accessed April 20, 2022.

[20] Nolan, note 14 and Kaplan F. A New, Chilling Secret about the Manhattan Project Has Just Been Made Public. Slate Magazine [Internet]. 2023 Aug 3 [cited 2023 Nov 14]; Available from: https://slate.com/news-and-politics/2023/08/oppenheimer-manhattan-project-radiation-atomic-bomb-declassified.html#:~:text=Finally%2C%20in%20a%20comment%20that, accessed September 3, 2023.

[21] Nolan, note 5, 101–3.

[22] Hersey J. Hiroshima [Internet]. The New Yorker. 1946. Available from: https://www.newyorker.com/magazine/1946/08/31/hiroshima, accessed September 3, 2023.

In the meanwhile, a remarkable phenomenon with long-term consequences began. Japanese medical experts began working with Americans in a Joint Commission to study radiation effects. While the Japanese physicians felt their contributions were not properly appreciated or acknowledged and the Americans were concerned about the quality of independent Japanese efforts, this quick cooperation still marks a stark contrast to the post-World War I contention between Allied and German scientists.[23] The World War I armistice left ambiguity about the war's outcome, allowing and even encouraging scientists to continue the conflict by boycott. Unconditional surrender and occupation proved a firmer basis than armistice for international scientific cooperation, even in the midst of continued mutual misunderstanding. It had taken years after World War I's more ambiguous outcome to produce far more tentative international collaboration.

Both the Japanese, to treat their own population, and the Americans, to protect their own military forces and prepare for civil defense, wanted to know the health effects subsequent to the bombing. Concern about longer-term effects of exposure led in 1946 to President Truman's approval for the formation by the U.S. National Research Council of the Atomic Bomb Casualty Commission (which in 1975 became the still operating Radiation Effects Research Foundation). Their work would produce important scientific results for decades. It was strictly limited, despite Japanese desires, to knowledge of radiation effects and excluded medical treatment of Japanese victims, to avoid the implication of American moral or legal liability.

Military requirements came into conflict with health and safety again during the Manhattan Project's last major effort, the "Crossroads" test of atomic weapons at Bikini Atoll in December 1946, just before turning over its responsibilities to the newly created civilian Atomic Energy Commission. United Nations and Congressional observers were present.[24] The Navy hoped the testing would demonstrate the survivability of its ships in nuclear warfare. It was planned with the pre-war radiation protection standards in mind, though again allowing higher

[23] On the origins and early history of the ABCC and its transformation into the RERF, see Lindee SM. American Scientists and the Survivors at Hiroshima. Chicago: University of Chicago Press; 1994.

[24] Shurcliff WA. Bombs at Bikini: The Official Report of Operation Crossroads. New York: William H. Wise, 1947;184–5.

single doses for personnel gathering data immediately after the test. The preparations aimed

> to reassure...that the safety measures adopted...were such as to attract no justifiable criticism, and to give what assurance was possible that no successful suits could be brought on account of the radiological hazards of Operation Crossroads.[25]

The first test with a bomb exploded above sea level went smoothly and yielded the desired data. But the second, conducted with a bomb exploded under the sea, did not. It contaminated the ships that had been placed nearby to determine the impact well beyond the levels that would be permissible for people to board. Radiation protection once again came into conflict with military requirements. This time, however, the tests were public and the urgency reduced. Radiation protection won. The ships were not boarded or decontaminated. A third planned test was canceled. General Groves feared "claims being instituted by men who participated in the Bikini tests."[26]

The testing and use of atomic bombs raised radiation protection to a far more public, and political, level. The issues no longer concerned only medical doctors and individual patients, or a relatively few women painting luminescent dials and uranium miners. Exposure of large numbers of people, the importance of atomic weapons to the post-war global balance of power, hopes for peaceful applications of the atom, and the involvement of government bureaucracies as well as scientists in many parts of the world beyond Europe and the United States defined a new landscape that stretched far beyond medical radiology.

The United States Takes the Initiative to Revive and Revise the Pre-war Norms

It would not have been surprising had the pre-war international radiation protection regime succumbed at this juncture. Government institutions, which in the United States and Britain now possessed large quantities of radioactive materials, might have shoved the physician radiologists and

[25] As quoted in Hacker, note 2, 119–120.

[26] Ibid., 149.

their health physicist colleagues aside and supplanted the professional organizations that generated the pre-World War II norms. Why did they not do so? The norms of the pre-war era survived and the institutions that generated them revived. What accounts for the apparent resilience of an international regime developed in a different context and for other purposes? World War II had devastated and divided Germany, arguably the leading force in the pre-war international radiation dosimetry and protection institutions. Britain and France were also devastated. America emerged unscathed at home and hegemonic abroad. The United States had invented dramatic new applications of radiation and radioactivity and caused a tremendous influx of new materials, problems, and experts with far more knowledge of the biological effects of radiation. Why did those changes not lead to a new regime and a different set of norms?

American experts took the initiative to revive pre-war national and international norm-setting institutions. Lauriston Taylor, a physicist who had initiated the National Bureau of Standards work on radiation protection before the war, returned to that role after serving in a different war-time capacity. Taylor reconvened the pre-war Advisory Committee on X-ray and Radium Protection informally in September 1946, with the intention of updating its more than decade-old recommendations, hitherto pertinent mainly to medical radiology.[27] The group quickly recognized that the war had dramatically changed the situation. Even in medical radiology, physicians were using far higher voltage X-rays as well as high energy electron accelerators (betatrons) and dozens of radioisotopes unknown before the war. Neutrons and protons were new factors, little considered in medicine previously but already recognized as biologically more "effective" (and damaging) than the X-rays, gamma rays, and alpha particles used before the war. In addition, both industry and the U.S. government were using X-rays and radioisotopes far more extensively for non-medical purposes. It was anticipated that the pre-war "tolerance dose" might need to be adjusted for different circumstances and different types of ionizing radiation. The Manhattan Project, the several branches of the armed forces, the Public Health Service, and the National Research Council were all now interested parties.

The Advisory Committee understandably decided to broaden its scope and its membership, on the assumption that doing so would encourage

[27] Taylor, note 3, 7-001.

acceptance of the committee's decisions.[28] The process and purpose were clear in this exchange between two of its pre-war physicist members at the first post-war meeting of the Advisory Committee:

> [Stanford Professor of Medicine and Biophysics Robert] Newell: Made the recommendation to broaden the base of the Committee to include any other organization having interest in the field.
>
> [Columbia Professor of Physics Gioacchino] Failla: Remarked that any such organizations would accept the decisions of the Committee if they felt that they were adequately represented on it.[29]

This was a co-optation strategy, as defined by Philip Selznick: "the process of absorbing new elements into the leadership or policy-determining structure of an organization as a means of averting threats to its stability or existence."[30] In radiation protection, the issue was reviving authority more than stability or existence. Taylor and other American participants in the pre-war institutions were determined to restore the independence and dominance over norm-setting for radiation and radioactivity that the Advisory Committee on X-ray and Radium Protection had begun to exercise within the United States. before World War II. Co-optation was not the only means available to the revived institution for regaining and maintaining authority over the norm-setting process, but it was an important one. The group would become post-war a driving force in regulation of radiation exposure not only in the United States but also internationally.

Reconstituted as the National Committee on Radiation Protection (NCRP) to reflect the broader applications of radiation beyond medical radiology, the group formed an Executive Committee as well as committees concerned with priority subjects. First priority was reconsideration of the tolerance dose (which the Americans now often dubbed the permissible external dose) as well as permissible internal doses, higher energy X-rays and electrons, heavy ionizing particles (protons and neutrons), and

[28] The re-assembly of the group by Taylor is described in detail in Whittemore, GF. The National Committee on Radiation Protection, 1928–1960: from professional guidelines to government regulation. Harvard University Ph.D. dissertation, 1986, 229–41.

[29] Ibid., 7-003a.

[30] Selznick P. Guiding Principles and Interpretation: A Summary TVA and the Grassroots. Berkeley: UC Berkeley Press; 1984.

radioactive isotopes (including both their handling and disposal). This was a far broader agenda involving many more committee and subcommittee members than would have been needed or even possible before the war. The experts came not only from the American Medical Association but also the National Electrical Manufacturers Association, the American Radium Society, and the new Atomic Energy Commission (AEC), which succeeded the Manhattan Project in January 1947. Enterprises using radiation were well-represented.

The AEC quickly followed the Manhattan Project in accepting the pre-war Advisory Committee recommendation (0.1 r/day) as its own "tolerance (maximum permissible exposure)" for its workers and in addition looked to the NCRP for a possible revision.[31] There were good medical and scientific reasons to tighten the norm. The impact on blood and blood-forming organs had already been a priority concern when the first ICRP tolerance dose was set in 1934, based on the many instances of leukemia and other blood ailments already evidenced by then.[32] There was pressure even before World War II from within the radiation protection community to cut the tolerance dose by a factor of five, as we have seen in Chapter 6. War-time animal "radiobiology" experiments, undertaken to determine the effects of whole-body radiation in war-time and means of countering them, had heightened concern in professional circles.[33] Experiments at the National Cancer Institute had demonstrated that the pre-war recommendation of 0.1 r/day

> ...produced no statistically significant changes in the peripheral blood counts of the animals, but ovarian tumors developed in many of the female mice after several years of exposure. All the other doses, which were higher

[31] Taylor, note 3, "Meeting of the Executive Committee, September 1947," 7-009–11, at 7-010 and Excerpt from AEC Isotope Branch B-1, August 1947, at 7-026.

[32] International Recommendations for X-ray and Radium Protection. British Journal of Radiology. 1934 Nov 1;7(83):695–9, Para 1 (b).

[33] Kraft A. Manhattan Transfer: Lethal Radiation, Bone Marrow Transplantation, and the Birth of Stem Cell Biology, ca. 1942–1961. Historical Studies in the Natural Sciences. 2009;39(2):171–218. https://www.jstor.org/stable/10.1525/hsns.2009.39.2.171, accessed April 22, 2023.

than 0.1 roentgen per day, produced significant effects on the blood counts and greatly increased the induction of tumors.[34]

This was too close for comfort.

In addition, the AEC wanted genetic factors considered and pushed for 1946 Nobelist H. J. Muller to be added to an NCRP subcommittee in 1947.[35] Muller and a second geneticist, Curt Stern (who like Muller had studied with T. H. Morgan at Columbia), on the committee pressed for tightening permissible doses based on the genetic effects. The AEC also rejected an initial NCRP proposal reconfirming the pre-war dose limits and convinced Canadian and British counterparts of the need to lower them.[36] Gioacchino Failla, who had before World War II successfully opposed considering mutation in setting radiation protection norms and who had prepared the proposal reconfirming the pre-war limits, now relented. The NCRP responded to the AEC before June 1948 with a recommendation to halve the daily rate but set the norm per week rather than per day, rounded up to 0.3 r/week of whole-body dosage, a time interval that corresponded to the usual monitoring on film.[37]

This quick post-war tightening of the NCRP-recommended norm was decided in the aftermath of the Crossroads test at Bikini Atoll, as Americans were belatedly recognizing, as a result of Hershey's book, that radiation had in fact caused many deaths at Hiroshima and Nagasaki. The AEC and the NCRP anticipated far wider human exposure to several additional types of ionizing radiation at far higher energy levels than had been common before the war. It would have been hard not to anticipate public concern. An AEC Board of Review in 1947 foresaw the need for "the further study of the biological effects of radiation and all forms of detection, protection and treatment, and for the protection of employees, the public if exposed, and the civilian population in case of war."[38]

[34] Jacobson LO. From Atom to Eve. Perspectives in Biology and Medicine. 1981;24(2):195–216. https://doi.org/10.1353/pbm.1981.0033, accessed August 16, 2023.

[35] Whittemore, note 28, 282–336.

[36] Ibid.

[37] Taylor, note 3, "New Permissible Dose," 7-034–7.

[38] Report of the Board of Review sent by Robert F. Loeb to AEC Chair David E. Lilienthal, June 20, 1947, in possession of the author.

By 1950, the NCRP had reached agreement not only on a permissible dose of 0.3 r/week (lowered from 0.5 r/week) but also on factors for the relative biological effectiveness of different types of radiation and specific limits for more sensitive organs in the human body, including the gonads. The AEC quickly adopted the new permissible doses for its own activities and they were circulated widely in professional circles, though the NCRP did not publish them for several more years.[39] The recommended norms were still all applicable to radiation workers, not the general public. There was no agreement within the NCRP on a genetically permissible dose to the general population, a subject that would remain controversial among the Americans and generate important professional and political consequences.

The AEC's reliance on a nongovernmental, interdisciplinary, epistemic group of experts to set norms is an example of "scientization," whereby a responsible government authority outsources a difficult and value-laden decision to an epistemic community.[40] The reasons boil down to confidence, convenience, and credibility. The NCRP had co-opted the right organizations from the AEC perspective, as Failla had suggested. Its prewar recommendations had held up well throughout the war, and it had quickly reorganized and expanded to confront post-war challenges. The AEC had inherited from the Manhattan Project 44,000 employees spread out across 13 states.[41] Use of radioactive material was also spreading quickly into the private sector, as the AEC was making radioisotopes widely available for research and industrial purposes. Perhaps most importantly: the AEC wanted uniform rules for both its own purposes and

[39] "Report of the Executive Committee, NCRP," June 23, 1948, Taylor, note 3, at 7-029. The new level was published only in Permissible Dose from External Sources of Ionizing Radiation. NCRP Report No. 17 (NBS-HB-59); 1954. https://nvlpubs.nist.gov/nistpubs/Legacy/hb/nbshandbook59.pdf, accessed April 19, 2023. See the explanation for the delay at Taylor, 7-081. Whittemore, note 28, delves more deeply into the complicated reasons for delay, 349–90.

[40] On "scientization," see Stone D. Global Governance: Depoliticized: Knowledge Networks, Scientization, and Anti-Policy. In: Anti-Politics, Depoliticization, and Governance. Oxford: Oxford Academic; 2017. https://doi-org.proxy1.library.jhu.edu/10.1093/oso/9780198748977.003.0005, accessed November 12, 2023.

[41] Hacker BC. Elements of Controversy: the Atomic Energy Commission and Radiation Safety in Nuclear Weapons testing, 1947–1974. Berkeley: University of California Press; 1994:10–11.

for others, thus circumventing the need for collective bargaining on protection issues with radiation workers.[42]

Faced with many other pending issues, the new civilian agency in charge of nuclear weapons as well as civilian applications found it convenient to off-load this potentially controversial decision about radiation protection to a credible, relatively independent organization with appropriate expertise and little competition. Keeping the norm-setting at arms' length gave at least the appearance of willingness to accept scientific conclusions about radiation protection. The AEC had representatives in the NCRP and its committees, so there could be no surprises. The Commission repeatedly asked the NCRP to address the tolerance dose, mentioning "the definite possibility...of designating [the NCRP] as the outside body to consider [the AEC's] problems of protection."[43] The NCRP however initially resisted even a semi-official designation that might put its independence in doubt, despite its interest in obtaining AEC travel funds for its experts.[44] Instead, it shared preliminary information with the AEC in order to stay on good terms and responded as quickly as it could to AEC requests for norms. There was no firewall between the two organizations, but the NCRP was concerned to maintain its independence from government and politics as well as its scientific focus and policy relevance.

The NCRP was also still hoping to sustain the informal monopoly on norm-setting that had characterized the pre-war recommendations applicable to medical radiology, when professionally validated guidelines sufficed to protect medical applications and their operators. It parried a takeover bid from the U.S. government-chartered National Research Council and initially did not favor legal adoption of its recommendations at the Federal or state level or want any official advisory role to the U.S. government. Taylor was pleased when the NCRP norms served informally as "legal guides," including in court cases, as had been the case pre-war.[45] He opposed involvement in radiation norms of the insurance industry's Underwriters' Laboratories and of the American Standards Association.

[42] Whittemore, note 28, 259–72.

[43] Taylor, note 3, "Meeting of the Executive Committee, September 1947," 7-010.

[44] Ibid., 7-010–11.

[45] Taylor, note 3, "Conversion of Recommendations to Regulations," Taylor to Dr. Warren, October 3, 1951, 7-127–9.

The NCRP declined to set stricter standards for the public than for workers in atomic facilities, claiming that its recommendations sufficed for both and fearing that labor groups and insurance companies would object to a double standard. Taylor believed this informal approach focused on radiation workers "resulted in a high degree of flexibility [for operators] and a high degree of confidence in the work of the committee." He added a claim to uniqueness via co-optation: "...the only qualified protection experts in the country are already members of this Committee."[46]. Epistemic domination, in addition to co-optation, supported authority.

That turned out to be correct, but Taylor's concept of operations for the NCRP was quickly superseded. Government regulation, both at the national and state levels, was inevitable.[47] Within a few years, the NCRP would be cooperating with the American Standards Association and the Underwriter's Laboratories as well as numerous state governments and Federal agencies in addition to the AEC. The NCRP dropped its opposition to legal regulation and tried instead to encourage uniform state regulations so as to avoid chaos within the United States.[48] It would also find itself in a storm of public controversy, focused on the effects of radiation on the general population, a subject Taylor, who supported nuclear testing, would have liked to avoid.

There was one systematic exception to the AEC's application of NCRP radiation protection standards: uranium miners. During World War II, the Manhattan Project had obtained most of its uranium from already mined tailings in the Belgian Congo, Canada, and the American West. After the war, the U.S. government became by law the sole customer for uranium and domestic sources blossomed. Starting in 1948, an AEC health and safety official documented levels of radon in Colorado mines higher than NCRP's norms. The AEC, however, decided that miners were not within its jurisdiction. Alerted to the risks, a state official leaked alarming test results to the Denver Post, but the two articles that appeared there did not light a fire. Higher up officials squelched the AEC health and safety

[46] Taylor, note 3, "Excerpts of a Letter of September 15, 1949, L. S. Taylor to W. G. Marks [U.S. Department of Labor]," 7-079–80.

[47] Taylor L. Radiation Protection Standards. London: Butterworths; 1971:43–5.

[48] Taylor, note 3, "General Communication No 29," May 20, 1954, Subcommittee No. 10, Taylor L, Chairman, 8-003–5 at 004.

official, and the media story died.[49] Informed of the need for control measures in mines by a Public Health Service (PHS) official, the acting chair of the AEC ignored the warning. He was more concerned with meeting the burgeoning demand for uranium for bomb-building.[50] The PHS kept its studies of Navajo miners' radiation-induced lung cancer in the 1950s secret.

Uranium mining, the radioactive tailings it left on the landscape, and water they contaminated are the proverbial exception that proves the general rule: public pressure is needed to generate regulatory action, even when scientific data and norms are available. That rule would be confirmed repeatedly in future decades. Only in 1967, a Washington Post expose', based in part on PHS studies, prompted Labor Secretary Willard Wirtz to order radon levels restricted to levels that would not cause "a higher risk of cancer than that faced by the general population."[51] A Federal standard (the equivalent of which is still in force) was set in 1969. Enforcement of that standard and eventual compensation came a decade and more later, after unsuccessful lawsuits, organization of support groups for miners, and Congressional testimony:

> For up to 2 decades after the harmful effects of uranium mining were known, protective safeguards were not implemented. The position of scientists in the government who were knowledgeable and who often argued for protection was seriously compromised.... Federal regulations for ventilation came nearly 20 years after the need was clear, and only when many miners were obviously sick and dying.[52]

The situation was no better on the international level. Although mining was raised as an issue within the ICRP in 1952, and radioactive material was used in construction in Sweden and elsewhere, the Commission

[49] This unfortunate tale is told in Pasternak J. Yellow Dirt: A Poisoned Land and the Betrayal of the Navajos. New York: Free Press; 2011:66–75. She documents in excruciating detail the Navajo struggle with uranium mining and its consequences.

[50] Ibid., 76.

[51] Ibid., 112.

[52] Brugge D, Goble R. The History of Uranium Mining and the Navajo People. American Journal of Public Health [Internet]. 2002;92(9):1410–9. Available from: https://www.ncbi.nlm.nih.gov/pmc/articles/PMC3222290/, accessed May 7, 2023.

first published on radiation protection in mines only in 1977.[53] No compensation schemes specifically for uranium miners exist in Europe, but after German reunification uranium miners from the East became eligible for compensation provided by the German Workers' Compensation Board.[54] In 1978, the U.S. Congress passed the Uranium Mill Tailings Radiation Control Act prohibiting use of uranium tailings in housing and construction projects. Under public pressure, especially from Navajo miners, Congress in 1990 provided a process for compensation of uranium miners as well as fallout victims living near nuclear testing sites that are still in force.[55] Compensation was upgraded in 2000.

The Hegemon Revives the International Norms as Well

At the international level in the early 1950s, the Americans were in an unavoidably hegemonic position. Because of the Manhattan Project, they knew far more about the biological effects of various radioactive isotopes, many of which were still unavailable in other countries, as well as newly relevant neutrons and protons than any European colleagues, who had led norm-setting efforts before World War II. Apart from Sweden, which remained neutral during the war, many leading European scientific establishments were still in ruins. War left American radiation-related laboratories and most scientists unscathed. Manhattan Project funding had vastly expanded some laboratories and clinics, in addition to research on biological effects at Oak Ridge, Hanford, and other newly established institutions.

Anticipating that the nuclear age would necessarily be one with international implications, the Americans looked first to their close allies and

[53] The 1952 discussion is mentioned fleetingly in Lindell B. The History of radiation, radioactivity, and Radiological protection. The Labours of Hercules, Part III (1950–66). Bo Lindell and Nordic Society for Radiation Protection. 2020;93. The 1977 ICRP report is ICRP, 1977. Radiation Protection in Uranium and Other Mines. ICRP Publication 24. Ann. ICRP 1 (1).

[54] Brugge D, Ifran A. Compensation for Uranium Miners world-wide: the Need for an Assessment and Action. The Extractive Industries and Society. 2020 April;7(2). https://doi.org/10.1016/j.exis.2019.01.011, accessed October 26, 2023.

[55] Dawson SE, Charley PH, Harrison Jr. P. Advocacy and Social Action among Navajo Uranium Workers and Their Families. In: Social Work in Health Settings: Practice in Context Second Edition. New York: The Haworth Press; 1997:391–7.

Manhattan Project partners in Canada and Great Britain, with whom they met in March 1948 at the AEC. The British had already activated a Medical Research Council Tolerance Doses Panel in 1946. The Canadians also expressed an interest in the American deliberations on what they too still termed "tolerance" levels.[56] Once the British and Americans had clarified a difference in their procedures used to measure X-ray exposures as well as the use of different units, they readily reached agreement in September 1949 at Chalk River, Canada, on norms that reflected the Americans' lowering of the maximum permissible external dose to 0.3 r/week, to specify the critical tissues most likely to be affected, and to consider dose rates more explicitly as well as lifetime exposure limits, which would be meant in part to prevent genetic effects.[57]

Taylor, who played a central role in the tripartite meetings with Canada and Britain, had been the pre-war Secretary of the International Commission on Radiological Units (ICRU) and had been asked to take on that role as well for the pre-war International Commission on X-ray and Radium Protection. In his account, it was the President of the 1937 International Congress of Radiology (the parent of both pre-war Commissions), the American physician and radiologist Arthur Christie, who prompted the reconstitution and reorganization of the two international commissions. The latter was renamed the International Commission on Radiological Protection to encompass its much-enhanced subject matter, but still maintain its link to medical radiology.[58] Medical

[56] Taylor, note 3, 7-072 and 7-205. Notably, the Canadians and British had not yet shifted to "maximum permissible limits" but continued to use nomenclature the Americans considered outmoded.

[57] These issues are reflected at length in documents available in Taylor, note 3, "Report of the United Kingdom, and United States Meeting, March 29 and 30, 1948," 7-033–4 and following as well as K. Z. Morgan's "Memorandum to the Subcommittee on Permissible Internal Dose" reporting on the same meeting, ibid., 7-082–6. The conclusions of the September 1949 meeting are in "Minutes of the Permissible Doses Conference held at Chalk River, Canada, September 29th-30th, R. M.-10, https://www.orau.org/health-physics-museum/files/library/warren1949_permissible_dose_conference_tripartite_conference.pdf, accessed December 5, 2023. Whittemore, note 28, argues that the resolution of the British/American difference in dosimetry procedures was a "tactful compromise to maintain the appearance of unanimity," 341–6.

[58] Taylor, note 3. ICRP Activities 7-205.

radiologists wanted to keep at least nominal control of radiation protection norms that affected and protected their profession, whose breadth and manpower had expanded greatly.

Taylor was willing. As most of the pre-war members of the two commissions had died, it fell to Taylor, Christie, and a British colleague (physician radiologist Ralston Paterson) to come to a consensus on ICRP membership representatives to the International Commission on Radiological Units were designated by national delegations to the International Congress of Radiology). Taylor, Christie, and Ralston Paterson decided on experts from the countries that had been represented pre-war: Sweden, England, France, Germany, Italy, and the United States. Canada was added later, in acknowledgment of its role in the Manhattan Project. This selection omitted the Soviet Union as well as the non-European world, most notably Japan. Presumably aware of this and other limitations, the Secretary of the ICRP wrote:

> The Commission's desire that the subcommittees be as widely representative as possible of the nations of the world can, I believe, be met if we think of the representation of the six committees together. I hope in this way we shall avoid any representation for political reasons.[59]

Protecting the independence of the epistemic group from political or governmental influence was still a priority. In practice, representation in the subcommittees was only marginally wider than representation on the Main Commission. Universality of representation, even from the relevant scientific world, was still far off, as we shall see.

The World War I boycott of German science was not however repeated in the aftermath of World War II. As with Japan, unconditional surrender permitted less hesitant, even if still delayed, regeneration of cooperation. Germany emerged from World War II with its scientific and medical institutions thoroughly destroyed and little research progress, including in nuclear energy. The Germans reconstituted their overall German Standardization Commission (Deutschen Normenausschuss) in 1947, but the radiological standardization committee of the German Röntgen Society was only reconstituted in 1949 and did not officially become active

59 Binks to Morgan, "International Commission on Radiological Protection," December 20, 1950, Taylor, note 3, 7-220.

until 1951.[60] Taylor in November 1949 invited German physicist Robert Jaeger, who worked at the Physical-Technical Institute as an expert on radiation measurements, to join the ICRP.[61] He had made his way into medical radiology during World War I, like other German physicists mentioned in Chapter 4.[62] Post-World War II, he had been quick to share with the Americans what he regarded as the then valid Deutsches Institut für Normung (DIN) standards for radiation.[63] Jaeger initially regarded the American-proposed tolerance dose as too high for prevention of genetic damage and thought it should be lowered by half.[64] But he yielded to the Americans he said after "polls and committee discussions" in Germany.[65]

When the ICRP met in 1950 in London for the first time after the war, the Americans were literally setting the agenda and dictating the norms. The committee structure decided was identical to the committee structure of the NCRP, with American chairs for the most important committees on permissible doses for external exposure and internal emitters. Based on a British proposal, the ICRP's first post-war recommendations corresponded to American preferences: the maximum permissible external dose was reduced to the level the Americans now preferred (0.3 r/week) and the British and Canadians had already agreed at Chalk River.[66] The

[60] Graf H. The Standardization of Radiological Technique, Its Origin and Development. Annex W, Item No. 7, in Taylor, ibid.

[61] Taylor to Dr. Jaeger, November 8, 1949, Taylor, note 3, 7-207.

[62] Robert Jaeger: Mainzer Professorenkatalog | Gutenberg Biographics [Internet]. Gutenberg Biographics, University of Mainz; Available from: http://gutenberg-biographics.ub.uni-mainz.de/personen/register/eintrag/robert-jaeger.html, accessed June 10, 2022.

[63] Jaeger to Taylor, September 13, 1949, quoted in Taylor, note 3, 7-208.

[64] Jaeger to Taylor, January 31, 1950, quoted in Taylor, note 3, 7-209.

[65] Jaeger to Taylor, June 23, 1950, quoted in Taylor, note 3, 7-210.

[66] "Proposal from the British Members," International Commission on Radiological Protection, VIth International Congress of Radiology, 1950, NP/P/64 and NP/P/TD/ in ICRP Archives, Box G042, 1950.pdf, 17–28. The Roentgen was a unit of what is now understood as exposure. The Americans sometimes preferred instead rem (roentgen equivalent man). It was intended to reflect the different biological effects of rays of different types in soft tissue: "that dose of any ionizing radiation which produces a relevant biological effect equal to that produced by one roentgen of high-voltage x-radiation." It is numerically equivalent to approximately .9 roentgen, which for our purposes is equivalent. To add to the confusion, the Americans also use a "rep" (roentgen equivalent physical). It originally represented an energy absorption dose in irradiated tissue of

Swedish and German representatives, who thought the norm should have been cut even further (to 0.1 r/week), lost that battle.[67] The reduction of the ICRP's pre-war recommendation, along with a recommendation that all types of ionizing radiation exposure be at the "lowest possible level," was justified on the same grounds the Americans had used: higher energy X-rays made for greater uncertainties about biological effects, especially in the blood-forming organs.[68] The Commission admitted it was not in a position to recommend maximum permissible limits for internal doses of radioactive substances and instead made reference to limits in use in the United States, Canada, and Britain.[69]

Why did the Americans bother with the international commission when they already had settled on what they wanted within the United States? The Cold War nuclear arms race heated up with a Soviet atomic bomb test in 1949. Expectations for peaceful applications of atomic energy were high. It was hoped that "the atom" would not only protect American and British national security from the Soviets but also provide vast quantities of cheap electricity in addition to expanding the medical and industrial uses of X-rays and radioactive isotopes. Medical radiologists, radiation-equipment manufacturers, nuclear energy companies, and the bomb-manufacturing and testing AEC were all represented in the NCRP and its committees. If their enterprises were to find public acceptance and continue to grow and prosper, they needed to protect at least their workers from harm and thereby avoid protest and dissension. International norms consistent with the NCRP's would reinforce their

93 ergs. See Parker HM. Tentative Dose Units for Mixed Radiations. Radiology. 1950 Feb 1;54(2):257. https://pubs.rsna.org/doi/epdf/10.1148/54.2.257, accessed August 22, 2022. Other units introduced later include the rad (absorbed dose in joules per kilogram), grays (joules of absorbed energy per kilogram = 100 rad), and sieverts (effective dose of absorbed radiation = 100 rems).

[67] Hercules, notes 53, 87. Lindell says that Rolf Sievert was already applying .1 r in Sweden, but the conversation he transcribed on this subject at 20 does not explicitly support that figure.

[68] This was discussed among knowledgeable experts in Stockholm in 1951, ibid., 20.

[69] International Recommendations on Radiological Protection: Revised by the International Commission on Radiological Protection at the Sixth International Congress of Radiology, London, July 1950. Annals of the ICRP/ICRP Publication. 1959 Jan;OS_1(1):1–8. July 17, 2022. The U.S., Canadian, and British norms had been discussed and decided in a tripartite "Permissible Doses Conference" at Buckland House, August 4–6, 1950, sponsored by the Medical Research Council Radiobiological Research Unit.

acceptance within the United States and strengthen the Committee's hand in a rapidly changing environment. Radiation protection experts did what the physicists and physician-specialists had done after World War I: they strengthened their own position nationally by means of an international epistemic group. That group sought not only to protect workers but also to protect beneficial enterprises from public concern and the prospect of more onerous regulation.

Taylor later wrote proudly that by the time of the first United Nations Atoms for Peace Conference in 1955 "all of the countries in the world were using the same basic radiation protection standards that had been recently recommended by the ICRP."[70] That may have been true for the most part in those countries using radiation and radioactivity, but with one important exception: the United States. The ICRP, as we shall see, recommended in 1953 a maximum permissible dose one-tenth the occupational level for prolonged exposure of the general population, in response to concerns about the genetic effects of fallout.[71] With its AEC compatriots testing atomic weapons in the atmosphere, the NCRP waffled about setting a limit for the general population for several years more. Only when public protest and the threat of losing its authority loomed did the NCRP bow to what others had already concluded was necessary. This would not be the last example of American exceptionalism to international radiation protection norms as American hegemony waned. The story of how the International Commission took the lead and the National Committee was pressured to catch up provides interesting lessons in the authority of international norms. The key factors were institutional competition and public concern, spurred by fallout from bomb testing and the genetic effects of radiation.

Bomb Testing Arouses the Japanese Public

The public controversies of the next decades would come in three waves, as recounted in Barton Hacker's admirably detailed and dispassionate, Department of Energy-sponsored account: radiostrontium in the 1950s,

[70] Taylor, note 40, at 46.

[71] Recommendations of the International Commission on Radiological Protection: Revised December 1954. Annals of the ICRP/ICRP Publication. 1959 Jan;OS_1(1):iii–x. https://journals.sagepub.com/doi/pdf/10.1016/S0074-27402880014-6, accessed July 17, 2022.

radioiodine in the 1960s, and American soldiers starting in the 1970s and 1980s, though the exposures had taken place in the 1950s.[72] This last controversy persisted into the 1990s, when a presidentially appointed Advisory Committee on Human Radiation Experiments reported that 2000–3000 service personnel were used as research subjects during bomb testing, only some of whom were asked to consent, as required by a 1953 "Nuremberg Code" memorandum from the Secretary of Defense. The experiments were conducted to determine the troops' psychological and physiological reaction to bomb blasts, not biological effects. Properly protected for the most part from acute radiation harm by the standards of the time, some may still have suffered longer-term effects.[73] The record for civilians was far worse. The AEC sponsored potentially harmful biological effects research on hospital patients and mentally retarded children for which informed consent was required, but absent public awareness the requirement was often ignored in the clinics conducting the studies.[74]

The first and second of the controversies were the more politically and internationally potent at the time. They occurred in reaction to the atmospheric testing of nuclear weapons in the 1950s, when the United States, Great Britain, and the Soviet Union were all testing thermonuclear weapons (hydrogen "super" bombs whose main blast was due to fusion rather than "atomic" bombs based only on fission). They did this above ground but away from their main population centers. The Americans chose to test in the Pacific, moving hundreds of people from test locations in the Marshall Islands to far less amenable areas, and in then still sparsely populated Nevada. The British tested at remote locations

[72] Hacker, note 41, 6–9.

[73] Advisory Committee on Human Radiation Experiments Final Report [Internet]. ehss.energy.gov. Washington, DC: Superintendent of Documents, 1995. Available from: https://ehss.energy.gov/ohre/roadmap/achre/report.html, accessed April 28, 2020. Rosenberg H. Atomic Soldiers. Boston: Beacon Press; 1980. Was one of the publications that raised the alarm.

[74] Ibid. and J. Samuel Walker. Permissible Dose: A History of Radiation Protection in the 20th Century. University of California Press; 2000:16. See also Human Radiation Experiments—Nuclear Museum [Internet]. Atomic Heritage Foundation Nuclear Museum. Available from: https://ahf.nuclearmuseum.org/ahf/history/human-radiation-experiments/, accessed September 21, 2023; and Creager A. Life Atomic: A History of Radioisotopes in Science and Medicine. Chicago: University of Chicago Press; 2013.

near and in Australia, without regard for the nearby indigenous population. The Soviet Union tested in Kazakhstan, where it moved thousands out of the way, and in the Arctic. Remote testing, it was thought, would help maintain operational secrecy and security as well as prevent major fallout problems in the general population.

What the U.S. military termed "rad safe" (radiation protection) continued in the 1940s to be based on the pre-war tolerance dose, with allowance for higher exposures during limited periods for urgent missions.[75] The focus of protection was the people gathering data after the tests at and near the test site. They were thought to be the people most at risk. Post-test data collection during Operation Sandstone in 1948 had exposed four workers to levels of radiation beyond the tolerance dose, but that incident was kept secret and hence not regarded as a major issue. Thereafter, the AEC allowed larger cumulative exposure (3 r) over a period of three months for people working on and monitoring the tests.[76] No labor protests ensued. Environmental testing for radioactivity beyond the immediate environs of the test sites focused primarily on gathering information useful for intelligence purposes, especially developing techniques to assess others' nuclear weapons tests, as well as predicting the possible impacts of nuclear war.

The bomb testers worried about acute effects to the general public, because they might prompt protests or lawsuits, but not about low-level radiation exposure or accumulation of radioactivity in the environment, a problem that was already well-known among experts trying to deal with the increasing quantities of radioactive waste.[77] At the same time, they were sensitive to public opinion. In preparation for the Ranger bomb tests in Nevada in 1951, discussion focused on radiation protection

> ...in order to make the atom routine in the continental United States and make the public feel at home with atomic blasts and radiation

[75] Hacker, note 41, 20.

[76] Ibid., 38 and 65–69.

[77] Parker to Morgan, "The Maximum Permissible Concentration of General Radioactive Contaminants Beyond the Area of Control," April 5, 1949, Taylor, note 3, 7-066–7. Environmental radiation levels remain an issue in the Marshall Islands: Hughes IN, Rapaport H. The U.S. Must Take Responsibility for Nuclear Fallout in the Marshall Islands [Internet]. Scientific American. 2022. Available from: https://www.scientificamerican.com/article/the-u-s-must-take-responsibility-for-nuclear-fallout-in-the-marshall-islands/#:~:text=Between%201946%20and%201958%2C%20the, accessed May 3, 2022.

> hazards….It appeared that the idea of making the public feel at home with neutrons trotting around is the most important angle to get across….It was agreed that adequate knowledge, if not control, of the radiological hazards involved should certainly be had before, during and after any shot. This means extensive monitoring activity.[78]

The public relations efforts were initially successful. By today's standards, the exposures permitted in the early 1950s were far too high, but the AEC norms were consistent with contemporaneous NCRP recommendations and initially aroused little concern either among people working on and monitoring bomb tests or among the general public.

As testing proceeded in a headlong arms race with the Soviets, the U.S. Defense Department was emboldened. Under the cloak of secrecy, pilots of Air Force planes monitoring post-test mushroom clouds and soldiers conducting maneuvers near test sites in Nevada were allowed higher exposures, and even those norms were sometimes exceeded. Again, no protests ensued. Sheep proved the bigger problem at the time, as the deaths of animals grazing near the Nevada test site aroused public rancher protest and eventually a failed lawsuit. This prompted some at the AEC to think about the difference between exposing workers at the test site and members of the general public, who had neither knowledge about nor any direct benefit from the bomb tests. One official suggested that the public merited more information about radiation risks, warnings about specific hazards, detailed reports after the fact, and reimbursement for losses.[79] But the AEC leadership insisted that radiation damage was not the cause of the sheep deaths, shrugged off rancher and political concern, and approved continued use of the Nevada Proving Ground.[80] Impact beyond the test site was still a public relations issue, not a radiation protection requirement. Without wider public protest, the AEC could continue to test without adjusting its procedures.

That began to change after the largest American thermonuclear test (Castle Bravo) at the Bikini Atoll in 1954. Post-detonation radiation levels near the test site and beyond were much higher than anticipated, prompting evacuation of both American test personnel and Marshall

[78] Hacker, note 41, 43.

[79] Ibid., p. 121.

[80] The deception was later revealed in court, see Scientists Implicated in Atom Test Deception. Science. 1982 Nov 5;218:545–7.

Islanders but minimal public acknowledgment by the AEC. Acting in secret, the Commission allowed some Castle test personnel higher exposures than originally permitted, which were already higher than the permissible doses the ICRP and NCRP recommended. Secrecy without urgency allowed those involved in the enterprise to avoid accountability.

It was the public and unanticipated international impact of the Castle Bravo test that foretold the political controversy to come.[81] The crew of a Japanese tuna fishing boat exposed to radioactive fallout from the test, unbeknownst to the Americans, was taken ill and one crewmember died months later (though the precise role of radiation in his death is not known). The exposed fish had already been sold before the public became aware of the situation. Once word got out, fish prices cratered. The Japanese public reaction was understandably swift and strong. At about the same time, Japanese scientists discovered radioactivity above background levels in rainwater and in agricultural produce. By the end of 1954, one-fourth of Japan's population had signed a ban-the-bomb petition. American officials feared the spread of anti-bomb sentiment to the U.S. Scientists in both the United States and Japan pointed to the NCRP's guidelines and the maximum permissible dose to quiet the furor. The U.S. government also made a small payment to the fisherman's widow and a $2 million ex gratia payment to the Japanese government, most of which got passed on to the fishing industry. Bomb testing in the Marshall Islands and Nevada continued. Once again, norms contributed to protecting an activity involving radiation, not only the people exposed to radiation.

The U.S. government continued to regard atmospheric testing of nuclear weapons as vital to staying ahead in the arms race with the Soviet Union. Rising Cold War anti-communist fervor supported continued testing. While the U.S. nuclear energy industry was not taking off as quickly as its proponents wanted, its proponents were determined to speed it up. The Congressional Joint Committee on Atomic Energy held five days of hearings in May 1956 on "Accelerating [the] Civilian Reactor Program."[82] Professionals concerned with radiation protection in the

[81] This story is recounted in more detail in Higuchi T. Political Fallout. Stanford University Press; 2020:77, and in Hacker, note 41, 148–58.

[82] Accelerating Civilian Reactor Program: Hearings before the United States Joint Committee on Atomic Energy, Eighty-Fourth Congress, second session, on May 23–25, 28, 29, 1956. Washington: U.S. G.P.O., 1956, [Internet]. HathiTrust. [cited

1950s thus faced strong governmental and nongovernmental pressures committed to atmospheric testing of nuclear weapons as well as use of nuclear power to generate electricity, in addition to medical radiologists who sometimes objected to what they regarded as excessive protection measures.

Mutation Takes the Limelight

Both political forces outside science and specialists within the scientific community drove the debate in the opposite direction. The specialty in question was genetics. American and British geneticists—though differing on how much long-term exposure might cause genetic harm—began to speak out publicly in the early 1950s about the risks of exposure to fallout. Taylor initially responded by trying to dilute the geneticists' influence in the key committee of the ICRP by adding physician radiologists.[83] But Muller's 1946 Nobel Prize had amplified his own voice, which was no longer alone. British biologist and geneticist J. B. S. Haldane took up the cudgels in Britain, quarreling in 1950 with radiation geneticist David Guthrie Catcheside, who was a member of the Tolerance Doses Panel of the Medical Research Council.[84]

Muller attended a Conference on Radiobiology and Radiation Protection in Sweden in September 1952 organized by the Swedish physicist Rolf Sievert, during which the ICRP also held a somewhat informal meeting, with only five members present (plus the Commission's Secretary).[85] Determining a permissible dose for genetic effects was a major

2023 Apr 30]. Available from: https://babel.hathitrust.org/cgi/pt?id=umn.31951d02097618f&view=1up&seq=3.

[83] Taylor wrote to the Secretary of the ICRP: "On the external dose committee that there was a little over-weight on the genetics side. This could be somewhat countered by putting on Dr. R. S. Stone and your Dr. Ellis as radiologists," see "Taylor to Binks," February 15, 1951, note 3, 7-223.

[84] J.B.S. Haldane to L. H. Gray, Medical Research Council Research Committee on the Medical and Biological Applications of Nuclear Physics, Tolerance Doses Panel of the Protection Sub-Committee, July 7, 1950, NP/P/TD/151. Haldane's protest led to the appointment of a panel of geneticists (Tolerance Doses Panel meeting July 13, 1950 reported in NP/PTD/152) and eventually to British support for a far tighter genetic dose limit than Catcheside had suggested. Copies of documents in the possession of the author.

[85] Taylor, note 3 above, 7-228–45. See also Hercules, note 53, 91–4. The meeting was originally intended to convene the ICRP, the ICRU, and the Mixed Commission on

focus of the conference. Muller argued on an ethical and cost/benefit basis to minimize exposure in general and for a permissible dose to the general public over a "reproductive lifetime" of 30 years, albeit one considerably higher (an average of 20 r) than ICRP Scientific Secretary Walter Binks advocated (3 r).[86] While primarily concerned with medical irradiation, Muller noted pointedly that

> ...a few of those in prominent positions connected with the development of atomic energy, and more in radiological practice, are promoting a policy of minimizing and casting doubt on the genetic damage produced by radiation, even though at the atomic energy installations themselves great care is used to protect the personnel. As a result, some editors of important American magazines refuse to publish discussions of the subject.[87]

Radiobiology of the International Council of Scientific Unions, but not all their respective participants were able to attend.

[86] Binks' proposal was on behalf of the British members, who thought .1 r per year (for 30 years) might increase the spontaneous mutation rate by 10 percent and was realizable "without any serious practical or economic difficulties," see Medical Research Council Committee on Protection against Ionising Radiations Report on The Conference on Radiobiology and Radiation Protection, held in Stockholm, 15th–20th September, 1952, PIRC/18, ICRP Archives, Archive Files 66–75, Archive Files 69, 1952 Radio Conference A.pdf, 55–60 at 56. Sievert, the Swedish ICRP Chair, thought 3 r too tight for his country because of the use there of concrete that contained radioactive shale, ibid. He preferred 5 r.

[87] Muller HJ. The Manner of Dependence of the "Permissible Dose" of Radiation on the Amount of Genetic Damage. Acta Radiologica. 1954;41(1):5–20, accessed August 24, 2022. When he later realized that his number was on the high side, Muller claimed: "I was afraid of so antagonizing those dealing with radiation in practice, by proposing a dose too low to be at all acceptable to them, that they would, in rejection, tend to continue in their almost complete disregard of the genetic damage," H. J. Muller, "The Permissible Dose in Light of Recent Developments," ICRP Archives, Box W-18, Archive Files 30, Munich 1959 re Genetic Somatic Rad. Effects.pdf, 43–48, at 43. The British and Americans, meeting with the Canadians in early 1953, were still perplexed what to do about genetic effects, see "Minutes of Tripartite Conference on Permissible Doses," March 30, 31 and April 1, 1953, ICRP Archives, Box 1163, Trip Conference 1953A.pdf, 5–41, at 11.

Taylor and K. Z. Morgan, an American health physicist from Oak Ridge National Laboratory and member of the ICRP, opposed setting a genetically permissible dose.[88] So too did the Associate Director of the AEC's Argonne National Laboratory Radiological Physics Division:

> The argument that both the cumulative genetic effects of radiation and the irreversibility of mutation dictate an immediate restriction on present day levels before adequate knowledge is available, appears to be unjustified. My preference would be to devote the cost entailed in such procedure to the acquisition of knowledge necessary to make a much wiser decision later.[89]

Researchers have an interest in doing more research. Muller had not yet convinced his American colleagues, each of whom had reasons to be friendly to the AEC. More than specialist expertise would be required to generate norms to prevent genetic effects.

The "informal" meeting of the ICRP on this occasion reconfirmed the then existing ICRP occupational norm of 0.3 r/week exposure of the blood-forming organs. But the five members present also concluded that even though then current radiation levels (above background) did not "constitute a significant genetic hazard," when exposure of large populations was in question "a considerable factor of safety" should be applied.[90] The ICRP also asked its committee chairs "to add industrial representation to their respective subcommittees. Those so invited to serve

[88] Binks prepared a summary of the conference for the ICRP, see Taylor, note 3 above 7-233–38, at 235. Bo Lindell also gives a first-hand account, Hercules, note 53, 89–94. The original of the Binks report is ICRP, "Report of the Conference on Radiobiology and Radiation Protection held in Stockholm, 15th–20th September, 1952 (Prepared by the Secretary of I.C.R,P. for the information of Members of the Commission and Chairmen of the International Sub-Committees)," ICRP/52/3, ICRP Archives, G051, Basic Anatomical and Physiological Data 1994.pdf, 430–5.

[89] Leonidas D. Marinelli to Sievert, July 14, 1952, ICRP Archives, Archive Files 66–75, Conf-Radiobiology and rad. protection in Stockholm 1952 B.pdf, 84–85.

[90] Ibid. The two questions posed to the Conference were these: (1) What doses per year and per capita of the population are, according to our present knowledge, permissible from a genetic point of view? (2) What radiation doses, under different conditions cause significant blood changes? Frank Ellis of the United Oxford Hospitals thought the genetic and blood changes might be interrelated, see Ellis to Sievert, September 8, 1952, ICRP Archives, Archive Files 66–75, Archive File 73, Conf-Radiobiology and rad. protection in Stockholm 1952 B.pdf, 73–5. Many responses from other recipients are in the same place.

should be persons actually engaged in industrial radiological work."[91] The Commission was prepared to tighten the dose limit for the general population but remained intent on ensuring that protection measures did not unjustifiably inhibit the applications of ionizing radiation.

The ICRP met again in Copenhagen in July 1953, still basing its deliberations and its recommendations mainly on reports of the NCRP.[92] But it adopted, over Taylor's objections but in the spirit of the Stockholm discussions the year before, a recommendation to limit non-occupational exposure to one-tenth the occupational level (the considerable factor of safety).[93] The NCRP did not follow suit. It remained out of sync with the ICRP for the next several years on both exposure of the general population and the unrelated (and less important) issue of the usefulness of blood counts for assessing occupational radiation exposure. This flexibility at the national level was a feature of the ICRP, not a glitch. National decisions remained the purview of national institutions. Allowing "local content" can be good for eventual adoption of international norms, especially in combination with a transnational epistemic community.[94] The Americans were not prepared to bolt from the ICRP entirely, as it was largely their own creature and generally served their interests well. Ultimately, they would have to either convince the ICRP it was wrong or bend to its norms. On blood counts they eventually did the former, but on the more important issue of exposure of the general population they did the latter. This would not be the last time American exceptionalism would appear as American hegemony receded.

[91] International Commission on Radiological Protection, "Meeting on 18th September 1952, in Uppsala, of Members of the Commission, attending the Stockholm Radiological Conference," ICRP Archives, Archive Files 46–54, Archive File 52, 7–8. There was a previous meeting the same day in Stockholm, see "International Commission on Radiological Protection, ICRP 52/1, ibid., 111–16.

[92] Sievert to Failla, June 10, 1953, ICRP Archives, Archive Files 46–52, Archive File 52, 1950–53.pdf, 2: "If your subcommittee should find it suitable to recommend 'the national report' to be used for the purpose of the international committee I should have no objection."

[93] Recommendations of the International Commission on Radiological Protection (Revised December 1, 1954). British Journal of Radiology. Supplement No. 6:10.

[94] See the case studies in Crowley-Vigneau A. The National Implementation of International Norms. Palgrave MacMillian; 2022. She attributes implementation to "transnational experience and expertise networks" (TEENs) who help with local adaptation of international norms. It is not clear to me how TEENs differ from an epistemic community.

Pressure on the Americans to conform on exposure of the general population came largely from within the United States. The NCRP kept genetic effects under study but decided not to publish ICRP reports in the United States until the differences were resolved.[95] But prominent American geneticists turned up the heat. CalTech professor Alfred Sturtevant, who like Muller and Curt Stern had studied under and worked with Thomas Hunt Morgan, aimed his presidential address to the American Association for the Advancement of Science in 1954 squarely at the AEC for its willingness to accept small increases in radiation exposure relative to the natural background. Sturtevant argued, as Muller had in Stockholm, that genetic effects were cumulative through generations and without a threshold.[96] This meant the harm to a large population might only be manifest many years in the future. The AEC was ignoring the possibility of long-term genetic effects of ionizing radiation, even if the studies of Japanese survivors of the bombings at Hiroshima and Nagasaki and their offspring were up to this point less than definitive.[97]

On the suggestion of the publisher of the New York Times, this elite but public clash with the AEC prompted the Rockefeller Foundation to fund a study on the "Biological Effects of Atomic Radiation" (BEAR) by the U.S. National Academy of Sciences.[98] Muller and Sturtevant both participated, along with AEC officials. The British Medical Research Council (MRC) undertook a comparable effort, in response to public concern and parliamentary inquiries.[99] In September 1955, the United Nations General Assembly created an intergovernmental Scientific

[95] Taylor, note 3 above, "Report on Meeting, Executive Committee, NCRP," December 5, 1954, 8-012–4 at 8-013.

[96] Sturtevant AH. Social Implications of the Genetics of Man. Science. 1954 Sep 10;120(3115):405–7. https://www.science.org/doi/abs/10.1126/science.120.3115.405, accessed July 8, 2022. And a lower one for others.

[97] Lindee, note 23, provides a deep dive into genetics research and results from the ABCC.

[98] National Academy of Sciences (U.S.), and National Research Council (U.S.). Biological Effects of Atomic Radiation, a Report to the Public from a Study by the National Academy of Sciences. Washington, D.C.: National Academy of Sciences—National Research Council; 1956.

[99] Medical Research Council. The Hazards to Man of Nuclear and Allied Radiations [Internet]. 1956 Jun. Available from: https://cipi.com/PDF/MedicalResearchCouncil1956HazardsToMan.pdf, accessed May 26, 2023.

Committee on the Effects of Atomic Radiation (UNSCEAR), "purportedly with the intention to deflect a proposal calling for an immediate end to all nuclear explosions."[100] The Americans and British intended it to deflect Swedish and Indian proposals they thought were anti-nuclear.[101]

While avowedly independent of each other, the American and British studies were in fact coordinated and eventually published on the same day in June 1956, not by accident.[102] The bottom line on genetic effects was ambiguous. As the AEC wanted, both reports suggested that bomb tests had not yet caused serious harm because the doses were still low compared to natural background radiation (between 0.02 and 0.04%). But the reports also underlined the long-term risk of genetic effects, as the geneticists advocated. In addition, the American study recommended tightening the long-term limits on exposure of workers and the general population due to genetic concerns, including a limit of 10 r for the "average exposure of the population's reproductive cells to radiation above natural background…from conception to 30 years." The new American suggestions were phrased as "operational guides" rather than maximum permissible limits "to forestall public concerns about slight overexposures."[103] The British report was more circumspect and looked to the ICRP to reconsider exposure of the whole population while suggesting it should not be allowed to exceed twice the natural background.[104]

[100] UNSCEAR. Historical Milestones [Internet]. United Nations: Scientific Committee on the Effects of Atomic Radiation. Available from: https://www.unscear.org/unscear/en/about-us/historical-milestones.html#:~:text=1955%3A%20The%20UNSCEAR%20established&text=Subsequently%20on%203%20December%201955, accessed October 15, 2023.

[101] Boudia S. Global Regulation: Controlling and Accepting Radioactivity Risks. History and Technology. 2007 Dec;23(4):389–406.

[102] Hamblin JD. "A Dispassionate and Objective Effort:" Negotiating the First Study on the Biological Effects of Atomic Radiation. Journal of the History of Biology. 2006 Jul 19;40(1):147–77, accessed July 8, 2022. Hamblin presents a thorough discussion of the coordination between the two reports and the geneticists' role, but he fails to note the normative conclusion in the American report, which would prove important.

[103] Hacker, note 41, 186.

[104] The Hazards to Man of Nuclear and Allied Radiations. Presented by the Lord President of the Council to Parliament: Her Majesty's Stationery Office; 1956 Jun para 355. https://cipi.com/PDF/MedicalResearchCouncil1956HazardsToMan.pdf, accessed July 9, 2022.

NCRP members had participated in the National Academy of Sciences study but did not control its outcome. The recommendation of an exposure limit for the general population was unwelcome but also not a surprise. Taylor had already anticipated a possible recommendation of a ten-fold lowering of the maximum permissible dose in January 1956 and thought it might be applied to radiation workers as well as the general population.[105] But the BEAR report threatened the NCRP's position as the unique, authoritative source of radiation protection recommendations inside the United States. Once the results of the study were known to its members who participated in it, the NCRP hastened to reassert its dominance by reconsidering the question of dose limits for genetic purposes both for radiation workers and for the general population. As Taylor put it, "the NCRP should make a decision on this question to maintain its leadership."[106] The BEAR public challenge to the NCRP's domination of the norm-setting process as well as the possible pending challenge from UNSCEAR were good reasons to reevaluate.

The NCRP had spent much of the previous five years debating the issue of protection from genetic effects, not to mention that it had already arisen in 1940. It would spend the better part of two more years figuring out how to adjust NCRP maximum permissible limits without changing its previous recommendations for maximum permissible doses to workers. But with public concern rising and the risk of competition from the National Academy of Sciences looming, they did adjust their recommendations, albeit in a different format from the NAS study. By the end of 1956, the NCRP had decided on tightened limits for long-term occupational exposures and exposures of the general population, based on genetic effects. It duly informed the AEC and issued a public statement.[107] The new limits included a "population gonadal dose" of 14 million man-rems per million Americans from conception to age 30 and half that amount thereafter. This obscure formulation was intended "to

[105] Taylor to the NCRP Executive Committee, January 20, 1956, Taylor, note 3, 8-037–8.

[106] "Extensive Notes, Meeting of the Executive Committee, NCRP," New York, N.Y., September 19, 1956, Taylor, note 3 above, 8-067–72, at 8-071.

[107] "Maximum Permissible Levels of Exposure to Man: A Preliminary Statement of the National Committee on Radiation Protection and Measurement," December 6, 1956, Taylor, note 3, 8-061–63. The NCRP had added measurements to its name but not to its acronym earlier that year.

draw attention away from the individual and to emphasize the statistical nature of the problem."[108] The NCRP did not however publish its final version, after much further discussion and revision, until August 1958.[109] It was at pains to emphasize that "the changes...are not the result of positive evidence of damage...but rather are based on the desire to...accord with the trends of scientific opinion."[110] The epistemic group wanted to be seen as responding to what we might term today "the science" rather than public concerns, which were rife in the midst of still frequent atomic weapons tests.

Less committed to allowing the AEC's bomb tests to continue than the NCRP and more subject to geneticists' influence, the ICRP hastened faster to pre-empt the NAS BEAR report as well as UNSCEAR, with some support from Americans involved in the less alacritous NCRP. Concerned that it would be "unwise to allow some other body to make such an important recommendation before the ICRP," two subcommittees of the ICRP in April 1956 considered a proposal to reduce the permissible dose for radiation workers by a factor of 3, to 5 rems per year, for the purpose of protecting genetic material, based on Muller's work.[111] Failla as chair made the motive clear:

> The alternative would be to leave things as they were. But there was then the possibility that other bodies [BEAR or UNSCEAR] might make recommendations on this point to the Commission: the Sub-Committees should take the initiative and not follow their [other] bodies.[112]

Morgan also worried that if the subcommittees did not act "some other body might do it for them." Taylor then warned explicitly that

[108] "NCRP Communication 35," December 14, 1956, Taylor, note 3, 8-060.

[109] "Maximum Permissible Radiation Exposures to Man," Taylor, note 3, 8-150–55. It was distributed first to scientific journals on April 15, 1958, but published four months later.

[110] Ibid.

[111] "Joint meeting of Sub-committees I and II of the ICRP on Friday, April 6, 1956," Taylor, note 3, 8-300–2, at 300. The existing norm of .3 roentgens per week was more or less the equivalent of 15 rems per year. The longer time period allowed for more day-to-day flexibility in meeting the norm.

[112] Ibid., at 8-301.

UNSCEAR might encroach, as it "was heavily weighted with geneticists."[113] Sievert's protégé, Bo Lindell, later said that the motive for acting quickly was to pre-empt not UNSCEAR but the BEAR report, which was expected to propose an annual limit of 5 rem per year for occupational exposure:

> This expectation worried ICRP members. It would not do for a national organisation to propose a lower dose limit before ICRP did. Sievert and others had also maintained that an annual dose limit of 5 rem...would be a consistent follow-up to Hermann Muller's proposal from the Stockholm meeting in 1952.[114]

The perceived encroachment threats from professionally competent organizations led the ICRP to adopt a statement in April 1956, even before the NAS report was published, suggesting that, in anticipation of the impending expansion of nuclear energy projects, doses to the general population not be allowed to rise above the level of natural background radiation, a notion that accorded with the British view:

> Until general agreement is reached, it is prudent to limit the dose of radiation received by gametes from all sources additional to the natural background to an amount of the order of the natural background in presently inhabited regions of the earth.[115]

This implied, American geneticist and ICRP member Curt Stern argued, no more than 4.3 r over 30 years, significantly less than the 10 r the BEAR study eventually recommended and far less than the 750 rems that a worker who received the then ICRP-recommended maximum permissible dose of 0.3 rem per week would accumulate in a 50-year career.[116]

Lauriston Taylor still opposed setting a dose limit for the general population, because he did not want to be "stampeded" by the geneticists.[117]

[113] Ibid.

[114] Hercules, note 53, p. 185.

[115] Report on the Amendments during 1956 to the Recommendations of the International Commission on Radiation Protection (ICRP). Radiation Research. 1958 Jun;8(6):539–42.

[116] Stern to Failla, August 21, 1956, Taylor, note 3, 8-055.

[117] Note 112, at 8-302.

In reporting on the April 1956 meetings, Taylor attributed the decision to recommend keeping public exposure to the level of natural background to "public clamor":

> There is an enormous amount of public pressure with regard to radiation exposure and I almost have the feeling that this limitation...may be regarded in some measure as slightly political.[118]

Political was not a nice word in Taylor's lexicon. It implied to him lack of independence and scientific integrity. Today his own relationship to the AEC might arouse similar doubts. But on genetic effects, Taylor was increasingly isolated. Failla—who had before World War II opposed a lowered limit to protect against genetic effects—differed. Now he thought radiation effects on the whole population needed to be considered, since "the genetic question was of worldwide interest."[119] Failla wrote to the incoming and outgoing Chairmen of the ICRP in August 1956:

> I regard it as very important for the future of the Commission to take the lead in such matters rather than be compelled to accept similar changes by the force of events later on. It is only in this way that we can command the respect of those concerned with radiation from an occupational point of view and a national or international point of view.[120]

In September 1956 he was even more explicit about the motivation, saying he

118 "Report on Meetings of the International Commission on Radiological Protection" (Transcription of tape recording of talk given to the Atomic and Radiation Physics Division staff by L. S. Taylor on June 1, 1956. This is an unedited discussion and is not for publication), Geneva, Switzerland, 1956, ICRP Archives, Box 040, Various 1954–59 A.pdf, 100–112.

119 "Minutes of the Plenary Session of the Commission and the Committees," April 9, 1956, Taylor, note 3, 8-306–14, at 8-306.

120 G. Failla to Sir Ernest Rock Carling and R.M. Sievert, August 10, 1956, ICRP Archives, Box W-18, Archive files 28, "ICRP Korrespondenz 1956.pdf, 131–2.

> ...knew of the NAS Genetics Committee recommendation and felt the International Commission should take steps in the same direction, thereby not losing stature by following instead of leading.[121]

Professional encroachment and public clamor were powerful motives, even though hard data on genetic effects were still lacking. Some worried that the cancerogenic effects like leukemia might in fact be due to mutations in the blood-forming organs.[122]

The ICRP, represented by Taylor, reported in August 1956 to the International Congress of Radiology in Mexico City that the average yearly occupational dose actually received of 5 rems (one-third the previously implied limit) "should be maintained" so as to limit the dose received up to the age of 30 to 50 rem (rather than the previously implied 150 rem). The Commission also reported that one of its committees recommended lowering the maximum permissible dose to the gonads as well as the whole bodies of radiation workers to 0.1 rem/week (which was implied, but not required, by the 5 rem annual limit, since with two weeks vacation 50 weeks/year × 0.1 rem = 5).[123] This suggested tightening of the occupational norm, one participant thought, would be "more of a hindrance to therapy than to energy projects," though vigorous objections were later registered by both the nuclear institutions at Chalk River (Canada) and Hanford (United States).[124]

Once the ICRP had moved, Taylor followed. In August 1956 he returned from Mexico City wanting the ICRP to publish something quickly because

> ...the release by the ICRP will give the radiologists a feeling that the Commission is providing some kind of leadership. I'm afraid that if we do not move in this direction fairly quickly, the feeling will grow that the ICRP has lost its leadership. This is important because of the possible effect

[121] Extensive Notes, Meeting of the Executive Committee. NCRP. September 19, 1956—New York, N.Y (Note 3, 8-067–72, at 8-068).

[122] See Ellis, note 90.

[123] ICRP, "Report of the Work of the Commission for presentation to the Executive Committee of the Eighth International Congress of Radiology (Mexico, 1956)," ICRP 56/17, ICRP Archives, Box G051, Basic Anatomical and Physiological Data 1994.pdf, 350–77.

[124] Note 112, at 8-301. The objections are in note 3, "Parker to Taylor, June 19, 1956," 8-317 and Taylor's retrospective note at 8-329.

on the future funding of the ICRP by some organization such as the Ford Foundation.[125]

The funding, as we shall see, would prove vital, but it was not the only factor at work. Taylor added that the AEC did not want to change its regulations until it heard from the NCRP, which in turn would want to base its work on the ICRP's statement.[126] The era of American hegemony in radiation protection was already over, due in large part to the threat of encroachment by the National Academy's BEAR report. That encroachment had been inspired primarily by American geneticists.

At this point, there was a great deal of confusion within the ICRP about precisely what had been agreed by whom, due in part to illness of the ICRP's scientific secretary. At Bo Lindell's suggestion, Failla tried to straighten things out with a revision of the ICRP's 1955 report in August 1956, though it was not published until 1958.[127] Still concerned about encroachment by other professional organizations, Taylor was annoyed with this delay, as it "makes it appear that we are following the U. S. [NAS] and U. K. [MRC] recommendations."[128] It included the general statement advising that the dose to the general population not exceed the natural background, because of concern about genetic damage. Failla however thought the Commission needed to go further and specify a definite figure. He himself favored a 10 r lifetime genetic dose from all sources, which he thought might not satisfy "the geneticists." With none in the Main Commission at this point, Failla polled the geneticists and

[125] Taylor to Rock Carling, Taylor, note 3 above, 8-823.

[126] Ibid.

[127] "Recommendations of Sub-Committee I—Revision of 1955 Report," Taylor, note 3, 8-325. Lindell gives an extensive account of the confusing discussion/negotiation of this revision, Hercules, note 53, 178–98. The suggestion to Failla is at 209. The final version was published as Report on amendments during 1956 to the Recommendations of the International Commission on Radiological Protection (ICRP) in both Radiation Research. 1958;8(6):539–42 and Radiology. 1958 Feb;70(2). https://doi.org/10.1148/70.2.261, accessed July 13, 2023. See also Failla's account of this and later confusion in his letters to Binks, July 10, 1958, and to Sir Ernest Mayneord and Binks, September 1, 1958, ICRP Archives, Box 039, ISO-ICU 1958.pdf, 47–50 and 40–44.

[128] Taylor to Sievert, October 21, 1957, ICRP Archives, Archive Files 12–22, Archive File 22, 1.8.57 to 31.12.57.pdf, 152–3.

others in Subcommittee 1, which he chaired.[129] Muller concurred by telegram with the 10r lifetime genetic dose suggestion, but in the end the ICRP preferred instead a 5 rem permissible genetic dose to the population (from conception to child bearing) that excluded medical exposure (and thus also excluded resistance from medical practitioners), and explicitly linking the decision to "proper planning for nuclear power programs."[130] The Commission also included the 5 rem/year occupational limit to the gonads of radiation workers, which had been favored by the Germans.[131]

The most senior member of the ICRP, German physician Hermann Holthusen, was in no doubt that genetic effects were driving the decision-making. He had already concluded that "genetics does dominate the permissible dose level so we cannot help it."[132] He therefore favored making the longer-duration limits, which biologists had agreed were the meaningful ones when it came to genetic effects, the fundamental ones and deriving shorter-term limits from them. That is what happened. There appear to have been no geneticists present when the decisions were taken, but two other specialists, an American and a British physicist, pressed for tightening of the weekly permissible dose for radiation workers to 0.1 rem (from 0.3).[133] For the general population, the limit (not

[129] Failla to Committee 1, June 25, 1958, ICRP Archives, Archive file 23, Sect. Correspondence 1.8.57-31.12.58.pdf, 1–3. Muller's response is ibid., at 4.

[130] ICRP. Recommendations of the International Commission on Radiological Protection: Adopted September 9, 1958. Annals of the ICRP/ICRP Publication. 1959 Jan;OS_1(1):iii–x, accessed August 3, 2023, https://journals.sagepub.com/doi/pdf/10.1016/S0074-27402880016-X. Failla's preference is in Failla to Binks, ICRP Archives, Box 039, ISO-ICU 1958.pdf, 47–50. Failla consulted Committee 1, which included two geneticists, before the new recommendations were written, ibid., 51–2.

[131] "Maximum permissible doses for occupational exposure," Sub-Committee on Radiobiology of the German Atomic Commission to Sievert, Bad Godesberg, February 6, 1958, ICRP Archives, Box 039, ISO-ICU 1958.pdf, 134–5.

[132] Holthusen to Sievert, "Recommendations of the ICRP," January 21, 1958, Taylor, note 3 above, 8-411-16 at 8-416. The English translation of the letter is also at ICRP Archives, Archive file 23, Sect. Correspondence 1.8.57-31.12.58.pdf, 64–71.

[133] "The question of the yearly limit was reopened by the members who arrived today." They were the physicists H. W. Koch and W. V. Mayneord, "Minutes of the ICRP Meetings, ICRU Officers Attending," ICRP/ICRU/NY/58/14, March 6, 1958, Box A788 Registry, ISO-ICU 1958.pdf, 128–33. Failla prepared a scoping paper for this unusually lengthy meeting: "Suggestions for discussion of Permissible Limits of Exposure by the ICRP at the Meeting of March 3–15, 1958, ICRP/ICRU/58/11, ICRP Archives, Box A788 Registry, ISO-ICU 1958.pdf, 143–60.

counting medical and background exposure) was set again at one-tenth the occupational figure (thus 0.5 rem per year) "for purposes of planning and design."[134] Fallout from bomb testing, still a small contributing factor and a politically sensitive one, was not explicitly considered. When delays in publication loomed, Failla argued forcefully for haste:

1. Numerical values are needed for planning purposes by engineers, governmental and private agencies, etc.
2. Owing to the publicity given to the genetic hazard of exposure to radiation, the public is afraid of <u>any</u> exposure to radiation. This attitude is detrimental to the proper practice of medicine, to the legitimate uses of radiation in industry and to the utilisation of nuclear power. The recommendation by an authoritative body such as ICRP of a permissible genetic dose would go far to allay these fears, since it would clearly indicate that something is being done to prevent undue harm.
3. The world is looking to ICRP to make such a recommendation as soon as possible.[135]

Professional, commercial, and public pressures all weighed heavily in the direction of publication.

The result became known as ICRP Publication 1, which recorded recommendations agreed in 1958 but not published until 1959.[136] The penultimate text was cobbled together, courtesy of World Health Organization funding, at Woods' Hole on Cape Cod in August 1958. The discussions involved Failla—by this time a strong advocate of taking genetics into account—and Lindell, along with Canadian physician David Sowby, who would become the ICRP Scientific Secretary a few years later, Columbia University biophysicist H. H. Rossi, and American physicist Elda Anderson, one of only a few women involved in radiation protection in the twentieth century. She had worked on the Manhattan Project at Los

[134] Note 130, 13.

[135] Failla to Sir Ernest Mayneord, September 1, 1958, ICRP Archives, Archive Files 1-11, Archive File 10, Draft recommendations 1958.pdf, 96–100, at 98.

[136] Note 108.

Alamos but was by this time at Oak Ridge National Laboratory.[137] Only physicists and a single nonpracticing physician were present. Lindell, who was at the time both Scientific Secretary of UNSCEAR and temporary Scientific Secretary of ICRP, did the drafting. The 1958 recommendations confirmed the 1956 reduction of the occupational permissible dose to 0.1 rem/week (down from 0.3/week in 1954) as well as the permissible dose for the general population at one-tenth the annual occupational dose limit (or 0.5 rem/year). And it added a maximum permissible genetic dose of 5 rems from birth to mean age of childbearing, assumed to be 30 years old. This would sometimes in the future be cited as 170 millirem per year (5/30 = 0.170 rem = 170 millirem).

This second post-World War II tightening of the ICRP's permissible doses confirms that science is a social enterprise in which scientists change their minds in response to other scientists' work and the social and organizational circumstances in which they are called on for expert judgment. Outside the epistemic community, public pressure was building due to the anticipated expansion of nuclear power and fallout from nuclear tests, which will be discussed next. Inside the epistemic community, the geneticists were pushing. Physicists and nonpracticing physicians like Sowby sympathized with their arguments. Encroachment by other professional organizations loomed. To the relevant epistemic community, those were all good reasons to tighten the norms and ensure continued ICRP dominance.

Notably absent from deliberations inside the ICRP in the mid1950s was much discussion of fallout from nuclear tests, which by then was a major subject of public controversy. Nuclear testing presented a political quandary for both the American and British participants in ICRP activities, who still dominated the Commission numerically. They and their other colleagues were sensitive to the national security requirements behind the bomb builders' efforts and anxious to stay on good terms with agencies that were also responsible for radiation protection. But at the same time, they could not help but be acutely aware of the public concern

[137] ICRP and UNSCEAR: some distant memories. Journal of Radiological Protection. 2001;21:57–62. https://iopscience.iop.org/article/10.1088/0952-4746/21/1/306/pdf, accessed May 21, 2023 Anderson, American physicist Edith Quimby (who worked with Failla at Memorial Hospital and Columbia University), and British epidemiologist Alice Stewart, who linked cancer in children to prenatal X-rays, were in the mid-twentieth century among the few women involved professionally in radiation protection.

not only about testing but also about nuclear war. Ignoring fallout was however still their preference. As late as September 1962 a meeting at the U.S. government Federal Radiation Council (FRC) concluded that "in spite of the relatively high levels of iodine-131 resulting from fallout, the situation did not appear to be critical enough to warrant the introduction of control measures."[138] Fallout would require political decision, not only expert advice.

Not everyone would have agreed with the American FRC. In Sweden, Soviet tests had increased radiation in food to levels Sievert thought close to the ICRP's norms for maximum permissible concentrations. Lindell worried that this imperiled the reindeer-consuming native Sami population. Sievert had written in December 1956:

> What will happen before we ascertain the levels at which the bomb tests begin to constitute a serious danger to mankind, and what will be the results when the first atomic war starts? I believe we will be forced to put monitors in the hands of everyone, in order to stimulate the general public to act against tests of atomic weapons and their use?[139]

In late 1956, Sievert floated the idea of an ICRP/ICRU-sponsored conference focused on the effects of nuclear war, hoping it would make that eventuality less likely.[140] Taylor condemned the idea by saying he was "a little concerned about the political aspects of a conference."[141] It never happened. Sievert continued to be concerned about fallout, which had been found in Sweden reaching levels twice the natural background.[142] Fallout, however, was still more a political issue than a health problem and would ultimately be settled outside the epistemic community by politicians rather than scientists and physicians.

[138] Conference—FRC—NCRP—NAS—on Fallout. Note 25, 9-093.

[139] Sievert to Reuben Gustavson, December 4, 1956, Archive Files 55–65, Archive File 56, 1955–1957 Sievert's Planner.pdf, 72–4.

[140] Confidential "Memorandum," ibid., 70.

[141] Taylor to Sievert, December 14, 1956, ibid.

[142] Sievert to A. Allen Lough at the U.S. AEC, December 17, 1957, ICRP Archives, Archive Files 12–22, File 22, 5.

Fallout: Radioactive and Political

The Americans and British had not agreed on everything in their 1956 reports. The BEAR and MRC reports of June 1956 differed on how to estimate the biological effects of radiostrontium (Strontium 90), which like radium behaves chemically like calcium and therefore accumulates in bones. The AEC knew its tests were producing radiostrontium and regarded that radioisotope as a major risk to the general population in the event of nuclear war. But it feared popular reaction and had kept its extensive worldwide survey (Project Gabriel), organized by Taylor during a leave from the National Bureau of Standards in 1948–49, a secret as long as possible.[143] The BEAR report suggested that the existing norm for radiostrontium, based on a threshold for cancer effects, was sufficient while the British did not. They had deemed more credible the evidence for linear no-threshold (LNT) cancer effects, analogous to genetic effects and presumably caused by ionization in somatic (as opposed to reproductive) cell chromosomes. Even before World War II, Muller had concluded likewise, but now there was evidence in the scientific literature.[144]

By the mid-1950s radiostrontium risks from fallout, along with those associated with Iodine 131 (which accumulates in the thyroid, especially of growing children), were widely discussed in public. The NCRP in late 1958 set up an Ad Hoc Subcommittee on Widespread Radioactive Contamination, in part to respond to an anticipated ICRP lowering of maximum permissible concentrations of radionuclides in the environment

[143] Taylor does not mention his personal role in Project Gabriel, note 3, but his Health Physics Society obituary does, see Nelson W. Taylor, Warren K. Sinclair, and Robert O. Gorson. In Memoriam: Lauriston S. Taylor. http://hps.org/aboutthesociety/people/inmemoriam/lauristontaylor.html, accessed July 18, 2022.

[144] On Muller, see Carlson EA. Genes, Radiation, and Society: The Life and Work of H. J. Muller. Ithaca and London: Cornell University Press; 1981:245 and 255. The extension of the LNT hypothesis to cancer effects still arouses opposition, see Calabrese EJ. LNT and cancer risk assessment: its flawed foundations part 1: Radiation and leukemia: where LNT began. Environmental Research. 2021;197(111025). https://doi.org/10.1016/j.envres.2021.111025, accessed May 21, 2022. https://doi.org/10.1016/j.envres.2021.111025, accessed May 21, 2022. Calabrese reviews the evidence existing in the mid-1950s in detail. He is correct about the leftist political influence he claims was at work, but the LNT hypothesis—even if it fits the data as badly as Calabrese claims—is still useful in considering scientific uncertainty and in avoiding the impossible task of attributing responsibility for exceeding a threshold. As for the hormesis Calabrese claims, the scientists should decide that issue. The evidence has been examined repeatedly without a favorable consensus emerging.

by a factor of 1/100 relative to occupational levels.[145] No longer confident of American hegemony, Taylor was anxious for the NCRP to be ready to respond, whatever the ICRP decided. While the ICRP tried to keep its focus on scientific issues, concern about the somatic effects of fallout did not arise in a political vacuum. Nobel prize winners Albert Einstein and Bertrand Russell, perhaps the most famous intellectuals of their day, had issued a "manifesto" in 1955 urging governments to renounce war, in particular war using nuclear weapons.[146] This required unusual courage and conviction because the mid-1950s were the height of the anti-Communist crusade in the United States. The U.S. government had deprived Oppenheimer of his security clearance in 1954, based on pre-war associations with Communists. Concern about Muller's politics caused the AEC to cancel his address on "the mechanism of production of mutations by radiation" to the UN Conference on the Peaceful Uses of Atomic Energy in 1955.[147] Nobel Laureate Linus Pauling (in Chemistry, only later for Peace) was deprived of his passport that year.

Many outlets for leftist politics were closed. Opposition to nuclear weapons signified Communist sympathies to many Americans, because Moscow trumpeted its opposition to nuclear weapons even while conducting an aggressive nuclear testing program to catch up with the United States. It was only a bit safer politically to campaign against nuclear testing than against nuclear weapons. Democratic candidate Adlai

[145] "Responsibilities of NCRP Ad Hoc Subcommittee on Widespread Radioactive Contamination," December 3, 1958, Taylor, note 3, 8-188–90. The idea of cutting public exposure to 1/100 of occupational exposure had been bruited for years, see "Minutes of the Plenary Session of the Commission and Committees," held on Monday, April 9, 1956, at 2.0 p.m. in Salle B, Maison des Congres (International Telecommunications Union) Geneva, ICRP Archive file 27, ICRP correspondence.pdf 1, 145–9, ICRP/56/11, at 3.

[146] Statement: The Russell-Einstein Manifesto [Internet]. Pugwash Conferences on Science and World Affairs. 1955. Available from: https://pugwash.org/1955/07/09/statement-manifesto/, accessed May 5, 2022.

[147] Carlson, note 136, 366. The specific concern in Muller's case was his opposition to development of the hydrogen bomb. It was at this conference, however, that Western scientists made their first contacts with Soviet counterparts, whom they viewed as on the same wavelength with regard to essential issues like maximum permissible concentrations of radioactive isotopes, see K.Z. Morgan to [F.G.] Krotkov, Taylor, note 3 above, 8-260. Morgan there opened the door to a participation by a Soviet scientist in the ICRP subcommittee on internal doses that he chaired. By 1956, M.N. Pobedinski had joined Morgan's committee and confirmed that the ICRP norms were already being applied in the Soviet Union, "Minutes," note 137, at 8.

Stevenson did so in his unsuccessful presidential campaign of 1956.[148] But the Eisenhower Administration even thereafter "blacklisted" theologian Albert Schweitzer, rated in 1956 as the fourth most admired person in the world. His crime? He spoke out against nuclear testing in 1957 in a "Declaration of Conscience" prompted by Norman Cousins, editor of the left-of-center weekly Saturday Review.[149] Schweitzer explicitly blamed continuation of nuclear testing on the lack of public opinion asking that it stop.[150]

That however was changing, as both the advocates and opponents of nuclear testing knew. The American Committee for a SANE Nuclear Policy and the British Campaign for Nuclear Disarmament (CND), responsible for many public demonstrations against nuclear testing and weapons, were both founded in 1957. The debate among geneticists on population exposures, though eventually resolved, and the divergence between American and British expert groups on radiostrontium, generated public controversy and further pressure to end bomb tests. While Prime Minister Winston Churchill had decided in 1955 to proceed with developing a hydrogen bomb, his successor, Harold MacMillan, had doubts, but continued mainly because the Americans refused to provide hydrogen bomb technology to the UK. American officials were still fully committed to nuclear tests, but it was difficult for them to hide the cognitive dissonance on radiostrontium. The British Atomic Scientists Association roiled the waters in public and in parliament with a statement on radiostrontium in April 1957.[151] In October, a fire at Britain's Windscale reactor, which produced both plutonium and electricity, heightened

[148] Wittner LS. Adlai Stevenson Had a Peace Proposal … Shouldn't Democrats Today? | History News Network [Internet]. historynewsnetwork.org, available from: https://historynewsnetwork.org/article/28611, accessed May 5, 2022.

[149] Wittner LS. Blacklisting Schweitzer. Bulletin of the Atomic Scientists. 1995 May;51(3):55. https://www.albany.edu/news/pdf_files/0903_Blacklisting_Schweitzer.pdf, accessed May 5, 2022.

[150] Ibid.

[151] Laucht C. Scientists, the Public, the State, and the Debate Over the Environmental and Human Health Effects of Nuclear Testing in Britain, 1950–1958. The Historical Journal. 2015 Dec 9;59(1):221–51.

public awareness of nuclear risks. The Federation of American Scientists and the Bulletin of the Atomic Scientists had long favored a testing moratorium, as did Pauling in an appeal published in early 1958.[152]

Other countries were increasingly engaged: Sweden, Norway, Canada, and India had begun pressing for constraints on nuclear testing and fallout. The Japanese had nothing good to say about nuclear testing, though they kept a relatively low profile to avoid provoking the United States. Japanese scientists demonstrated that exposure to strontium 90 from rice and other foods was far higher than exposure in the United States and Britain, where it was due primarily to milk. The Soviets had for several years favored a moratorium on testing, to slow the Americans from widening their thermonuclear lead. In March 1958 the newly empowered Chairman of the Soviet Union's Council of Ministers, Nikita Khrushchev, took the initiative and announced a unilateral testing moratorium, to bring international public pressure to bear on the United States and Britain.[153]

It was in this contentious atmosphere that UNSCEAR issued its first report in June 1958.[154] It rejected a Soviet proposal to recommend ending nuclear tests, but it mentioned the possibility and credited the argument that testing exposed people, including in future generations, to risks though they received no benefits from the tests. The Americans had even voted in favor of an Indian draft that failed to pass but acknowledged even more explicitly the growing contribution of nuclear testing to population exposures:

[152] The Right to Petition—Linus Pauling and the International Peace Movement [Internet]. scarc.library.oregonstate.edu. Available from: http://scarc.library.oregonstate.edu/coll/pauling/peace/narrative/page27.html, accessed May 6, 2022.

[153] Evangelista M. Unarmed Forces the Transnational Movement to End the Cold War. Cornell University Press; 1999:56.

[154] Report of the United Nations Scientific Committee on the Effects of Atomic Radiation. General Assembly Official Records: Thirteenth Session 1958 Supplement No. 17 (A/3838) (New York: United Nations) [Internet]. United Nations: Scientific Committee on the Effects of Atomic Radiation. Available from: https://www.unscear.org/unscear/en/publications/1958.html, accessed April 30, 2023. See especially para 54 and associated footnotes, on p. 41. See also Lindell B, Sowby D. The 1958 UNSCEAR Report. Journal of Radiological Protection. 2008;28:277–82. as well as Hercules, note 53, 218–22 for Bo Lindell's first-hand account of the meetings leading up to the report.

> ...it is undesirable to allow any general rise in the level of world-wide contamination because of its harmful effects and that any activity which produces such a rise should be avoided. Nuclear tests are the main source at present which produce such a rise.[155]

Even if fallout was still far from breaching a permissible dose, the LNT hypothesis meant that some portion of the world's population would be harmed. That harm and the numbers of people affected would increase with long-term accumulation of radionuclides. Most of the people exposed would not benefit from the exposure or have a say in controlling it.

This argument is not fundamentally scientific. It is ethical and political. The irony is manifest: a UN committee the British and Americans insisted be intergovernmental so that they could control the membership and thereby the outcome reached conclusions inimical to the nuclear tests the two governments had intended to protect. The outcome vindicated, even if it did not recommend, the Japanese and Soviet interest in suspending nuclear tests. President Dwight Eisenhower shared with MacMillan that he considered that "public opinion is a most important element." As Higuchi puts it,

> It was this interplay between the reconstruction of biological knowledge [through the LNT hypothesis, which may or may not have been correct] and the transnational activism that guided the UNSCEAR toward a consensus that deemed global fallout contamination as unacceptable.[156]

Spurred by UNSCEAR, the United States and Britain announced in August 1958 that they would join the Soviet-initiated moratorium on nuclear testing.

The NCRP's Ad Hoc Committee report on Population Exposure was published in May 1959 in this highly charged political context. It shifted the American position and concluded that the LNT hypothesis should be used for norm-setting, as this was more conservative (from the perspective of avoiding harm) and practical than resorting to unknown and uncertain

[155] The (darkly) comedic rejection of the Indian draft is recounted in Sowby D. ICRP and UNSCEAR: Some Distant Memories. Journal of Radiological Protection. 2001;21:57–62. https://iopscience.iop.org/article/10.1088/0952-4746/21/1/306/pdf, accessed May 21, 2023.

[156] Higuchi T. Political Fallout. Stanford University Press; 2020:134.

thresholds. The Committee also suggested that levels in the environment (not including medical and occupational exposure) should be kept low enough that they would not approach the natural background level of about 0.1 rem per year, a figure below the then current ICRP recommendation.[157] The U.S. Congress held multi-day hearings on fallout in 1957 and 1959 and on radiation standards in 1960 and 1962, with the last focused on Strontium 90 and Iodine 131.[158] Public concern was having an impact.

As Higuchi documents, there ensued in the early 1960s a period of local fallout surveys in the United States and Britain focused on "hot spots." In the United States, the progressivist state of Minnesota and the nongovernmental Consumer's Union surveyed radiostrontium in milk. Mothers and Dr. Benjamin Spock, the leading U.S. expert of the time on children's health, were a highly effective lobby against atmospheric testing of nuclear weapons. Minnesota also discovered elevated levels in wheat. In Britain, the focus of concern was mainly on sheep in Wales, where elevated radiation levels and nationalist politics were conducive to protest. Throughout, it was the International Commission norms on radiation protection, specifically the permissible internal doses, that were the yardstick for concern. What had begun as a scientific debate about remote genetic risks to the human race among scientists had turned into a public debate about radiostrontium in children's teeth and bones, as well as radioiodine in their thyroids, that could not fail to arouse scientific and medical as well as public concern. Though his declared moratorium had ended in September 1959, Eisenhower concluded "no free country can go back to atmospheric testing because [world] opinion—the adverse effect of alienating free world countries—would stop it."[159] MacMillan had concluded likewise.

The Soviet Union, certainly not a free country, ironically proved them right by announcing in August 1961 an end to the moratorium, followed

157 "Permissible Somatic Dose for the General Population (Report of the Ad Hoc Committee to the NCRP), May 6, 1959, Taylor, Appendix P.

158 Hearings Before the Subcommittee on Research, Development, and Radiation of the Joint Committee on Atomic energy of the Joint Committee on Atomic Energy, 87th Congress, Second Session, on Radiation Standards, including Fallout, JUNE 4, 5, 6, AND 7, 1962, https://www.osti.gov/opennet/servlets/purl/16367058.pdf, accessed August 13, 2023.

159 Higuchi, note 156, 158.

by a massive thermonuclear test in October 1961.[160] The Americans followed suit, initially testing mostly underground. There followed more than a year of accelerated weapons testing in the atmosphere, but both in the United States and in the Soviet Union scientific and popular opinion had won the thinking of political leadership over the preferences of those who saw national security at risk if testing were stopped. After maneuvering around substantial domestic political opposition in each of their countries, President Kennedy, Chairman Khrushchev, and Prime Minister MacMillan signed the Partial Test Ban Treaty in December 1963. Prohibition rather than balancing of risks and benefits was the ultimate solution to the fallout problem. Political rather than epistemic authority resolved it.

The political and moral arguments prevailed, but the arms race continued. France continued atmospheric testing, China conducted its first atmospheric test in 1964, and the United States, Soviet Union, and Britain did theirs underground. Their weapons testing would continue until the early 1990s, but no longer play a major role in debates about radiation protection. The ICRP would find it necessary to explain itself and adjust its 1958 recommendations in sometimes excruciating detail, but major changes in radiation protection norms lay decades in the future.[161] As discussed in the next chapter, the main arena for radiation protection debates shifted to the nuclear power industry, when two major incidents would challenge the prevailing normative regime.

The Institutions Gain Legitimacy

Throughout the 1950s and into the early 1960s, the ICRP was a self-perpetuating, nongovernmental, epistemic group of experts. It was concerned with maintaining its independence from "politics" and its dominance over norm-setting as well as solidifying its institutional character. Sievert averred in 1960:

[160] Comprehensive Test Ban Treaty Organization. 30 October 1961—the Tsar Bomba [Internet]. www.ctbto.org, available from: https://www.ctbto.org/specials/testing-times/30-october-1961-the-tsar-bomba/, accessed June 24, 2022.

[161] Recommendations of the International Commission on Radiological Protection (As Amended 1959 and Revised 1962). ICRP Publication 6. 1964; Oxford: Pergamon Press. The next revision, Recommendations of the International Commission on Radiological Protection (Adopted September 17, 1965). ICRP Publication 9. Oxford: Pergamon Press was largely a codification of the two previous ones.

> It must be obvious for everyone that the most competent group to decide upon the members needed for the work of the ICRP will be the commission itself and that this will safeguard - as far as this is possible - against political considerations....[162]

Co-optation was still a key to independence and authority. As Lindell explained later:

> Every ["Any"] election of members which was controlled by outsiders risked increasing the number of members and adding members who had been elected for some immaterial reason such as nationality or prestige, members who appeared to increase the Commission's authority but who in reality reduced its competence. A safety valve lay in the fact that ICRP could exist only for as long as its recommendations were good enough to be accepted by the outside world.[163]

The ICRP was knowledge-based, even if not indifferent to outside opinion. It would decades later open up to nominations for membership in the Commission and its subcommittees and task forces from outside its own membership, but it remains even today focused on professional credentials as the primary qualification.

Particularly important to the ICRP were the views of national radiation protection institutions, which were well-represented in the Commission's membership. Apart from the United States, countries participating in the ICRP, like Great Britain and Sweden, had national radiation protection organizations more definitively associated with their respective governments. In 1964, the American Standards Association cataloged 16 other countries and 12 international organizations with published nuclear standards.[164] Unlike most of these however, the American NCRP had no official status even within the U.S. government's National Bureau of Standards, which on an informal basis provided most of its administrative and organizational support. Even in the midst of American hegemony, the legal status of the NCRP and ICRP was ambiguous and

[162] Sievert to Pochin, May 4, 1960, ICRP Archives, Box W-18, Archive files 25, 180–181.

[163] Hercules, note 53, 97.

[164] American Standards Association, Subcommittee N6.9, 1965 Compilation of National and International Nuclear Standards, (Excluding U.S. Activities), ICRP Archives, Box W-18, Archive Files 29, 11–25.

their financial situations were precarious. The ICRP remained a creature of the International Congress of Radiology, which was a nongovernmental organization focused on medical radiology, not the far broader scope radiation protection post-World War II required. The NCRP was *sui generis*: a norm-setting organization with secretariat support from the U.S. Government's National Bureau of Standards and broad participation by interested governmental and nongovernmental organizations, including the AEC, industry, and academia, but no official status.

The ICRP repeatedly considered dissociating itself from the triannual International Congress of Radiology (ICR), which still focused on the applications of radiation in medicine. The post-World War II international order offered several other possible affiliations: UNESCO, the International Labor Organization, and WHO in the first instance, then later the IAEA and the International Standards Organization, among others. But leading members of the ICRP repeatedly preferred independence, in particular from governmental and political influence, as well as scientific focus. The ICR permitted that, if only by neglect. The members of the Commission and its subcommittees were chosen by the existing members (when necessary by voting), ideally without regard to nationality, politics, or policy. The Main Commission members were invariably approved *pro forma* by the Executive Council of the ICR. This independence, based on co-optation of experts whom the existing members thought most qualified, the ICRP Main Commission members wanted to preserve. They put it bluntly:

> A strength of the ICRP and the ICRU is that they are completely independent of political and other influences. In practice they are self-perpetuating; making it possible to co-opt, without consideration of nationality, the best available specialists to take part in the work. The leadership they have maintained in their field for many years has been made possible by their freedom to carry out their work independent of non-technical influences.[165]

This exaggerated their independence, as public controversy and perceived competition with other institutions had clearly affected the norm-setting process, but it properly expressed their preference that the ICRP remain

165 "Statement of the need for an enlarged scope of activity for the ICRP and ICRU," Taylor, note 3, 8-399.

a strictly professional, scientific group based in the epistemic community studying as well as using ionizing radiation and its biological effects.

While they disavowed any intention of interfering in "national freedom in this field," as Taylor put it later, Failla said at the time "The organizations [ICRP and ICRU] had to be able to act as a world authority in the field of radiation protection."[166] Some would have liked the ICRP to have its own research capability, rather than depending on the research of Commission and subcommittee members. Rolf Sievert had served as the first chair of the pre-World War II International Committee on X-ray and Radium Protection and was re-elected to chair the ICRP in April 1956. He successively prepared proposals to convert the ICRP, along with the ICRU and eventually including UNSCEAR, into an academy, an association, an organization, an institute, or a foundation, but he failed to find the financing required to support the permanent secretariat, national affiliates, and research capacity he and others thought necessary.[167]

Sievert was also chosen to chair UNSCEAR in 1958. While his grand institutionalization efforts failed and some feared UNSCEAR might undermine the ICRP, Sievert steered UNSCEAR, which commissioned a major international study of radiation doses to the gonads due to medical radiology from the ICRP and ICRU, clear of norm-setting and focused mainly on the biological effects of radiation and their relationship to bomb testing in the atmosphere.[168] Throughout the 1950s, the ICRP was sustained on minor contributions, mainly for travel, from the International Society for Radiology, set up to plan the triennial International Congresses of Radiology, the National Association of Swedish Insurance

[166] Taylor, note 3, 7-244; for Failla's ambition, "Minutes of the Opening Session of the International Commission on Radiological Protection," April 3, 1956, ICRP/56/9, 8-294.

[167] Taylor, note 3, 7-253–8 and 8-271–5 (Academy), 8-243 and 8-288–90 (Organization), 8-389–94 (Institute) and 8-460 (Foundation). Sievert originally hoped to find the financing from insurance companies, which had an interest because the ICRP's "recommendations have hitherto been widely accepted as the basis of national 'codes of practice.' Where such codes are adopted, responsibility for accidents can often be repudiated." But his efforts succeeded only modestly with the Swedish insurance companies, so he refocused on the Ford and Rockefeller Foundations.

[168] The ICRP/ICRU study commissioned by UNSCEAR was published as Exposure of Man to Ionizing Radiation Arising from Medical Procedures. Physics in Medicine & Biology. 1957;2(2):107–51. https://doi.org/10.1088/0031-9155/2/2/301, accessed August 22, 2023.

Companies as well as private Swedish sources, and occasionally from the WHO, especially for publication of its reports. But it continued to have perpetual problems funding its publications or finding someone to publish them at no cost. That was at least part of the reason for its delays in publishing its recommendations.

By the mid-1950s, the informal arrangements inside the United States were raising questions within the National Bureau of Standards.[169] In addition, the Congressional Joint Atomic Energy Committee was not comfortable with basic radiation protection standards set by an organization without a clear identity.[170] The NCRP was neither a government committee nor a nongovernmental organization. At least three-quarters of its budget came from the Federal government, though it was aiming for no more than one-third.[171] It had organizational rules, but no constitution or other founding document.[172] It relied on technical people who in part represented their employers, whether governmental or nongovernmental, but was increasingly called upon to make value judgments that lay beyond the remit of the National Bureau of Standards. NBS had no biological expertise or mandate to take responsibility for safety standards, especially those that extended well beyond the confines of radiation-using establishments to the general population. The NCRP had no research capabilities of its own but relied on those of its committee and subcommittee members. The AEC and Public Health Service relied on the NCRP when it came to radiation measurements and radiation protection standards, but they were under no obligation to do so.

The NCRP Executive Committee met in May 1959 with the Director of the NBS and others to discuss these and related legal and organizational issues. Their goal was to "get the NBS off the hook" but allow the NCRP to continue operating without interference. Options included formal NBS sponsorship, joint NBS/PHS/AEC sponsorship, a Presidential Executive order, an entirely independent nongovernmental body, and a Congressional charter, similar to that of the National Academy of

[169] Meeting of the Executive Committee of the NCRP with the Director of the National Bureau of Standards, May 12, 1959, Taylor, note 3, 8-219–26.

[170] Ibid., Comment by LST, 8-228.

[171] Annual Meeting of the Executive Committee (1962), note 3, 9-099–100.

[172] Organization and Operational Procedures of the National Committee on Radiation Protection and Measurements. Ibid., 8-218–19.

Sciences.[173] While an NBS lawyer pressed for changes to formalize the NCRP's status, the Executive Committee of scientists and medical doctors preferred any option that left things as close to the status quo as possible. As one put it:

> ...the success of the NCRP is due entirely to the fact that although while enjoying official sponsorship of a sort, it in fact had been able to operate as if it were a completely unofficial body and could leave problems of official pronouncement to those agencies which were statutorily responsible.[174]

Another emphasized the recognized professional and scientific integrity of the NCRP:

> ...the strength of the NCRP is essentially a moral one deriving from the fact that no individuals profit personally from operations of the Committee except in an intellectual sense. Furthermore, he did not think of any areas where there were any conflicts of interest between the members and their organizations. He stressed that this was a very strong point in favor of making as little change as possible from the standpoint of how the scientific public in particular regards the operations of the Committee.[175]

While far from today's standards on conflict of interest, the NCRP of the 1950s and early 1960s represented most interested scientific institutions, including not only government agencies but also medicine, academia, and industry. It was far less interested in participation by organizations representing the lay public. It rejected a proposal to include organized labor (AFL-CIO) among its "sponsoring" organizations, on grounds that would open the door to other interested groups ("mental health or ministry").[176] But at the same time it welcomed the American Veterinary Medical Association and the Industrial Medical Association as sponsors, because of their scientific interests and capacity. The NCRP's participation in 1959 included 150 people coming from a broad range of professional

[173] Note 169, at 8-221.

[174] Ibid., at 822.

[175] Ibid.

[176] "Minutes of the NCRP Executive Committee Meeting, November 16, 1959," Taylor, note 3, 8-238–41.

disciplines, but no one from outside the epistemic community associated with radiation protection in one way or another.[177]

In the midst of the fallout controversy, President Eisenhower in August 1959 established an interagency Federal Radiation Council (FRC) to advise him among other things on establishing radiation protection standards. This move appeared to threaten the existence of the NCRP, not least because a Commerce Department lawyer maintained that no government officials should participate in the NCRP and its subcommittees to avoid any potential conflict with Administration policies. At the time, 16 of 45 members of the NCRP main committee were government employees or contractors, though in the subcommittee dealing with basic radiation protection criteria only the chair was a government contractor.[178] The FRC was supposed to be responsible for value judgments weighing social, economic, and security factors against the biological effects of radiation, but in practice it relied on the NCRP's recommendations, which were regarded as authoritative despite their lack of legal force or even foundation.[179] The relationship between the NCRP and the FRC became a subject of extensive discussion, both within the Administration and in the Congressional Joint Committee on Atomic Energy. Legislation giving a statutory basis to the FRC required it to consult the NCRP chair, among others, but the NCRP still lacked a clear relationship to the FRC and even to the National Bureau of Standards, whose Commerce Department superiors were resisting the idea that it could sponsor an independent advisory body.

Taylor, a seasoned and savvy bureaucrat, raised half a dozen options in response to criticism, including terminating the NCRP. That proposition met with opposition both in the Administration and in Congress. The

[177] "NCRP Activity Report (1959) and Membership," Communication No. 59, October 6, 1959, Taylor, note 3, 8-233.

[178] "Discussion of NCRP Organization Problems," NCRP/M-E/60/10, May 12, 1960, in Taylor, note 3, at 9-021. Overall, 1/6 of NCRP committee and subcommittee members were government employees, see the memo from Lauriston Taylor to the NCRP Main and Executive Committees, NCRP/M-E/60/14, June 10, 1960, 9-027–30, at 9-029.

[179] "Legislative Aspects of Radiation Standards—Role of NCRP and Government," Address of Congressman Chet Holifield, Chairman of the Special Radiation subcommittee of the Joint Committee on Atomic Energy—presented at the fifth Annual Meeting of the Health Physics Society, Boston, Massachusetts, June 30, 1960, Taylor, note 3, 9-039–43.

Commerce Department lawyer reversed his position on officials participating in the NCRP. Taylor fended off suggested absorption into the National Academy of Sciences, the University of Chicago, or a new radiation institute. He also underlined that the NCRP, unlike the ICRP, dealt exclusively with "controllable" sources of radiation, which conveniently excluded nuclear weapons testing and fallout from its purview as well as the associated political controversy.[180] After years of uncertainty, discussion, and lobbying, Congress ended the bureaucratic struggle in 1964 by granting the NCRP (as the National *Council* on Radiation Protection and Measurements) a Congressional Charter.[181] The NCRP then gave itself bylaws and formalized its relationship with collaborating organizations.[182]

The ICRP was no better established in the 1950s than the NCRP. This was in part intentional. Like the NCRP, the Commission wanted to maintain its scientific focus and independence. The minutes of its informal meeting in Stockholm in 1952 noted:

> The general view was that it was not desirable to establish the Commission under Government Control [capitalization in the original] as, for example, under UNESCO. The Commission wished to maintain as much freedom as possible, though it was realized that it might be legal and other obligations that prevent complete freedom.[183]

By the early 1950s, its sole formal connection to the governmental world was "consultative" status as a nongovernmental organization with WHO. That entailed no substantial constraints on the ICRP, which lacked even

[180] This was implicit earlier in the NCRP's reluctance to set a maximum permissible limit for the general population, but Taylor made it explicit in a note of September 27, 1963, to Secretary of Health Education and Welfare Anthony Celebrezze, who chaired the FRC, see Taylor, note 3, 9-126–7. It had become largely irrelevant by then, because of the Partial Nuclear Test Ban Treaty signed the month before.

[181] For the lawyer's reversal of position, see "Synopsis of Conference on the Problems of NCRP - NBS - FRC Relationships," July 21, 1960, in Taylor, note 3, 9-044–45. For the takeover propositions, see Taylor, note 3 above, 9-045–51. For one weighing of the options, Taylor, 9-078–85. For the final legislation, "Public Law 88-376, 88th Congress, H.R. 10437, An Act to incorporate the National Committee on Radiation Protection and Measurements," Taylor, note 3, 9-145–9.

[182] The "Bylaws," Taylor, note 3, 9-153–60 and the Policy on Collaborating Organizations, 9-204–15.

[183] Ibid.

the tax-exempt status in the United States or Great Britain required to receive foundation grants.

But radiation protection had become a high-profile, worldwide issue, with many national governments and international organizations competing for resources, prestige, and attention. Failla even suggested at an ICRP meeting in 1956 that discussed Sievert's proposal for a bigger and better organization:

> ...it was now time to expand our affiliations to include all groups interested in radiation protection...to safeguard the interests of the common people with regard to radiation protection, and these people should be represented.[184]

A WHO Study Group in April 1958 challenged the competence of the ICRP to recommend maximum permissible doses, on the reasonable grounds that they required a "moral" rather than scientific judgment:

> In the example of the maximum permissible dose, it will be the duty of scientists to find out and make known what risks the public and the workers in atomic industries will suffer from present and foreseeable plans. They must also describe the probable effects of doses of radiation of whatever size, and under whatever circumstances, upon workers, the population of other countries that might conceivably be affected. But to indicate a maximum permissible dose is entirely another matter. It is doubtful if this is a proper question to put to scientists for it appears to the Study Group to be a moral problem of extremely wide and important implications as to what risks and dangers perhaps quite unconnected people may be forced to undergo as a result of human actions.[185]

Sievert as ICRP chair circulated this excerpt from the WHO Study Group report to its members along with three weighty questions:

> Why are the recommendations of the ICRP at present recognized all over the world?

[184] International Commission on Radiological Protection, Minutes of the Opening Plenary Session, April 3, 1956, ICRP/56/9, Taylor, note 3, at 8-294.

[185] "Excerpt from Report of Study Group on Mental Health Aspects of the Peaceful Uses of Atomic Energy," WHO/MH/AE/2, 1 April 1958, p. 42, as reproduced in Taylor, note 3, 8-468.

> Does the situation in the fields relevant to the work of the ICRP appear changed basically during the last 5-10 and, if so, in what respects?
>
> What must be done by the ICRP in order to enable the Commission to continue its work in the future?[186]

Having tried for years to establish the ICRP and ICRU on a firmer basis, Sievert went further and questioned whether the Commission could long survive without a better institutional foundation:

> Frankly speaking, I always feel concerned when we speak of the world-wide recognition of the ICRP and the ICRU and of our leading position.
>
> If we continue on the present scale of our work I am sure we will soon lose our reputation because we have not sufficiently realized the new order of importance of our task. Do you really think that the ICRP with its limitation in specialists and means can take the responsibility of establishing MPL 's [maximum permissible limits] affecting the entire atomic energy work? I am convinced that this will, within a few years, be impossible if we are not closely linked to a powerful safety organization working on a very broad basis.[187]

Sievert wanted the UN to organize a new, well-funded body based on UNSCEAR, the ICRP, and the ICRU, so as to ensure adoption of their radiation protection recommendations by a body more representative of all relevant fields, not just medical radiology.

The answers to Sievert's questions that Taylor preserved were long and varied, but they agreed it was the combination of expertise and independence that incentivized the world to accept the Commission's recommendations, along with its long historical record and first mover advantage.[188] They saw nothing profoundly new in recent developments,

[186] Sievert to Members of the Main Commission of the ICRP, ICRP/58/21, Stockholm, May 17, 1958, in Taylor, note 3, 8-467.

[187] Sievert to Taylor, Stockholm May 3, 1958, Taylor, note 3, 8-466.

[188] Originals of some of the replies are in ICRP Archives, Archive Files 55–65, Archive File 57, part 1.pdf, 2-146. Radiologist Sir Ernest Rock Carling, a former ICRP chair, stated: "Unless it be possible to induce the United Nations Organization to recognise I.C.R.P (as attached to W.H.O.) as the authoritative body, I can see no hope for its continuance, unless the ten million dollars of which you speak can be found." Sievert's own views are there too.

only the emergence of radiation risks on a much wider geographic scale and longer time horizon than ever before. They wanted more money for the Commission, mainly for travel and secretariat support, but resisted Sievert's effort to create a more elaborate institutional mechanism connected in some way to governments.[189] The UN Secretary General also resisted, though he was prepared to make UNSCEAR more permanent and strengthen its mandate.[190] Undermined both within the ICRP and with the UN, Sievert conceded in a meeting with Secretary General Hammarskjold that "the Commissions are expert in a limited field and therefore should not attempt to create a large laboratory or world center."[191]

Sievert also reported to the Rockefeller Foundation, which had provided funds for a meeting of the chairmen and vice-chairmen of UNSCEAR, ICRP, and ICRU in New York in June 1958 to discuss institutional issues and in 1959 for a Munich meeting of the ICRP, that the Commissions would not relinquish their independence and recruitment of their members would continue to be exclusively on their scientific merits.[192] After an informal meeting of the ICRP with delegations from other UN agencies, Sievert made a last-ditch effort with a draft Swedish UN General Assembly resolution proposing an International Co-operation Council for Radiation Safety, but even that watered-down version of his hopes met with U.S. State Department opposition and was never passed in the General Assembly.[193]

[189] The responses from Rock-Carling, Binks, Holthusen, Jaeger, and Stone are at Taylor, note 3, 8-468–76.

[190] "Report of the Secretary-General on the strengthening and widening of scientific activities in the field of the effects of atomic radiation," A/3864, 6 August 1958, in Taylor, note 3, 8-487.

[191] "Minutes of ICRP Meeting, ICRU Officers Attending," New York, N.Y., Saturday, March 8, 1958, ICRP/ICRU/NY/58/16, ICRP Archives, Box A788 Registry, ISO-ICU 1958.pdf, 117–23.

[192] "Report on the informal meeting of the chairmen and vice-chairmen of the United Nations Scientific Committee on the Effects of Atomic Radiation (UNSCEAR), the International Commission on Radiological Protection (ICRP) and the International Commission on Radiological Units and Measurements (ICRU) in New York, June 2-7, 1958," in Taylor, note 3, 8-489–90.

[193] "ICRP Meeting with Delegations from Other Agencies," Taylor, note 3, 8-497–8 and 8-501–6, the "2nd draft of Swedish Resolution to UN," September 11, 1958, Taylor, note 3, 8-488–9, and "Comments on Sievert Proposal," in a memorandum from John A. Hall, Acting Assistant General Manager for International Activities, to Philip J. Farley,

The ICRP found the solution to institutionalization in financing. The Pergamon Press agreed to publish its reports at the Press's own expense and risk.[194] The Ford Foundation in 1960 granted $250,000 over five years, passed through the Royal Swedish Academy of Science.[195] That was in addition to the usual but far smaller amounts ($10,000 or less) that the ICRP had begun receiving for specific purposes from WHO, the International Society of Radiology, UNSCEAR, and the IAEA, which by 1959 had agreed in principle to provide funding comparable to that of WHO ($10,000) and to base its own recommendations "fundamentally on the recommendations of the ICRP."[196] While the Ford grant was far less than the millions Sievert had originally hoped to get from either the Ford or Rockefeller Foundations, it was enough to enable the ICRP to continue to play a central role in international norm-setting. It hired its first full-time Scientific Secretary, David Sowby, in 1962. He would provide continuity, intellectual rigor, and institutional memory for the next 24 years.

The Commission would remain an independent, nongovernmental entity with no legal force behind its recommendations. That would prove irrelevant—and perhaps even advantageous—in meeting the need for radiation protection standards in the coming era of multi-billion-dollar power plants that would expose the world's entire population to low levels of radiation produced in routine operations and more limited numbers of people to higher levels in nuclear accidents. While Sievert contributed enormously to the ICRP's revival and vitality, he was wrong in believing that only a big institutional supporter could protect the ICRP from the

Department of State, October 23, 1958, Taylor, note 3, 8-494–5. A version of Sievert's proposal is also in ICRP Archives, Box 040, Various 1954–59 A.pdf, 192–7.

[194] "Conditions for the publication by the Pergamon Press of Reports of the International Commission on Radiological Protection and Its Committees," October 14, 1958, Taylor, note 3, 8-508.

[195] News from the Ford Foundation, for release October 10, 1960, Taylor, note 3, 9-307.

[196] The finances are reported in ICRP Publication 6. Recommendations of the International Commission on Radiological Protection (as Amended in 1959 and Revised 1962). Oxford: Pergamon Press; 1964:2. https://journals.sagepub.com/doi/pdf/10.1016/S0074-27406480004-0, accessed September 18, 2022. Henri Jammet reported the IAEA's agreement in "Representation of the ICRP at the General Conference of the International Atomic Energy Agency" (Translation from the French), ICRP/59/22 Appendix, ICRP Archives, Box A788 Registry, "Report on Decisions at 1959 Meeting.pdf," 12–14.

competition it faced from more formal and legally empowered organizations. While the Commission had written rules and standard procedures, it lacked even a constitution until 1987.[197] Funded, scientific domination and organizational independence sufficed.

Thus the NCRP and ICRP, each in its own way, had both acquired by the mid-1960s firmer institutional foundations, just as commercial nuclear power plants began to become a reality. Their construction would peak in the 1970s, around the time of the 1979 Three Mile Island accident in Pennsylvania, then tail off and eventually slow to a trickle by the time of the 1986 Chernobyl accident in Ukraine, haunted by public concern. The nuclear energy industry would test, once again, the strength of an international regime that relied on an independent, professional, epistemic group of experts seeking to protect the public from radiation and the enterprises that used radiation from publics that were alternately, and sometimes simultaneously, enthusiastic and fearful. The international regime would survive as it again tightened norms once thought adequate, as we shall see in the next chapter.

[197] Constitution of the International Commission on Radiological Protection. Approved at a meeting of the Commission at Como, Italy in September 1987; https://www.icrp.org/docs/Constitution.pdf, accessed August 11, 2023.

CHAPTER 8

Tightening Norms Again and Opening to the Public, 1965–2023

> The responsibility of those who have to decide what maximum permissible doses are appropriate will...be very large. They have to navigate between the Scylla of the hindrance of development and the Charybdis of the risks of injurious effects. A mistake may result either in unnecessarily costly protection measures or damage to large population groups.[1]
>
> —Rolf Sievert, Director of the Swedish Radiophysics Institute and ICRP Chair

Although medical applications have remained the major source of human exposure worldwide, low levels of radiation exposure from nuclear power plants rather than medical applications would dominate the discussion of radiation protection norms after the mid-1960s. Continued epidemiological monitoring of biological effects at Hiroshima and Nagasaki provided vital data. In addition, the U.S. Atomic Energy Commission (AEC) contemplated applications that were later abandoned and are now mostly forgotten but played roles in arousing public debate about radiation protection. These applications included the use of underground explosions to release natural gas from rocks (and create the cavity in which the gas could be stored) as well as nuclear explosions in outer

[1] Rolf M. Sievert, Chairman, "The International Commission on Radiological Protection," ICRP Archives, Archive Files 12–22, Archive File 22, 1.8.57 to 31.12.57.pdf, 182–8, at 182.

D. Serwer, *Strengthening International Regimes*, Palgrave Studies in International Relations, https://doi.org/10.1007/978-3-031-53724-0_8

space to counter ballistic missiles. In the end, though, it was concern over long-term biological effects, especially cancer, that led to tightening of ICRP's basic radiation protection norms, which would remain the main basis of standards throughout the world.

There were other sources of exposure to ionizing radiation that might have generated public and professional attention. As early as 1948, concern grew in the United States about the possibility of a major nuclear reactor accident. In response to an insurance company request, the NCRP declined to undertake a study of the probable effects of a large-scale release of radioactive material.[2] That prospect would remain a daunting one. But the NCRP did agree to study the rapidly enlarging problems of waste disposal and decontamination, with the understanding that at least half the people so engaged would not come from the AEC, in order to ensure as much independence as possible. The AEC had been doubling its distribution of radioisotopes every six months between June 1946 and January 1949.[3] The AEC's own national laboratories (especially at Hanford and Oak Ridge) as well as many universities, hospitals, and companies were rapidly accumulating substantial volumes of radioactive waste. The isotopes of primary interest included Iodine 131, Phosphorus 32, Carbon 14, Iron 55 and 59, Gold 198, Cobalt 60, Sodium 24, and Potassium 42.[4]

The AEC was still also concerned about workers in atomic installations, who might demand compensation, disability payments, or other special benefits for exposure to radiation hazards. The Commission again sought NCRP advice. Chair Lauriston Taylor responded in detail, but on a personal basis, that he saw no reason for any special provisions for workers in atomic installations, so long as the proper procedures were followed, as the NCRP recommendations were intended to reduce harm to readily acceptable levels. He was unequivocal: "I feel quite confident

[2] "Insurance Against a Nuclear Accident," in Lauriston Taylor, Organization for Radiation Protection: the Operations of the ICRP and NCRP, 1928–74, published by the U.S. Department of Energy, DOE/TIC-10124, 1979, 7-057.

[3] "Committee on Waste Disposal and Decontamination," ibid., 7-063–6, at 7-063.

[4] "Organization and Activities of the Subcommittee on Waste Disposal and Contamination," ibid., 7-069–71, at 070.

that today we know how to cope with all the known hazards in the radiation field."[5] Apart from individual cases resulting from negligence, there was no longer any reason, Taylor thought, for special treatment of atomic workers, which he had long opposed. He thought the NCRP and ICRP recommendations sufficed to protect both the workers and the public.

Some industries using and generating ionizing radiation welcomed ICRP and NCRP norms. Already in 1952, the Netherlands Electrotechnical Committee, after a meeting of the International Electrotechnical Commission (IEC), approached the ICRP about setting radiation standards for television sets that would make them "intrinsically safe," which meant no special measures would be required on the part of the viewer. A TV manufacturer would not have to be unusually enlightened to want to meet that requirement. While objecting to that terminology, the ICRP Secretary offered appropriate guidance in response.[6] In 1953, a delay in publication of the ICRP's recommendations led to a quandary: X-ray manufacturers wanted to know about any new requirements as soon as possible, to ensure that their equipment would comply. Those manufacturers who had representatives in the ICRP or its subcommittees would be advantaged over others. Despite concern about releasing the recommendations piecemeal, the decision was taken to share at least the most relevant recommendations.[7] Fifteen years later, Taylor for unstated reasons denied a similar GE request for draft NCRP reports the company regarded as vital to its X-ray business.[8] At least some radiation-related industries had bought into the idea that radiation protection would be good for business, and failure to protect the public would expose them to public criticism and lawsuits. Radiation protection standards would also help to cull less technically competent manufacturers from the marketplace.

The nuclear power industry was initially in a more equivocal position. Its profitability in the 1950s and early 1960s was still in doubt.

[5] Lauriston S. Taylor, Chairman NCRP to Donald B. Straus, Executive Secretary, President's Commission on Labor Relations in Atomic Energy Installations, "Guidance in Establishing Benefit Policy for Hazardous Occupations in Atomic Energy," ibid., 7-060–3, at 7-063.

[6] "X-rays from Television Sets," ICRP/53/6, ibid., 7-275–8.

[7] Oosterkamp to Taylor, November 9, 1953, ibid., 7-284–5.

[8] Kirke Malone letter March 26, 1968 at Taylor 10-071–2 and Taylor to Malone, May 15, 1968, ibid., 10-072–3.

Utilities then still believed nuclear power would depend on recycling plutonium, which required expensive and potentially dangerous chemical reprocessing of radioactive spent nuclear fuel. Industry proponents of civilian nuclear power worried more about tightened radiation protection standards than television and X-ray manufacturers. As we shall see, power industry people would express their concerns bluntly to ICRP and NCRP insiders, though ultimately nuclear power (without reprocessing) would achieve previously unanticipated low levels of radioactive emissions and the emission standards would be made significantly tighter without much industry protest. Already in 1972, Bo Lindell had reason to believe that "The nuclear power critics did not like the fact that the protection was kept at such a level that it became difficult to criticise."[9] Norms, he and others associated with the ICRP believed, could protect both the public and the nuclear power industry.

Civilian Applications Arouse More Public Concern Than Military Accidents

Civilian nuclear power relies on the same physical phenomenon, nuclear fission that produced both the controlled chain reaction at Fermi's Chicago "pile" and the explosions at Hiroshima, and Nagasaki. Used to boil water, the heat from a controlled nuclear fission reaction can drive turbines to power a ship or generate electricity. Controlling fusion, the phenomenon that produces even larger, "thermonuclear" explosions, in a way that produces substantially more energy than it uses has proven infeasible so far, despite decades of effort.

The Americans and Soviets mastered controlled fission quickly. The Americans provided proof of concept in 1951 with the startup of an Experimental [Plutonium] Breeder Reactor, one that could produce not only more energy but also more plutonium fuel than it consumed. But the main initial U.S. effort at power production was military. Admiral Hyman Rickover had built an operating naval propulsion reactor by 1953. The first U.S. nuclear submarine launched in 1954. President Eisenhower initiated international cooperation on civilian applications with

[9] Lindell B. The Toil of Sisyphus, Part IV. (1967–1999+): The Labours of Hercules, Part III (1950–66), Nordic Society for Radiation Protection; 2020.

his "Atoms for Peace" speech to the UN General Assembly in 1953.[10] The Soviets were not far behind. Their "Peaceful Atom" reactor was completed in 1954. Both the United States and the Soviet Union claimed to have produced electricity using nuclear power at the first UN Atoms for Peace Conference in 1955. The British followed at Windscale in 1956. Today, about 10% of the world's electricity generation (about 19% in the United States and 22% in the EU) is produced from nuclear power plants, which number around 440. Worldwide, about 160 military ships are today nuclear powered.

In the United States, the electric utility industry recognized early the risk of a nuclear accident, which posed a serious barrier to commercialization of nuclear power. As the NCRP had no doubt understood when it declined to undertake a study of the probable effects of a large-scale release of radioactive material, such an accident could be catastrophic. No American utility would have been able to foot the bill if the containment structure of a nuclear power plant were breached and all its radioactive material were released. Responding to the President's Atoms for Peace initiative, Congress in 1954 explicitly charged the AEC with promoting civilian nuclear power, in addition to its regulatory responsibilities. Three years later Congress enacted the Price-Anderson Act, which limited liability for public claims for personal injury and property damage caused by a commercial nuclear power plant accident, while streamlining the claims process. A total insurance pool of more than $13.5 billion currently exists for this purpose.[11] Similar limits on liability exist in other countries with nuclear power plants. In 1977, minimal standards for such

[10] International Atomic Energy Agency. Atoms for Peace Speech | IAEA [Internet]. Iaea.org. 2014. Text available from: https://www.iaea.org/about/history/atoms-for-peace-speech and video available from: https://www.iaea.org/newscenter/multimedia/videos/atoms-peace-speech, accessed November 8, 2022.

[11] Congressional Research Service. Price-Anderson Act: Nuclear Power Industry Liability Limits and Compensation to the Public After Radioactive Releases [Internet]. CRS Reports. 2018. Available from: https://crsreports.congress.gov/product/pdf/IF/IF10821#:~:text=Congress%20responded%20in%201957%20by, accessed October 23, 2022.

arrangements were adopted internationally in the Vienna Convention on Civil Liability for Nuclear Damage.[12]

Major accidents in nuclear facilities, though the subject of much concern, speculation, and dramatization, have proven frightening and deadly but few. During the 1950s they occurred in relatively small, sometimes experimental, installations. The worst happened in 1957 in Kyshtym (USSR), where a waste tank at a military plutonium-production facility exploded, but that incident was not widely known in the West until the 1970s (and not confirmed by the Soviets until 1990). A far less serious accident at the plutonium-production reactor at Windscale in Great Britain occurred in the same year, another at Vinča near Belgrade, Yugoslavia killed a student in 1958, and a third at the Reactor Test Station in Idaho Falls, Idaho in 1961 resulted in three deaths. This prompted the U.S. Army to define Emergency Radiation Protection Guides for rescue parties and property salvage.[13] Already by the mid-1960s these and other incidents had also generated substantial popular literature, both fiction and non-fiction, focused on the consequences of nuclear war and accidents.[14]

The two most serious civilian incidents between the mid-1960s and the mid-1990s were at Three Mile Island in central Pennsylvania (USA) in 1979 and at Chernobyl in northern Ukraine (USSR) in 1986. Less than two weeks after the film China Syndrome premiered in the United States based on a fictional core meltdown, operator errors and poor control room design at one (of two) Three Mile Island reactors combined to cause most of the highly radioactive core to melt down, but it remained contained in the pressure vessel and little radioactivity escaped the concrete containment structure.[15] Days of public tension generated serious issues, focused on whether to order a mass evacuation. In the end,

[12] IAEA. Vienna Convention on Civil Liability for Nuclear Damage | IAEA [Internet]. Iaea.org. 2014. Available from: https://www.iaea.org/topics/nuclear-liability-conventions/vienna-convention-on-civil-liability-for-nuclear-damage, accessed October 23, 2022.

[13] Taylor participated in this effort, see "Radiation Exposure in Reactor Emergencies," Taylor, 9-160–70.

[14] Lindell B. Depictions of Disasters in the 1950s. In: The Labours of Hercules, Part III (1950–66). Nordic Society for Radiation Protection; 2020:250–1.

[15] The Need for Change: the Legacy of TMI, Report of the President's Commission on the Accident at Three Mile Island. Washington, DC. 1979 Oct; http://large.stanford.edu/courses/2012/ph241/tran1/docs/188.pdf, accessed May 16, 2023.

the Governor decided on only a limited evacuation.[16] At Chernobyl, plant operators conducting unauthorized experiments destabilized a reactor of a different design and caused a major release of radioactive material, as the Soviet plant lacked a containment structure. Heroic efforts prevented a complete meltdown of the reactor core but several hundred people were killed and more seriously injured in the immediate aftermath. Europe was on tenterhooks for weeks as a radioactive cloud drifted north and west.[17] A Soviet radiation protection expert claimed that early interventions undertaken with international norms in mind reduced the health impact in the nearby area dramatically.[18] Twenty years later there was a "dramatic increase in thyroid cancer in children" (due to the accumulation of radioactive iodine in their thyroids) in addition to indications of "increased leukaemia incidence in Russian clean-up workers." The mental health impact eventually also caused long-term public health problems.[19] But there has not been an overall accounting for the health impacts, which may have been far more extensive.[20]

The Three Mile Island and Chernobyl disasters heightened public alarm and led to ferocious debates on nuclear power, including an advisory referendum in Sweden and an eventual prohibition of new nuclear power plants there. Norway abandoned its nuclear power plans in 1980 and Denmark in 1985, even before the Chernobyl incident. Italy phased out nuclear power after the Chernobyl meltdown, based on a referendum. Germany followed suit in 2000. But the accidents

[16] Walker JS, U.S. Nuclear Regulatory Commission. Three Mile Island: A Nuclear Crisis in Historical Perspective. Berkeley: University of California Press; 2004.

[17] Park CC. Chernobyl. London and New York: Taylor & Francis; 1989. See also Chernobyl Radiation Live Map 2022 [Internet]. Surveying Group. 2022. Available from: https://surveyinggroup.com/chernobyl-radiation-map/, accessed May 4, 2023.

[18] Llyin L, Pavlovskij O. Nuclear Power & Safety Radiological Consequences of the Chernobyl Accident in the Soviet Union and Measures Taken to Mitigate Their Impact Analysis of Data Confirms the Effectiveness of large-scale Actions to Limit the accident's Effects [Internet]. IAEA Bulletin. April 1987. Available from: https://www.iaea.org/sites/default/files/publications/magazines/bulletin/bull29-4/29402791724.pdf, accessed May 17, 2023.

[19] Sumner D. Health Effects Resulting from the Chernobyl Accident. Medicine, Conflict and Survival. 2007 Jan;23(1):31–45. https://doi.org/10.1080/13623690601084583, accessed December 12, 2022.

[20] These are the main points in Brown K. Manual for Survival: a Chernobyl Guide to the Future. S.L.: W. W. Norton; 2020.

did not arouse professional alarm about the basic radiation protection norms, in particular the permissible dose limits. Radiation protection professionals continued to believe they provided appropriate criteria for deciding whether serious harm to health had been done. Swedish ICRP Chair Bo Lindell commented after addressing a public symposium on the Three Mile Island incident at Penn State University:

> The many radiation measurements that had been carried out after the accident by scientists from a large number of scientific institutions had clearly shown that the reactor accident had not caused any worrying doses of radiation in the surrounding area. Yet there were locals who had come to the meeting not just worried but panic stricken.[21]

Lindell was still concerned about a major reactor accident that might contaminate a large area with significant amounts of radioactive material. He postulated one in the Swedish government report on "More Effective Emergency Preparedness" issued at the end of 1979, in the aftermath of Three Mile Island.[22] But he and most other radiation protection experts knew the existing norms for public exposure had not been breached at Three Mile Island. They were prepared to accept even higher doses in emergency situations and were pleased when that proved unnecessary.

There was thus no concerted scientific challenge to the notion that the existing norms provided adequate protection from the releases of radioactivity during the Three Mile Island incident. Without that ingredient, even the dramatic public concern in the immediate aftermath of the accident had no route into the process for setting radiation protection norms, which remained in the hands of the epistemic community of radiation protection professionals satisfied that they had set the norms at reasonable levels to protect both the public and the nuclear energy industry. The Chernobyl incident was more serious but still did not arouse professional alarm about the ICRP's dose limits. Bo Lindell and Dan Beninson, his Argentine successor as ICRP Chairman, would during the 1980s become proponents of tightening the ICRP norms. But even they, working with WHO, concluded within two weeks of the Chernobyl meltdown that

[21] Lindell, note 9, "The Harrisburg Meeting with Very Concerned People," 282–3.

[22] "More Effective Emergency Preparedness," ibid., 249.

"high enough doses of radiation to involve a tangible risk to the irradiated person could not really be expected outside the Soviet Union."[23] Longer-term environmental contamination nevertheless required some action, they thought, based on the existing ICRP norms.[24]

Military nuclear accidents had even less direct relevance to radiation protection norms than civilian accidents. Already before 1965 there had been 28 American "Broken Arrow" incidents (defined as an unexpected event involving nuclear weapons that result in their accidental launching, firing, detonating, theft, or loss) within the United States and abroad.[25] There were another 15 or so in the next 15 years.[26] Most of these weapons lacked the mechanisms needed to trigger a nuclear explosion. There would be another 16 American Broken Arrows before 1995.[27] None detonated. Six U.S. nuclear weapons have never been recovered. The total number of Broken Arrows in other countries is uncertain, but the Soviets lost 30 nuclear weapons aboard a single submarine in 1986.[28] Many of these incidents were known at the time, but important data was often kept secret. Public concern was evanescent and did not translate to professional alarm, because the established permissible doses for the general public were unlikely to be exceeded. The norms again served their dual purpose: to protect the public as well as the military applications of nuclear technology.

The same was not true for routine emissions from nuclear power plants. While in normal operation most radioactivity remains in the reactor core of a nuclear power plant, radioactive airborne and liquid

[23] Lindell, note 9, "Guests of WHO in Copenhagen," 331–3, at 332.

[24] Lindell reports the 20-year consequences of Chernobyl, ibid., 334–45.

[25] For one Broken Arrow incident, see Dobson J. The Goldsboro Broken Arrow: the B-52 Crash of January 24, 1961, and Its Potential as a Tipping Point for Nuclear War. Lulu Publishing; 2013.

[26] Oskins JC, Maggelet MH. Broken Arrow: The Declassified History of U.S. Nuclear Weapons Accidents. Michel H. Maggelet and James C. Oskin; 2007.

[27] Broken Arrows: Nuclear Weapons Accidents | atomicarchive.com [Internet]. www.atomicarchive.com. Available from: https://www.atomicarchive.com/almanac/broken-arrows/index.html, accessed October 23, 2022.

[28] National Security Archive. Soviet Nuclear Submarine Carrying Nuclear Weapons Sank North of Bermuda in 1986 | National Security Archive [Internet]. nsarchive.gwu.edu. George Washington University; Available from: https://nsarchive.gwu.edu/briefing-book/environmental-diplomacy-nuclear-vault-russia-programs/2016-10-07/soviet-nuclear, accessed October 23, 2022.

effluent is produced from leaks from fuel rods, activation of materials in reactor cooling water, and erosion of materials in mechanical systems as well as leakage from storage of spent fuel and other waste. That effluent was the issue that drove tightening of radiation protection standards for twenty-five years of epistemic challenges to the existing radiation protection regime in the United States and elsewhere. Both public and professional concern focused in these decades not primarily on genetic effects, as had been the case in the 1950s and 60s, but rather on the effect of low levels of radiation over long time periods on somatic (as opposed to reproductive) cell DNA. Cancer returned as a major issue in determining radiation protection norms. The normative regime shifted toward tightening with the dual purpose of protecting the civilian nuclear power industry as well as the public.

The Experts Expect No Tightening of Norms

The norm-tightening was not anticipated or welcomed among radiation protection professionals or industrial experts in the early 1960s. Some thought the standards could even be loosened in order to accommodate national security and economic interests. Before the signature of the Partial Test Ban Treaty, Harald Rossi, a Columbia University biophysicist and member of the NCRP, argued that somatic effects would likely follow a "modified threshold" (rather than the linear, no-threshold hypothesis) and that "it may occasionally be necessary to permit radiation levels that represent a larger risk, simply because of over-riding considerations of national interest."[29] He and other radiation protection experts believed that taking into account the benefits of radiation would necessarily lead to loosening, not tightening, of the NCRP and ICRP recommendations. He proposed increasing the maximum permissible levels by a factor of 100. He must have been supremely disappointed by the tightening that ensued decades later.

The nuclear industry was still concerned about possible tightening of the radiation protection norms. A General Electric official working at Hanford and NCRP member, H. M. Parker, had written to Taylor in 1956 to protest a rumored tightening of the ICRP maximum permissible dose by a factor of one-third. He was "horrified" and thought "the

[29] Rossi to Taylor, September 14, 1962, Taylor, note 2, 9-094.

effects on the atomic energy program could be extremely drastic" because of "the needless waste of funds" required to meet a lower permissible dose.[30] A Canadian counterpart at Chalk River likewise protested, but to Sievert.[31] Dow Chemical, which was planning to reprocess plutonium from nuclear power plants, was concerned that the ICRP and NCRP recommendations would make it uneconomical to do so and urged Taylor and Sievert to "...do what you can to see that permissible limits of radiation are not further reduced without adequate justification."[32]

As the NCRP prepared to update its basic radiation protection recommendations in the early 1960s, it faced many technical issues, including some that involved the relationship between its recommendations and those of the ICRP.[33] But there was no sign of any major impending revision to the recommended maximum permissible doses.[34] An epidemiological study confirming life-shortening among American radiologists generated more curiosity than alarm.[35] Taylor suggested in 1967 that "permissible dose" be defined as the "dose of ionizing radiation accumulated under specified conditions that, in the light of present knowledge, is not expected to cause appreciable bodily injury to a person at any time in his lifetime." He continued to emphasize that "there has not yet been

[30] "Parker to Taylor," June 19, 1956, Taylor, note 2, 8-317.

[31] Taylor, note 2, 8-329.

[32] To Taylor from the Director of the Health Physics and Medical Section, Dow Chemical, "ICRP and NCRP Recommendations," January 8, 1960, note 2, 9-313.

[33] Karl Z. Morgan, "Some Topics for Consideration by the Executive Committee of NCRP from Subcommittee 2," August 10, 1964, Taylor, note 2, 9-194–6.

[34] "Revision of Handbook 59 (to Members SC-1)," NCRP/64/19, July 30, 1964, Taylor, note 2, 9-172–9.

[35] Seltser R, Sartwell PE. The Influence of Occupational Exposure to Radiation on the Mortality of American Radiologists and Other Medical Specialists. American Journal of Epidemiology. 1965 Jan 1;81(1):2–22, accessed July 12, 2023. Life-shortening had been reported more than 10 years earlier by Warren S. Longevity and Causes of Death from Irradiation in Physicians. Journal of the American Medical Association. 1956 Sep 29;162(5):464. https://doi.org/10.1001/jama.1956.72970220006007, accessed July 12, 2023. The Shields Warren paper at the time did arouse questions inside the ICRP, but no changes to the recommendations: "Minutes of Joint Meeting ICRP-ICRU Revised," ICRP/56/28 and ICRU/56/10, October 31, 1956, ICRP Archives Box W-18, Archive files 33, 177–8.

established any causative relationships between any radiation exposure at permissible levels and any injury."[36]

On the international level there was also no anticipation of tightened norms. The ICRP, ICRU, and UNSCEAR had jointly initiated in 1959 a major study of somatic effects.[37] By the 1960s, all three organizations were newly concerned with environmental monitoring in the vicinity of nuclear power plants and other radiation-producing installations. But the ICRP, like the NCRP, anticipated no major revisions, and even considered watering down its recommendation that members of the general public not be exposed to more than one-tenth the maximum permissible dose to workers in radiation establishments.[38] H. J. Muller, who had to resign from the ICRP in 1965 for health reasons, was anxious to ensure that his replacement on the Commission would be a geneticist who shared his concerns.[39] The Commission also considered maximum doses in the event of an incident at an atomic energy establishment that were many times higher than those permitted in routine operations, following the precedent set for military applications.[40] In April 1969, the ICRP's main subcommittee concerned with basic radiation norms was focused on dose limits to the lens of the human eye, quality factors applicable to different forms of radiation, and "uses and limitations of further refinements of data for purposes of protection." These included whether to raise its recommended dose limits. The ICRP itself rejected the committee's narrow focus, but without initiating a broader effort.[41]

[36] Taylor, quoting himself, note 2, 9-414.

[37] The ICRP/ICRU/UN Study plans are documented at note 3, 9-314–23. The report appeared in 1961, ICRP-47.

[38] The then-existing recommendations are helpfully summarized in "ICRP Recommendations on Maximum Permissible Doses for Non-Radiation Workers and Members of the General Public," note 2, 9-340–42. The potential watering down is referred to in H. J. Muller's note "to All Members of the Main Commission," August 13, 1962, 9-372.

[39] Muller to Pochin, February 12, 1065, ICRP Archives, Box W-18, Archive Files 29, 168–170.

[40] Report from Committee V to the Commission. "The Application of the Recommendations of the ICRP to the Control of Activities Resulting in Environmental Contamination," ICRP/62/S-9, May 11, 1962, note 3, 9-342–5.

[41] "Report on the Meeting of the International Commission on Radiological Protection (ICRP), April 1969," Taylor, note 2, 10-338–40.

Controversy Brews

Controversy would brew by 1970 within both the NCRP and ICRP. It was rooted in the ambiguity of what was meant by "maximum permissible dose." While Taylor was correct in believing no specific diseases in specific people had been traced to radiation exposure at that level, others were concerned about what later came to be known as "stochastic" effects, that is chance events at lower doses.[42] If the linear no-threshold (LNT) hypothesis were correct and the probability of a particular biological effect at higher doses known, then it was possible to extrapolate, using a straight line, how many people might suffer that effect at lower doses. This from Taylor's perspective was hypothetical, not real, but from the point of view of someone contracting leukemia it was real, not hypothetical. The AEC, charged with promoting uses of nuclear energy, naturally took Taylor's perspective: no biological effects had been observed below the maximum permissible dose. But the Secretary of the ICRP observed at the time:

> The individual effects are really 'probabilities' of effects, and in this case the probability is very low for any particular individual. But in a population there will be some effects, and this load to society may be too great, even though the individual risks are acceptable. We have this situation today with road accidents.[43]

The issue of effects at lower doses was raised within NCRP/ICRP circles by Oak Ridge health physicist K. Z. Morgan in 1965. He supervised monitoring the accumulated doses of 4500 employees at Oak Ridge and had worked on estimating the radiation doses at Hiroshima and Nagasaki. From that data, he estimated the then current ICRP recommendation of maximum permissible dose for the general population (0.5 rem/year) could lead to 300,000–3,000,000 deaths worldwide. He was understandably reluctant for the NCRP to publish this estimate.[44] But such population risk calculations were readily made. He offered an example in

[42] The earliest sign I have seen of this sort of calculation is in "[K.Z.] Morgan to [Leonard] Hamilton," August 26, 1965, Taylor, note 2, 8-319–21.

[43] Sowby FD. Survey of Comments on Third Draft of 1965 Recommendations. ICRP/65/MC-11, note 2, 9-463–4.

[44] K. Z. Morgan comments on ICRP/64/MC-14, note 3, 9-441–3.

testimony in late 1969 and then became in the 1970s a critic of the ICRP even while sitting on its Main Commission.[45]

He was not alone in his concerns. The public controversy had its origins in the publications of University of Pittsburgh professor Ernest J. Sternglass. Trained at Cornell in applied engineering and physics, Sternglass moved from Westinghouse to the University of Pittsburgh School of Medicine to develop electronic imaging in medicine. He became a professor of radiology and director of radiation physics, as well as a professor of radiological physics in the Graduate School of Public Health.[46] So Sternglass by all appearances was a medical radiation professional. A strong proponent of banning atmospheric testing of nuclear weapons, in 1963 he had suggested that fallout in the 1950s correlated with pauses in declining infant mortality in parts of the United States. He claimed that fallout from nuclear weapons testing may have caused 400,000 infant deaths and 2 million fetal deaths in the United States.[47] Sternglass, however, was an outsider to the tightly knit scientific community centered on the NCRP and ICRP. Shut out of access to data he wanted by the AEC, Sternglass chose to publish and speak in what professionals regarded as unworthy public fora, including Esquire magazine and NBC's Today show.[48]

Despite his media presence, Sternglass would have gained little traction on his own. As an outsider and individual with little professional reputation or following, he presented no serious threat to the authority of the

[45] Congressional Hearings on the Health and Safety Act of 1968, Taylor, note 2, 10-388. Morgan was later voted off the main ICRP commission but made an emeritus member, "ICRP in Brighton," Lindell, note 9, 133–43.

[46] Fitzgerald M. The High Resolution Life: Ernest Sternglass, Nuclear Reductionist. PittMed. 2015; https://www.pittmed.health.pitt.edu/story/high-resolution-life, accessed November 6, 2022. A second University of Pittsburgh professor, epidemiologist Edward P. Radford, later joined those who thought risk estimates for radiation exposure should be raised and chaired a controversial NAS BEIR III report, see "NAS Study Takes the Middle Road," Science, Vol. 204, May 18, 1979, 711–4.

[47] Boffey PM. Ernest J. Sternglass: Controversial Prophet of Doom. Science. 1969 Oct 10;166(3902):195–200. https://doi.org/10.1126/science.166.3902.195, accessed September 12, 2023.

[48] Hacker BC. Elements of Controversy: the Atomic Energy Commission and Radiation Safety in Nuclear Weapons testing, 1947–1974. Berkeley: University of California Press; 1994:253. See also Lindell, note 9, "Sternglass," 57–8 and "The Nordic Society for Radiation Protection in Copenhagen," 103–106 for Sternglass' reception in Britain and Scandinavia, where openness turned quickly to rejection.

NCRP and ICRP. His work all too obviously conflated correlation with causation. His critics dismissed what they regarded as his mostly spurious correlations between radiation and health effects. The ICRP Scientific Secretary in 1971 wrote to Lindell:

> Perhaps like the monkeys at the typewriters he may occasionally produce something worthwhile, but his performance so far has been such that I for one find it extremely irksome to delve any more into his writings.[49]

But one of Sternglass' critics, physicist Arthur R. Tamplin, saw merit in the idea of tightening the existing radiation standards. Tamplin, a physicist who was a research associate at the AEC's own Lawrence Livermore Laboratory, joined forces with John Gofman, who had been invited to join a scientific committee of the NCRP but declined.[50] Gofman also worked at Livermore but was a professor of medical physics with both a doctorate and a medical degree at the University of California, Berkeley. Far more credible than Sternglass working alone, Tamplin and Gofman based their work on data that the NCRP and ICRP also used. They focused their critique on the AEC and Federal Radiation Council (FRC) standards, which were however essentially identical to the norms recommended by the NCRP and the ICRP.

The two AEC-affiliated scientists advocated reducing by a factor of 10 the "maximum allowable radiation dosage to the population from peaceful nuclear activities."[51] They declared to the Executive Director of the FRC, in a note distributed widely to scientists, government officials, and members of Congress:

> You have stated so well publicly that we have made a direct frontal attack on all radiological biology and on all standards, including those of the Federal Radiation Council, the International Commission on Radiological

[49] David Sowby to Bo Lindell, November 26, 1971, ICRP Archives, Archive Files 66–75, Archive File 66, Misc Docs 1.pdf, 84–6 at 85.

[50] "Report Review Procedures," Taylor, note 2, 10-102. In light of later developments, Taylor regarded Tamplin's refusal to join the committee a "lucky break" for the NCRP.

[51] Tamplin AR, Gofman JW. The Radiation Effects Controversy. Bulletin of the Atomic Scientists. 1970 Sep 1;26(7):2–8. https://www.tandfonline.com/doi/pdf/10.1080/00963402.1970.11457836, accessed November 8, 2022.

> Protection, and the National Committee on Radiation Protection. We do indeed make this direct frontal attack.[52]

Their testimony before the Senate Subcommittee on Air and Water Pollution in late 1969 prompted a letter from Senator Edmund Muskie to Lauriston Taylor at the NCRP.[53] Taylor responded at length, with the approval of the NCRP Board, by pointing to the conservative character of the LNT hypothesis. He claimed that the limits were "probably excessive by substantial factors."[54] He noted as well that the NCRP had revived its Committee on Somatic Dose for the General Population, originally established in 1959 (which had previously recommended no downward revision in the maximum permissible dose). This revival was intended to "explain the problem in a manner which can be understood by the lay public and by scientists who are not familiar with radiation protection history and philosophy."[55] Taylor was not only dismissive of Gofman and Tamplin's technical arguments, but also criticized them for failure to publish in professional refereed journals and to submit proposals for changes to the NCRP, ICRP, or FRC. He suggested that Senator Muskie and his committee had a vital role in weighing the risks of radiation against the economic and social consequences of limiting their use. Taylor and others were convinced that weighing the benefits of radiation would make the NCRP and ICRP permissible limits look entirely reasonable.

The leadership of the American epistemic community focused on radiation protection was mostly cohesive and rallied around Taylor, publishing

[52] John W. Gofman and Arthur R. Tamplin to Dr. Paul Tompkins, Executive Director, Federal Radiation Council, "The Federal Radiation Council Review of Radiation Standards for Population Exposure," December 26, 1969, ICRP Archives, Archive Files 66–75, Archive Files 66, Misc Docs 1.pdf, 57–61.

[53] John W. Gofman and Arthur R. Tamplin, "Federal Radiation Council Guidelines for Radiation Exposure of the Population-at-Large—Protection or Disaster?" Testimony presented before the Sub-Committee on Air and Water Pollution, Committee on Public Works, United States Senate, 91st Congress, November 18, 1969, ICRP Archives, Box 054, Circular letters 1970.pdf, 11–32.

[54] "Political Activity," which includes Muskie's December 1, 1969 letter and Taylor's January 23, 1970 reply, note 2, 10-106–10. Taylor was even more annoyed when Senator Muskie wrote directly to the ICRP, note 2, 10-356–60: "As you can see I am not very happy."

[55] Ibid., at 10-109. The new report was never officially published by the NCRP but sought to justify, once again, the existing norms, see "Radiation Dose to the General Population: Ad Hoc Committee Report," March 1971, Taylor, note 2, 10-156–62.

in two different journals a statement that vaunted, “At present FRC recommendations are directly derived from those of the ICRP, an international body that draws upon the accumulated wisdom of experts from the entire world.”[56] The norms reflected shared values that the American expert community, which had played a major role in their evolution, was prepared to defend. Even Gofman and Tamplin tipped their hats to the authority of the ICRP, while attacking its recommendations. In a joint note to its Main Commission members in March 1970, they declared, emphasizing their commonalities with the ICRP:

> The ICRP, to its lasting credit and honor, has always taken the conservative approach requisite to protection of the public health in every area where direct data are unavailable.....We thank our lucky stars that the ICRP has existed and exists today. And we wish to do everything possible to be of help, to the extent of our limited abilities, to the ICRP in the continued effective guidance it has provided.[57]

They also defended their presentation to a meeting of the Institute for Electrical and Electronic Engineers and to the U.S. Senate, said their work would be submitted to refereed journals (as it subsequently was), and criticized the AEC for reluctance to take long-term risks into account. Above all, they wanted the promotional and regulatory functions of the AEC separated. Gofman also wanted all release of all pollutants limited to zero and only allowed after a public process demonstrated the need to run the associated risks.[58]

Unlike Sternglass, who had offered his own often dubious data, the Gofman and Tamplin critiques of the existing norms were based on data that the NCRP and ICRP had also used. While sometimes aggregating

[56] “Reprinted from the ACR Bulletin of June 1970,” Taylor, note 2, 10-366–7.

[57] John W. Gofman and Arthur R. Tamplin to The Members of the ICRP, “An Earnest Request for Our Mutual Cooperation in Furtherance of the Understanding of Radiation Carcinogenesis,” March 2, 1970, ICRP Archives, Archive Files, Archive Files 66–75, Archive File 66, Misc Docs 1.pdf, 54–56.

[58] A Congressional Seminar: (A) the History of Erroneous Handling of the Radiation Hazard Problem in Atomic Energy Development (Presented by John W. Gofman); (B) A proposal for a Rational Future Protection Policy with Respect to Radioactivity and Other Forms of Pollution (presented by Arthur R. Tamplin,” April 7–8, 1970, GT-119-70, ICRP Archives, Archive Files 12–22, Archive File 12, 401–26, at 425.

data differently, the underlying research basis was the same.[59] This heightened the impact of the criticism. Gofman and Tamplin differed mainly in their guesstimates of dose, not effects. That would prove prescient. But the value proposition also differed. It was not sufficient, Gofman and Tamplin believed, that stochastic effects at low levels of exposure and low dose rates were undetectable. Nor was it sufficient to suggest the LNT hypothesis might not hold at low doses and dose rates. At any dose, people might die. There were still real human beings at risk. To them, the risks were not real, not hypothetical.

The newly prominent American critics would continue their public campaign to tighten the ICRP norms. Tamplin soon faced off against Taylor in an unsuccessful Federal court challenge to an AEC plan to release radionuclides at Rulison, Colorado after detonation of a small nuclear bomb underground to stimulate release of natural gas from the surrounding rock and store it in the cavity created by the explosion (Project Ketch).[60] This was part of the Atoms for Peace program, which included "Project Ploughshare" for nonmilitary applications of nuclear explosions. Taylor won this round. The court found that the existing AEC standards (based on the NCRP and ICRP recommendations) embodied an adequate risk–benefit evaluation based on "the best available scientific knowledge" and that no compelling evidence had been presented that they should be lowered by a factor of 10, as Tamplin and Gofman wanted.[61] Once again, radiation protection standards had been found adequate to protect both health and an application utilizing radiation.

Norms on the Defensive

The AEC and NCRP success would not last long. Again the main push for tightening norms would come from within the United States. Amidst a wave of environmental activism, President Richard Nixon in 1970 proposed creation of the U.S. Environmental Protection Agency (EPA),

[59] Sowby D. ICRP Secretary, "Gofman/Tamplin Reports," March 31, 1970, Taylor, note 2, 10-359.

[60] "Rulison Detonation," quoted from the Health Physics Society Newsletter of December 1970, Taylor, note 2, 10-036–40.

[61] Taylor also faced off against Gofman and K.Z. Morgan in various court cases in the 1980s, "Lauriston Taylor v Karl Morgan," Lindell, note 9, 309.

which took over the radiation protection functions of the Federal Radiation Council, thus fulfilling one of the goals of Gofman and Tamplin.[62] The EPA did not maintain the FRC's explicit link to the NCRP and quickly contracted with the National Academy of Sciences for an updated version of its report on biological effects of ionizing radiation. Senators Muskie and Mike Gravel were expressing openness to Gofman and Tamplin's critiques. Well before the NAS report was ready, the AEC preempted it by hastening in 1971 to lower its limits on radioactive effluent from nuclear power plants by a factor of 100, which it had come to regard as technologically and economically feasible.[63]

This unanticipated move worried Taylor, who continued to think the permissible limits sufficient to protect human health. While acknowledging that the AEC was correct in tightening its standards for nuclear power plants to minimize radioactive effluent to the lowest practicable level, Taylor was concerned that the AEC's move would lead to pressure to reduce the overall dose limits to the general population.[64] This the NCRP opposed, because nuclear power plants were only one source of radiation exposure of the general population. They still contributed a negligible dose received by the general population (less than 2% of the total from man-made sources other than medical exposure). Accelerating its work, the NCRP set up no less than five different expert committees under the aegis of an "ad hoc" committee to assess public radiation exposure from consumer products, nuclear power generation, natural background radiation, medical examinations, and occupational exposure. It also issued in January 1971 a defense of its basic radiation protection recommendations.[65] This in turn was followed quickly by a report of the ad hoc committee, which again defended the NCRP's basic radiation

[62] Brinkley D. Silent Spring Revolution: John F. Kennedy, Rachel Carson, Lyndon Johnson, Richard Nixon, and the Great Environmental Awakening. HarperCollins; 2022.

[63] Walker JS. Permissible Dose, A History of Radiation Protection in the Twentieth Century, J. Samuel Walker, 2000. Berkeley: University of California Press; 2000:47.

[64] "Taylor to McCool," August 6, 1971, Taylor, note 2, 10-173. Taylor was reacting to the proposed rulemaking, published in the Federal Register, Vol. 36, No. 111, June 9, 1971. Taylor later testified in favor of the AEC's tightening of the power plant standards, while expressing concern about the implications of requiring all radiation sources to meet a "lowest practicable" standard, see Taylor, note 2, Annex T, "Testimony at AEC Hearings on ALAP [as low as practicable], 1972.

[65] The text of this Report 39 is no longer readily available, but it was the subject of a press conference at the Mayflower Hotel, January 26, 1971, see Taylor, note 2, 10-152–4.

protection recommendations while suggesting that the Council adopt in the future a risk/benefit approach to each category of radiation exposure.[66] Even with pressure from the AEC reduced, the foot dragging in the NCRP persisted. The epistemic group was committed to maintaining its norms and reluctant to acknowledge that they might be too lax.

There was moreover an institutional problem, recognized even before the ad hoc committee was constituted. As the risks were imposed on the general population, should it not be somehow represented in weighing risks and benefits? Should there not be "outsiders" involved, in keeping with the environmentalist and consumerist spirit of the times?[67] The general membership of the NCRP formally approved a proposal to the Board of Directors to constitute another ad hoc committee on "social responsiveness" of the Council, but the Board deferred on that question.[68] The NCRP instead proposed a project to assess risks and benefits in one or more of the five sources of exposure, including people from outside radiation biology and related areas of expertise to evaluate broader social and economic factors with a "judicial" objective "of weighing carefully and dispassionately how much the benefits of certain technological advances must be to outweigh potential risks to life and health." The draft report on these issues, never formally published, justified the existing NCRP maximum permissible dose for the general population while suggesting that the NCRP would need a far more elaborate, "rational" process seriously to evaluate benefits and compare them to known and extrapolated risks.[69]

Events would not permit that process to be undertaken. Instead, the National Academy of Sciences would intervene, as it had in 1956, though with far less effect. Word reached the public before the end of 1972 that the NAS Committee on Biological Effects of Ionizing Radiation (BEIR in this iteration) would describe the existing norm of 170 millirem per

[66] "Radiation Dose to the General Population," Ad Hoc Committee Report, March 1971, Taylor, note 2, 10-156–62.

[67] Sixth Annual Meeting of Members, March 19, 1970, Taylor, note 2, 10-110–12.

[68] Seventh Annual Meeting of Members and 21st Meeting of the Board of Directors, March 18, 1971, Taylor, note 2, 10-162–7. The idea died in the hands of Russell Morgan, who constituted a "one-man committee" to prepare to give the matter further consideration, Taylor, note 2, 10-172.

[69] The report's main recommendations and conclusions are reflected in a 1972 proposal for foundation funding, Taylor, note 2, 10-211–4.

year (equivalent to 5 rem over a 30-year generation) as "unnecessarily high."[70] Adopting a risk/benefit framework, the NAS report suggested societal needs could be met at lower levels of risk. NCRP members who participated in the BEIR Committee had not been permitted to review the "Summary and Conclusions," where this statement appeared. Already concerned that its "position of leadership" had "been definitely slipping in the past decade," the NCRP undertook a "crash evaluation" of maximum permissible doses.[71] An UNSCEAR report complicated the situation, because it accepted the notion of "population dose," that is "the product of the number exposed and the dose to which each is exposed" (expressed as man-rads), a product that permitted calculation of risks to the general population on the basis of the LNT hypothesis. That was precisely the kind of calculation that Sternglass, Tamplin, and Gofman advocated as a basis for tightening the maximum permissible doses.

The issues that led the NCRP, BEIR Committee, and UNSCEAR to different conclusions arose from different understandings about the LNT hypothesis, which was accepted in principle by all three. The science was ambiguous, or at least left room for different interpretations. The NCRP regarded the LNT hypothesis as specifying *maximum* biological effects and thought the low rate at which doses normally accumulated in members of the public as well as natural repair mechanisms would make the carcinogenic and mutagenic effects to the general population significantly less than the hypothesis suggested. The Council would eventually conclude that it would not use the term "sum of individual doses to members of the general population" (which UNSCEAR called "population dose") or calculate "population risk". The NCRP instead averred that

> ...risk estimates for radiogenic cancers at low doses and low dose rates derived on the basis of any extrapolation from the rising portion of the

[70] National Academy of Sciences and National Research Council. The Effects on Populations of Exposure to Low Levels of Ionizing, report of the Advisory Committee on the Biological Effects of Ionizing Radiation [Internet]. 1972 Nov. https://inis.iaea.org/collection/NCLCollectionStore/_Public/37/004/37004410.pdf, accessed February 4, 2023.

[71] Proposal that the NCRP Initiate a New Activity Concerned with Reassessment of the Maximum Permissible Dose Equivalent Levels. Taylor, note 2, 10-218–9.

> dose incident curves at high doses and dose rates have such a high probability of overestimating the actual risk as to be of no value for risk/benefit analysis.[72]

The BEIR Committee and UNSCEAR, while agreeing with the NCRP that the LNT hypothesis likely overestimated biological effects, preferred an excess of caution.

A More Receptive International Response

While their work fell on deaf ears at the NCRP, Gofman and Tamplin got a more mixed reaction among non-American radiation protection experts. The UNSCEAR Secretary, Francesco Sella, was dismissive: "I do not believe that anyone who is in the slightest bit used to risk estimates, and the problems they bring, ought to concern themselves with Gofman and Tamplin's argument."[73] But it had not been the ICRP's intention to allow nuclear reactors to increase radiation in the environment to the level specified by ICRP as a genetically permissible dose to the general population (5 rem over a 30-year generation). As Vice Chair of the Main Commission, Lindell wrote to ICRP colleagues that Gofman and Tamplin's one-tenth proposal, applied only to radiation from nuclear power reactors, was reasonable:

> I have realised that Gofman and Tamplin have demanded that the share for this purpose [nuclear power] be 0.017 rem per year and I find that this concurs with what we think ourselves and with ICRP's philosophy and, last but not least, also with the actual safety planning that is currently taking place.[74]

Lindell lamented further the Commission's defensive posture toward Gofman and Tamplin:

> I was somewhat disappointed with the Commission's attitude during the meeting, and Dan [Beninson] told me, at his own initiative, that he was too. We had the impression that the main goal now seems to be guarding

[72] Radiation Quantities—Population Dose (II), Taylor, note 2, 10-308–9.

[73] Lindell, note 9, Gofman and Tamplin. pp. 71–75, at 73.

[74] Ibid.

> a status quo and that any statement or action might, by definition, be a change to the worse. My impression is that Gofman and Tamplin are doing some of the work that the Commission might be expected to do and I find some quite fresh arguments in their book, even though I find its title [Population Control Through Nuclear Pollution] disgusting, their language uncivilized, their arguments often weak and biased and some of their thinking quite naive. Nevertheless they tell some truths which are true also to us except that we have been too cautious to tell them. And, again, overcautiousness may result in greater hazards, also for ICRP.[75]

He was no less agitated six months later:

> …we react like mechanical puppets or like insects shown a stimulus triggering aggressive reactions, when we are faced with statements or ideas which are not branded with the mark of the old truth. Should we not instead be curious and appreciative?[76]

Lindell was particularly concerned about the use of nuclear explosions for excavation, but he was also concerned about nuclear power plants, which were being treated differently in different countries.[77] Citing different standards in Germany, Sweden, and the United States, Lindell wrote:

> Most of these policies are incompatible and the situation seems to become what it has not been in other cases: a chaos of national norms while the resulting radioactive contamination does not respect national borders. Why has not ICRP been ahead of this development?[78]

[75] Lindell to Sowby, May 4, 1971, ICRP Archives, Archive Files 35–45, Archive File 43, SOWBY July 1972.pdf, 127. This and other more technical points about risk estimates and dose limits are discussed in Lindell to Sowby, March 10, 1970, ICRP Archives, Archive File 43, SOWBY July 1972.pdf, 202–5.

[76] Lindell To Sowby, November 25, 1971, Taylor note 2, 10-389–93. This extraordinary letter deals not only with Sternglass, Gofman, and Tamplin but also with other controversial issues like radiation exposure in supersonic aircraft and for pregnant women. Lindell, who was ICRP Vice Chair, had other complaints about the ICRP's mode of operation, see Minutes of the Commission Meeting in Ottawa: March 1972, ICRP Archives, Box W-10, in "Minutes 1953–72.pdf," 4–16, at pp. 11–12.

[77] Ibid.

[78] Ibid.

The American NCRP, still beholden to the AEC and uncertain for its own future with the newly empowered EPA, did not ask this kind of question. The ICRP, less subject to U.S. hegemony than in the past, quietly appointed in May 1970, at more or less the height of the Gofman/Tamplin controversy, a small group, chaired by Argentine physician and biophysicist Dan Beninson, to report to the Main Commission on the possibility of modifying its recommended dose limits.

Beninson and Lindell were by this time best friends. They had met in 1956 at the United Nations and would constitute what Lindell later acknowledged as the "Beninson-Lindell mafia."[79] Both were specialists in the sense that their main professional focus was radiation protection. They were government officials, not practicing radiologists or laboratory scientists, though Lindell had laboratory scientists who worked with him. Technically competent and mathematically inclined, Lindell and Beninson viewed themselves as working to protect people from radiation as well as to allow medical radiology, nuclear energy, and other beneficial applications of radiation to progress and benefit the world. Despite Lindell's concern about the variability of emissions from nuclear power plants, he was convinced of their virtues for producing electricity and prepared to defend their use with numbers, as he believed that they could be used consistent with even tightened ICRP norms.[80]

Beninson and Lindell would remain best friends as their lives intertwined with the international institutions concerned with radiation protection. Lindell was an engineer who became head of the Swedish radiation licensing authority in 1965. A protégé of Rolf Sievert, he had served temporarily as Scientific Secretary of UNSCEAR in 1958 in addition to assisting Sievert as Secretary of ICRP, a position he left in 1962 to become a member of the Main Commission. Following Sievert's retirement, he would become Swedish representative to UNSCEAR 1965–88 and serve as its Chair 1970–71 and 1987–88. He also chaired the ICRP for two terms, 1977–81 and 1981–85. Beninson, trained as a physician in Buenos Aires, studied radiation physics and biology at the University of California,

[79] Lindell B. Tribute to Dan Beninson. Journal of Radiological Protection. 2004;24:91–2. https://iopscience.iop.org/article/10.1088/0952-4746/24/1/L01/pdf, accessed August 20, 2023.

[80] Lindell to Charles B. Meinhold, June 11, 1969, ICRP Archives, Archive File 35, Comm 3 Task Group Grande 1965–70.pdf, 8–10.

in addition to playing "blitz" chess with Bobby Fischer.[81] He worked in and later directed Argentina's Nuclear Regulatory Authority and eventually chaired its National Atomic Energy Commission. He was a member of the Main Commission of the ICRP for more than three decades (1968–2001) and its chair 1985–93. He, too, served on UNSCEAR, where he was rapporteur in 1979–80, Vice Chair in 1981–82, and Chair in 1983–84.

These two men from lesser powers in the geopolitics of the Cold War were key influential figures in the international radiation protection regime from at least the early 1970s for more than two decades. They expressed themselves and exercised influence in different ways. More reserved in person, Lindell was a prolific letter-writer who corresponded with dozens of experts, including many of the ICRP's critics in Sweden and abroad. There is little Beninson correspondence in the ICRP Archives, but he was ebullient in person, as well as a good listener and inveterate smoker. He wrote unsigned papers that presaged changes in the Commission's concepts and recommendations. Both devoted seemingly unlimited time and energy to their ICRP and UNSCEAR roles, which they treated as at least as important as their national responsibilities. Relishing travel, they thrived on the stimulus of their international colleagues. Certainly the shaping of the international regime for radiation protection gave them far more influence, and satisfaction, than the often routine regulatory responsibilities they both exercised at home.

In a memorandum subsequently rejected by the Main Commission, Beninson's committee charged with recommending maximum permissible doses suggested acknowledging bluntly that radiation protection was stretching the limits of science:

a. That protection criteria especially when applied to individuals, which are capable of practical implementation, can never have a completely scientific basis.
b. That all such limitations cannot be overcome either by experimental studies or by recalculation from existing data.
c. That consequently, for the purposes of radiological protection, the utilization of new data is likely to be profitable in the future only if

[81] Taper B. Prodigy [Internet]. The New Yorker. 1957. Available from: https://www.newyorker.com/magazine/1957/09/07/prodigy-3, accessed August 20, 2023.

> carried out with great discrimination and if directed toward aspects on which there is both a clearly established need and reasonable ground for anticipating a practically useful outcome.[82]

This discussion of the limits of science for establishing radiation protection norms arising from the difficulty in establishing biological effects at low doses, especially for genetic risks, was too much for the Main Commission. The doubts were never published.

The Beninson group was sent back to work to fulfill the charge of presenting "a definitive proposal on either maintaining or changing the present system."[83] The basis of the existing norms was a longstanding interest of Beninson's. Lindell recounts that when they first met Beninson

> ...began bombarding me with Spanish inquisition-style questions. On which basis had ICRP chosen its dose limit? If it was not obvious that there were threshold values for dangerous doses of radiation, the choice had to reflect a view of which risk could be acceptable. How had they arrived at such a risk?[84]

While recognizing the authority and utility of the existing ICRP norms, Beninson's group did not like their basis, which the group described as a threshold supplemented by a safety factor. It produced a report

[82] "Uses and Limitations of Further Refinements of Data for Purposes of Protection," ICRP/69/0:C1-13, April 17, 1969, note 3, 10-339–40.

[83] The never published Beninson report "ICRP Task Group on Dose Limits Report to Main Commission" is in ICRP Archives, Archive Files 1–11, Archive File 11, 65–6 B.pdf, 119–91. Taylor provides a brief summary "Report of the Task Group on Dose Limits," note 2, 10-427, and in Appendix V he gives the bulk of the report. The date appears to be 1973. A draft of the full report, presumably the one discussed in 1972 at the ICRP meeting at Great Fosters appears in ICRP Archives, Box G044, Discussed at meeting at Great Fosters Engl. 1972.pdf, 1–72. David Sowby regarded the results as fortuitous: "Our present approach is to discuss levels of risk considered to be acceptable for non-irradiation conditions, and then to use these levels to arrive at a dose limit. In the case of whole body exposure it turns out that the dose limit based on this method exactly equals the one we have had for the past two decades," Sowby to Lindell, October 21, 1974, ICRP Archive Files 34, Sowby 1974–76, at 216. The idea of comparing radiation risks with those in other occupations was not new, see E. E. Pochin, "Biological Bases for Standards and Maximum Radiation Levels Under Normal Conditions," Scheveningen, December 1961, ICRP Archives, Box 039, C1 TG Spatial Distribution 1965–1969.pdf, 61–70. Pochin was an ICRP Main Commission member and became its Chair in 1962.

[84] Note 14, 205.

not intended for publication that proposed a new approach, rooted in previous ICRP publications on risk estimates.[85] Agreeing with BEIR and UNSCEAR, it concluded "There are no grounds for using anything but a linear relationship in making decisions in radiation protection at levels of dose at or below the dose limits."[86] It would no longer suffice to assert that there were no known effects below the level of the dose limits, as Taylor had repeatedly done, echoing the tolerance dose concept while claiming not to rely on it. Instead, Beninson's group wanted the ICRP to establish a more coherent, logical basis for its norms. It did this using the concepts of population dose and population risk that the NCRP had forbidden, even though the risks might be overestimated due to the LNT hypothesis.[87] Since quantitative balancing of risks and benefits was not possible, the group suggested relying instead on quantitative comparison of the occupational risks due to radiation with the risks in other occupations and on comparison of the risks to the general population from radiation to other risks in everyday life. On this basis, it concluded that the existing dose limits were still adequate.[88]

For some Main Commission members, including Lindell and Beninson, that conclusion weakened in the next few years. While genetic risk estimates were revised downward based on clinical human genetics as well as from relevant theoretical and experimental studies, new data were becoming available from studies of Japanese survivors (*hibakusha*) at Hiroshima and Nagasaki on leukemia.[89] Its implications were not yet as clear as they would become in the 1980s, but in 1975, K. Z. Morgan,

[85] ICRP. The Evaluation of Risks from Radiation: A report prepared for Committee I of the International Commission on Radiological Protection and received by the Committee on April 20th, 1965. Pergamon Press. 1966; Publication 8. https://journals.sagepub.com/doi/pdf/10.1016/S0074-27406580002-2, accessed July 30, 2023 and Radiosensitivity and Spatial Distribution of Dose: Reports prepared by two Task Groups of Committee 1 of the International Commission on Radiological Protection. Pergamon Press. 1969; Publication 14. https://journals.sagepub.com/doi/pdf/10.1016/S0074-27406980001-2, accessed July 30, 2023.

[86] Ibid., V-13.

[87] ICRP Task Group on Dose Limits Report to Main Commission. Taylor, note 2, Appendix V.

[88] Ibid.

[89] "Report on Meeting of ICRP Committee 1," Harwell, England, November 18–21, 1975, in ICRP Archives, Box G054, Circular letters 1976 and Whiteshell 1976.pdf, 120–7.

who had moved to Georgia Tech but was still an Emeritus Main Commission member, wanted the occupational limit halved and dose limits to individuals tightened, partly on the basis of the Hiroshima and Nagasaki data.[90] In 1976 doubts about the adequacy of the occupational dose limit were forwarded to the Main Commission by its Scientific Secretary.[91] An unpublished paper on dose limits prepared for the Main Commission the same year, presumably by Dan Beninson, confirmed those doubts. It suggested, on the basis of comparison with other risks of everyday life, that the acceptable risk of death from radiation for an average member of the general public should be five in a million.[92] That would have required a significant reduction in the ICRP's recommended dose limit for the general population.

While that calculation received support from the head of the "Soviet NCRP," the draft recommendations proposing a consequent reduction in the dose limits ran into stiff resistance.[93] The Commission responded by convening a "special" meeting at Woodstock (England) that decided not to change either the occupational limit or the limit to the general public.[94] Beninson and Lindell were still arguing in favor of tightening the 0.5 rem/year norm (of committed effective dose equivalent), now called five "millisievert" (mSv). But the then dominant British and Canadians in the Commission–led by physician Sir E. E. Pochin–were opposed,

[90] K. Z. Morgan to David Sowby, February 19, 1975, ICRP Archives, Box #29, Archive Files 35–45, Archive files 34, Sowby 1974–76.pdf, 175–8.

[91] F. D. Sowby to Members of the Main Commission, April 14, 1976, "Quality Factor for Neutrons," ICRP/76/MC-151976-04-14, ICRP Archives, Circular letters 1976 and Whiteshell 1976.pdf, 34, forwarding a paper prepared by Harald Rossi that had been sent to the Chair by A. C. Upton, which is at 35–40.

[92] "Report on Dose Limits," ICRP/76/MC-13, Box G054, Circular letters 1976 and Whiteshell 1976.pdf, 19–29.

[93] See, for example, G. W. Dolphin, "ICRP 29," ICRP Archives, Archive Files 35–45, Archive File 41, Cirk 1977–1978.pdf, 252, Charles B. Meinhold, ibid., 265–7, Liniecki, Comments, ICRP/77/MC-4, ibid., 268–70, H. J. Dunster to Sowby, January 5, 1977, ibid., 272–3. The Soviet support is in a paper by L. A. Ilyin, who in the 1990s became a member of the Main Commission, see "Comments of the NCRP of the USSR to Draft 4, Recommendation of the International Commission on Radiological Protection," ICRP/75/B.MC-2, ICRP Archives, Archive Files 35–45, Archive File 44, Circular MC-G- 1975.pdf, 245–53.

[94] "Minutes of Special Main Commission Meeting, Woodstock, 1977," ICRP/77/MC-13, ICRP Archives, Archive File 41, Cirk 1977–1978.pdf, 205–6. Beninson himself moved the adoption of the unchanged recommendations.

forcing Lindell to offer a compromise that preserved the official numerical norm but conditioned it in ways that he hoped would limit actual doses to no more than 20% of that figure (0.1 rem or 1 mSv/year).[95] Without either compelling new data or more intense public pressure, an epistemic group like the ICRP had little reason to undermine its own previous judgment, and much reason to maintain constancy in its recommendations, though at least three of its more specialist, non-physician members had been prepared to make the change.

Beninson's unpublished paper on risks, which had suggested a reduction in the permissible dose was needed, was redrafted in 1977. The new draft confirmed that the existing 0.5 rem/year dose limit to the general public would result in a risk of death in the range of one in 10,000, higher than other acceptable risks to the public, but it also noted that the average radiation dose to the general public had in fact been found to be an order of magnitude less. On that shaky basis, it confirmed that the existing limit was adequate to ensure the risk of death from radiation would be in the acceptable range of one in a million to one in 100,000.[96]

While the 1977 recommendations of the ICRP did not change the previous numerical dose limits, they included other major reforms.[97] Lindell explained to British physicist Joseph Rotblat, who had worked on the Manhattan Project but left it and became a vigorous opponent of nuclear weapons, that the maximum permissible dose was no longer to be treated as a planning device but rather as an absolute limit, not to be reached year after year: "the MPD is transformed from a planning level to an absolute annual ceiling."[98] The recommendations abandoned the earlier notion of critical organs and established procedures for aggregating doses of different radionuclides to an individual, arousing controversy

[95] Lindell, note 9, "ICRP in Woodstock," p. 194.

[96] "Report on Dose Limits," ICRP/77/B:MC-5, May 5, 1977, ICRP Archives, Box G054, Circular letters 1996.pdf, 109–121. Resistance to lowering the occupational dose limit came from several Commission members, see.

[97] These are discussed in detail and defended in Lindell DB, Sowby FD. International radiation protection recommendations. Five years experience of ICRP Publication 26 (IAEA-CN-42/15). Nuclear Power Experience, Proceedings of an International Conference, Vienna, 13–17. 1982 Sep;Volume 4: Nuclear Safety:3–22. https://inis.iaea.org/collection/NCLCollectionStore/_Public/14/779/14779115.pdf?r=1, accessed August 24, 2023.

[98] Lindell to Rotblat, January 17, 1978, ICRP Archives, Archive Files Box 81, Archive Files 81 part 2.pdf, 92–3.

because they allowed higher limits than previously for some radionuclides (and imposed lower limits for others).[99] The 1977 recommendations also codified what would become an enduring strategy for radiation protection. The main principles were these:

a. no practice shall be adopted unless its introduction produces a positive net benefit;
b. all exposures shall be kept as low as reasonably achievable, economic and social factors being taken into account; and
c. the dose equivalent to individuals shall not exceed the limits recommended for the appropriate circumstances by the Commission.[100]

These principles were not a departure from past practice. Avoiding unnecessary exposures to ionizing radiation had, in one formulation or another, been part of the recommendations since before World War II. The ICRP had long been thinking of its recommendations as balancing costs and benefits, even if it could not quantify them. The purpose of the ICRP dose limits had always been to protect individuals. But this is the first time the Commission codified its approach so simply and directly. The principles eventually became known as (a) justification, (b) optimization, and c) limitation. They would remain the basis for the ICRP's work until the present, with (a) and (b) regarded as satisfying Jeremy Bentham's and John Stuart Mill's "utilitarian ethics" and (c) as an example of Immanuel Kant's "duty ethics."[101]

[99] See, for example, Dickson D. Radiation: ICRP Rules Row. Nature. 1980 Jun 1;285(5764):350. https://doi.org/10.1038/285350a0, accessed August 9, 2023. The ICRP received voluminous responses to its request for comments on practical applications of the 1977 recommendations, ICRP Archives, Box 815, Task Group reviewing Pub. 26.pdf, 31–354. Lindell received a scathing critique from Edward Radford, a colleague of Sternglass at the University of Pittsburgh, November 14, 1979, ICRP Archives, Archive Files 81, Archive Files 81 part 1.pdf, 68–71.

[100] Recommendations of the ICRP. Annals of the ICRP. ICRP Publication 26(Oxford: Pergamon Press):3. reprinted 1987.

[101] Clarke RH, Valentin J. The History of ICRP and the Evolution of its Policies, invited by the Commission in October 2008 and published in Annals of the ICRP 2009.

The ICRP Tightens the Norms

The more formal tightening of ICRP numerical norms awaited three developments: the arrival of new data, a push from within the Commission from members who were specialized in radiation protection (especially Lindell and Beninson), and renewed public concern.[102] The new data came in the early 1980s from an old source: close to 80,000 Japanese survivors exposed to ionizing radiation at Hiroshima and Nagasaki. Continuing study of this group led to reevaluation of stochastic risks. The biological effects, mainly leukemia, were not in doubt. The dosimetry was: the suspicion started as early as 1981 that the *hibakusha* had been exposed to fewer neutrons at Hiroshima than had previously been estimated.[103] The recalculation of doses resolved an outstanding quandary that had suggested different rates of radiation-induced death at Nagasaki and Hiroshima.[104] Data also became available on people who were children at the time of the Hiroshima and Nagasaki bombings, causing an increase in the overall risk previously estimated for older people since the children would be exposed for more years to ionizing radiation.[105]

Much of this was known in the early 1980s, but the ICRP only gradually moved to reduce the maximum permissible dose for the general population. In 1983, the Commission tightened its wording to put more emphasis on a reduced limit for those repeatedly exposed for long periods:

[102] The tightening of the basic dose limits discussed here was only one of many changes from 1977 to 1990. These are reviewed in Clarke RH. Changes in Underlying Science and Protection Policy. Nuclear Energy Agency (OCSCE), Evolution of ICRP Recommendations 1977, 1990 and 2007. NEA No. 6920, 2011. https://www.oecd-nea.org/upload/docs/application/pdf/2019-12/6920-icrp-recommendations.pdf, accessed August 25, 2023.

[103] Working Group "Report to the Thirtieth session of UNSCEAR UNSCEAR/XXX /9", Vienna, 6 to 10 July 1981 (7 July 1981), Chairman: Prof. Z. Jaworowski (Poland) and Rapporteur: Dr. K.H. Lokan (Australia), ICRP Archives, Box 26, Archive files 90, "C-1.pdf," 10–11. See also "New A-Bomb Studies Alter Radiation Estimates," Science, Vol. 212, May 21, 1981, 900–903 and Science, Vol. 214, October 2, 1981, 31–2. The impetus for the recalculation of doses came from researchers at Lawrence Livermore Laboratory, the same lab where Gofman and Tamplin had worked.

[104] Preston AV, Prentice RL, ass. Koda M. Possible Between-City Inconsistency of Dose-Mortality Relationship in A-Bomb Survivors Using T65DR and LLNL Dose Estimates. Radiation Effects Research Foundation, approved 31 March 1983, printed September 1985. https://www.rerf.or.jp/library/scidata/tr_all/TR1983-06.pdf, accessed February 27, 2023.

[105] Lindell, note 9, 358–61.

> For stochastic effects in members of the public the Commission recommends that the committed effective dose equivalent from exposure to radioactive materials in any year be limited to 5 mSv, and, for repeated exposures over prolonged periods, that it would be prudent further to restrict this to 1 mSv from each year of lifelong exposure.[106]

In 1984, the Commission clarified how to calculate the effective dose commitment but made no further change in the numerical norm.[107] A committee of the ICRP had already examined the implications of the revised doses at Hiroshima and Nagasaki as well as twenty-five papers in the epidemiological literature but had concluded that reports of excess cancers at low or undetermined doses were "at best questionable." It issued a statement saying: "no changes in current cancer risk estimates are required at the present time."[108]

Beninson however was not satisfied. He revisited his risk calculations in an unsigned paper prepared at the end of 1984, while Lindell was ICRP chair. It demonstrated once again, as he had in 1976 before redrafting, that 1 mSv was closer to the region of acceptable every day risk for members of the general public than 5 mSv.[109] With Beninson newly elected to chair in 1985, the ICRP shifted its position in the direction his unsigned paper suggested, emphasizing 1 mSv (which Beninson and Lindell had advocated at least since 1977) rather than 5 mSv as the principal limit for the general population:

> The Commission's present view is that the principal limit is 1 mSv in a year. However, it is permissible to use a subsidiary dose limit of 5 mSv in a year for some years, provided that the average annual effective dose

[106] ICRP Publication 26, note 100. Statement from the 1983 Meeting of the International Commission on Radiological Protection, at 67.

[107] Ibid., Statement from the 1984 Stockholm Meeting of the International Commission on Radiological Protection, at p. 75.

[108] Report of Committee 1 to the Main Commission, Stockholm, May 14–18, 1984, ICRP/S: C1-01, 1984-5-16, para 1.1 and the appended report ICRP/84/S:C1-04, ICRP Archives, Box W-10, Minutes 1962-96.pdf, 165–82.

[109] "The Dose Limits," ICRP Archives, Archive Files 46-53, Archive File 53, part 1.pdf, 143–50.

equivalent over a lifetime does not exceed the principal limit of 1 mSv in a year.[110]

This shift was rooted in a critical examination of the risks associated with the ICRP's dose limits, prompted by concerns that its previous recommendation was confusing and relied on rounded numbers in ways that were hard to justify. This argued for a new set of basic recommendations. John Dunster, the Director of the UK Radiation Protection Board who would become the principal author of the 1990 recommendations, was already offering ideas for how the Commission should approach the process in 1985.[111] By then, the 1977 recommendations had been amended dozens of times in Commission statements and committee reports.[112] The moment had come for a comprehensive revision.

This time, tightening of the permissible limits was anticipated. The Three Mile Island accident had heightened public concern. By 1984, the ICRP had drafted a major report on planning protection for the public in the event of major radiation accidents.[113] Beninson, a supporter of nuclear energy, had long preferred to err on the side of caution. Several years later, he responded to a question about so-called "de minimis" (small) doses of radiation that some wanted to ignore:

...if you were to overlook all doses/risks which did not lead to significant evidence in the injury statistics, you would obtain different 'de minimis' values depending on the size of the population. Even doses of radiation exceeding current dose limits would be negligible, but it would scarcely be

110 ICRP Publication 26, note 100 above. Statement from the 1985 Paris meeting of the International Commission on Radiological Protection, at p. 79.

111 H. J. Dunster, "The Basic Objectives and Policy of the Commission: A Discussion Note," ICRP/85/MC-35, ICRP Archives, Archive Files 48–54, Archive File 48 (54), PartB.pdf, 215–7.

112 Nineteen amendments in Commission statements and forty-seven in Committee reports are listed in "Policy Statements Issued Since ICRP Publication 26," ICRP/86/MC-04, ICRP Archives, Archive Files 48–54, Archive file 48, PartA.pdf, 23–30.

113 ICRP, "Principles for Planning Protection of the Public in the Event of Major Radiation Accidents," ICRP/84/C4-5/1, ICRP Archives, Box 26, Archive Files 89, "Committee 4 Task Group 1984.pdf," 64–109. This appeared later in the year as ICRP, 1984, Protection of the Public in the Event of Major Radiation Accidents - Principles for Planning. ICRP Publication 40. Ann. ICRP 14 (2).

a pleasing protection ambition to wait until you could 'count the bodies' before providing the protection.[114]

Ignoring the biological effects of low doses, as Taylor effectively had advocated when he suggested no detectable health effects below the maximum permissible limits, would no longer do. Lawsuits in the United States, some won and some lost by plaintiffs against nuclear employers, were attracting public attention.[115] So too did the legal maneuvering after the death of Karen Silkwood, a nuclear worker contaminated with plutonium who was suing her employer when she died in a mysterious auto accident in 1974. Her family won its case in the U.S. Supreme Court in 1984.[116] While that incident and some others were unrelated to nuclear electricity, the public increasingly needed reassurance if nuclear power and other applications of ionizing radiation were to survive. Then the Chernobyl accident in April 1986 dramatically underlined the need for such reassurance, as it understandably shifted European public opinion against nuclear power.[117]

In addition, tightening the norms had epidemiological support. The U.S.-Japan Atomic Bomb Radiation Dosimetry Committees, established in 1982 to re-examine the doses delivered at Hiroshima and Nagasaki, concluded in March 1986 that a new dosimetry system should replace the

[114] Note 2, "IRPA in Sydney," 370–72, at 372. The Secretary of the ICRP, David Sowby, and Bo Lindell, its Chair, had already argued against the "de minimis" advocates in 1984, Memorandum to Members of the Main Commission, "The question of trivial or de minimis levels," January 20, 1984, ICRP/84/MC-01, ICRP Archives, Box 26, Archive Files 89, "Committee 4 Task Group 1984.pdf," 2–7. The issue of "de minimis" levels was also the focus of an exchange of letters between Bo Lindell and Walter Marshall in 1982, ICRP Archives, Box W-10, Commission Correspondence 1996.pdf, 26–34. Beninson was best friends with Lindell and would have known about these exchanges.

[115] These were reviewed by Ralph E. Lapp, "Cancer Risk and Litigation," AIF Conference on Insurance and Legal Issues in the 1980s," New Orleans, January 23, 1985, ICRP Archives, Archive file Box W-10, Commission Corespondence 1996.pdf, 86–105.

[116] Silkwood v. Kerr-McGee Corp., 464 U.S. 238 (1984) [Internet]. Justia Law US Supreme Court. Available from: https://supreme.justia.com/cases/federal/us/464/238/ accessed September 24, 2023.

[117] Verplanken B. Public Reactions to the Chernobyl Accident: a Case of Rationality? Organ. Environ. 1991 Dec;5(253):253–69. https://journals.sagepub.com/doi/epdf/10.1177/108602669100500402, accessed March 4, 2023.

one previously used.[118] Donald Pierce and Dale Preston at the U.S.-Japan Radiation Effects Research Foundation determined cancer risks based on the recalculated doses of neutrons and gamma rays at Hiroshima and Nagasaki.[119] The effects were greater than had previously been thought. Beninson, Lindell, and others in the ICRP likely knew of this result before its publication and would have anticipated public concern. They had already begun asking fundamental questions about the Commission's existing recommendations and how they might be revised.[120] Beninson in his 1987 charge to the committee preparing what would become the 1990 ICRP recommendations stated that the 1 mSv/year (0.1 rem/year) figure for public exposure (down by a factor of five from the 1977 recommendations) would be their basis.[121] This was equivalent to "the radiation dose that person would receive from natural background radiation," a dose limit that both NCRP and ICRP had cited as an aspiration 32 years earlier. The committee, which Beninson chaired, accepted his charge.[122]

By the time the ICRP met at Como, Italy in September 1987, the Preston-Pierce report was a major issue, as noted in a public statement after the meeting and in Lindell's trip report on the meeting.[123] There

[118] US-Japan Atomic Bomb Radiation Dosimetry Committees (US Committee Chairman: Frederick Seitz Japanese Committee Chairman: Eizo Tajima), "Joint Statement on the Reassessment of the Atomic Bomb Radiation Dosimetry and the Establishment of a New Dosimetry System," 17 March 1986, Hiroshima, ICRP Archives, Archive Files 48–54, Archive File 49 (54), PartA.pdf, 385–6.

[119] Preston DL, Pierce DA. The Effect of Changes in Dosimetry on Cancer Mortality Risk Estimates in the Atomic Bomb Survivors. Radiation Effect Research Foundation. 1987. This paper was later published in *Radiat Res.* 1988 Jun;114(3):437–66. An abstract is available at https://pubmed.ncbi.nlm.nih.gov/3375435/, accessed March 4, 2023.

[120] "Revision of the Commission's Basic Recommendation," ICRP/87/MC-05, ICRP Archives, Archive Files 46–53, Archive File 53 part 1.pdf, 543–70.

[121] ICRP Archives, W-18 Archive Box 32, ICRP Como 1987, "Minutes of the ICRP Meeting Washington USA 1987," March 18, 1987, 190–95. Beninson reiterated the 1 mSv figure in a note to the Main Commission dated August 18, 1987: "The value of the limit for members of the public should be based on risk considerations and be equivalent to the dose received from the 'usual' natural background (about 1 mSv)," Beninson to Dear Colleague, ICRP 87/C: MC-02 in ICRP Archives, MCTG 1987.pdf, 178–83 at 181.

[122] Ibid., ICRP/87/MC-1/71987-06-10, "Minutes of a meeting of a Main Commission Task Group (previously a drafting group) held at N.R.P.B.," Chilton, Oxon, United Kingdom from 27–29 May 1987.

[123] "ICRP meeting with the Committees in Como," Lindell, note 9, 358–61, at 359. The minutes of the Committee 1 meeting in Como summarize the discussion of the

was still public pressure to reduce the norms further. Friends of the Earth organized a campaign for lowering the occupational dose limits, including a petition signed by 800 scientists from around the world.[124] The Como meeting attracted far more public attention than previous ICRP gatherings. Lindell reported:

> The meeting aroused international attention for the first time in the history of ICRP, with German television on site and petitions from a number of environmental organisations, including Friends of the Earth, and critical scientists like Alice Stewart and John Gofman.[125]

Papers submitted by Stewart, a British epidemiologist and longstanding nuclear critic who had campaigned against prenatal radiological exposure, and by Friends of the Earth (UK) advocating tightening of dose limits were discussed in an ICRP committee.[126] The committee agreed with a memorandum received from an unidentified French source in which Gofman suggested that a revision of the risk estimates was a matter of priority, due to the data from Hiroshima and Nagasaki.[127] But the Main Commission also thought its recently tightened norm for the general population sufficient and preferred to await the report of yet another NAS Committee on the Biological Effects of Ionizing Radiation (BEIR V) expected in 1988 (but not actually published until 1989).[128] The

Preston-Pierce report, see ICRP Archives, Box W-10, "Minutes 1962–96.pdf," 96–113. It is also referred to in "Statement of the 1987 Como meeting of the International Commission on Radiological Protection," Archive Files 96, MC 1987.pdf, 32–42.

[124] The Friends of the Earth efforts and critique are presented in a letter to the editor from Patrick Green, "The response of the International Commission on Radiological Protection to calls for a reduction in the dose limits for radiation workers and members of the public," International Journal of Radiation Biology. 1988;53(4):679–82, https://www.tandfonline.com/doi/pdf/10.1080/09553008814551001, accessed August 1, 2023.

[125] Lindell, note 9, "ICRP meeting with the Committees in Como," 358–61, at 359.

[126] ICRP Archives, Box W-10, Minutes of ICRP Committee 1 Meeting Como, Italy: 7–11 September 1987, "Minutes 1962–96.pdf," 96–113.

[127] Ibid.

[128] ICRP. Statement from the 1987 Como Meeting of the International Commission on Radiological Protection. Radiation Protection Dosimetry. 1987 Jul 1;19(3):189–92. https://doi-org.proxy1.library.jhu.edu/10.1093/oxfordjournals.rpd.a079941, Environmental groups were not happy. UK Friends of the Earth registered its objection to the ICRP's decision not to lower dose limits at Como, Green P. The Response of

Commission then concluded neither it nor the 1988 report of UNSCEAR provided additional reasons to tighten the norm for public exposure further.[129]

At least some portions of the nuclear industry did not object to the tightened permissible limits. British physicist John Dunster forwarded to fellow Main Commission members in July 1987 a note from Amersham International that he thought "most clearly stated the views expressed by the major users of radioactive materials and radiation."[130] Amersham, a radiopharmaceutical manufacturer, had no comment on specific dose limits but urged that the ICRP base its recommendations on risk estimates (compared to those of other occupations) rather than "social judgements" and "give greater emphasis to justifying de minimis levels of dose below which it is not sensible to attempt to achieve further reduction."[131] The international dose limits were needed, Amersham said, to help protect the industry: "If different standards were applied in different countries it would only provide more ammunition for the anti-nuclear lobby." The ICRP later credited Dunster with being the principal author of the 1990 recommendations, so the Amersham note may well have been influential.[132] Dunster certainly welcomed it.

the International Commission on Radiological Protection to Calls for a Reduction in the Dose Limits for Radiation Workers and Members of the Public. International Journal of Radiation Biology. 1988;53(4):679–82. https://doi.org/10.1080/09553008814551001. So too did H. Stockinger for the Austrian Naturschutzbund Salzburg Regional Section in a letter to Beninson, ICRP Archives, A805, Comments on draft 90-G01.pdf, 57. See also Read "Health Effects of Exposure to Low Levels of Ionizing Radiation: BEIR V" at NAP.edu [Internet]. nap.nationalacademies.org. Available from: https://nap.nationalacademies.org/read/1224/chapter/1, accessed March 6, 2023. No doubt Beninson knew its conclusions well before 1990, as Arthur C. Upton, then chair of an ICRP committee, also chaired BEIR V.

129 UNSCEAR. Sources, Effects and Risks of Ionizing Radiation 1988 Report to the General Assembly, with annexes United Nations [Internet]. Available from: https://www.unscear.org/unscear/uploads/documents/unscear-reports/UNSCEAR_1988_Report.pdf, accessed March 6, 2023.

130 John Dunster to Dr. D.J. Beninson, Dr. H. Jammet, Prof. J. Liniecki, Mr. C.B. Meinhold, and Dr. W.K. Sinclair, July 14, 1987, ICRP Archives, Box A801 Registry, MCTG 1987.pdf, 184.

131 The Amersham note is from A. McNair, Safety Controller, ibid., 185–9.

132 ICRP, "H John Dunster CB ARCS BSc FSRP 1922–2006," May 12, 2006, https://www.icrp.org/page.asp?id=101, accessed August 8, 2023. Dunster's note asking for employer input prior to the 1987 Como meeting as well as a summary of the replies

The 1990 recommendations stuck with the 1 mSv/year number for exposure of the general population.[133] It has remained the norm for limiting the dose to the general population ever since. The Commission at the same time reduced the maximum permissible limit for occupational exposure to 20 mSv/year (down from 50 mSv/year) averaged over five years. This was less stringent than Friends of the Earth had sought. The British National Radiation Protection Board had preferred 15 mSv/year.[134] The competent French authorities strongly protested the reduction of the occupational dose limit, but the German authorities concurred because the new figure was more consistent with existing German regulations.[135] One American member of the Main Commission received from Oak Ridge Associated Universities a strong objection to the tightening of the norms, but less due to the dose limits and more due to the increasing attention to optimization, which required keeping emissions "as low as reasonably achievable."[136]

The Commission attributed the tightening to "New data and new interpretation of earlier information," which indicated "with reasonable certainty that some risks associated with ionising radiation are about three times higher than they were estimated to be a decade ago."[137] As usual, it focused on the immediate scientific rationale, omitting mention of public

is at ICRP Archives, Archive Files 96, MC 1987.pdf, 77–90. He also received input from the Trades Union Congress.

[133] 1990 Recommendations of the International Commission on Radiological Protection. ICRP Publication, 60. https://journals.sagepub.com/doi/pdf/10.1177/ANIB_21_1-3, accessed March 4, 2023.

[134] Clarke RH. Interim Guidance on the Implications of Recent Revisions of Risk Estimates and the ICRP 1987 Como Statement. www.ostigov [Internet]. 1987 Nov 1; Available from: https://www.osti.gov/etdeweb/biblio/5544248#fullrecord, accessed August 1, 2023. This is an abstract of the document, which I have not found.

[135] "Position of the French Competent Authorities on the New ICRP Recommendations (February 1990 draft)," ICRP/90/MC-W/07, June 18, 1990, ICRP Archives, Box G043, "Minutes of C 1 -Bethesda Maryland 1990.pdf," 51–4. The French predicted "disastrous effects both on the public and the workers involved" due to fear and disavowal of the previous limit. For the German position, see Heinrich Joachim Hardt of the Bundesminister für Umwelt Naturschutz und Reaktorsicherheit Geschäftszeichen to O. Ilari of the NEA/OECD, March 8, 1990, ibid., 94–5.

[136] William A. Mills to Warren Sinclair, May 29, 1990, ICRP Archives, Archive Files 1–11, Archive File 9, MC-1-18-1988.pdf, 119–24.

[137] ICRP, "Statements and Annual Reports part 2.pdf," Press Release, November 12, 1990, Statements and Annual Reports Part 2.pdf, ICRP Archives, Misc Box 4, at 97.

pressure in the wake of the Chernobyl incident, the suggestions and petition from the Friends of the Earth, and the long effort by Beninson, Lindell, K. Z. Morgan and others to tighten the norms. An early draft had acknowledged not only new biological information but also the Commission's effort "to maintain as much stability in the recommendations as is consistent with the new information and thus to minimise the problems of authorities and operating managements in implementing the new recommendations."[138] Protecting the applications of radiation was still a major concern.

Geographic Diversity Grows, but Slowly

As discussed in the previous chapter, the ICRP was far more secure as an institution by the early 1960s than it had been in the 1950s. It had financing from the Ford Foundation as well as WHO, the IAEA, and UNSCEAR. It also had working cooperation with the ILO and FAO. But the Commission was still predominantly West European and North American in membership. In 1956, only a single member of one of the Subcommittees (A.R. Gopal-Ayengar, India) was from what was termed then a "Third World" country, out of a total of about 60 members. At least one of the ICRP committees in 1959 still had essentially the same membership as its American NCRP counterpart. As a result, the NCRP committee chose to publish an "expurgated" version of the ICRP report.[139] In 1962 the Main Commission included a Swedish Chair and a Swedish Secretary, four Americans, three Brits, two Germans, and one expert each from Denmark, Canada, and France. This was little changed from the 1930s.

Rumblings of dissatisfaction with the ICRP's geographic basis had begun in the 1950s. The International Congress of Radiology (ICR), which formally appointed the ICRP's members, suggested that the nominees selected by the Commission, who were invariably approved, should be more representative. In 1955, the ICRP Scientific Secretary told Rolf Sievert that

138 ICRP, "DRAFT - IN STRICT CONFIDENCE, RECOMMENDATIONS OF THE COMMISSION 1990,"ICRP/88/MC-1/32, 1988-11-08, ICRP Archives, Archive files 94-102, "97 MC1988-90 A.pdf" 167–8. I have not found this frank statement in the final version.

139 "Committee II Report on Internal Dose," Taylor, note 2, 9-264.

> The radiation-protection problems which have to be faced concern all nations and we must, therefore, envisage some expansion of the membership of the Commission and its Subcommittees in order to include other experts in the world.[140]

He hastened to add however that recent retirees from the Commission could be invited to meetings, to "maintain the scientific contacts and the friendships which we all value so highly." Sievert in 1960 considered a proposal from Failla to

> ...reorganize the Commission in that way that all the present members of the Committees are included in the Commission and the Main Commission is transformed into the Executive Board of the ICRP. It would thus be easier to cover more nations in the Commission itself than at present.[141]

While this particular stratagem was never used, other devices would keep the Commission's decision-making firmly in the hands of North Americans and West Europeans for decades in the future.

Concerns about radiation were unquestionably spreading worldwide. In 1962, the League of Arab States invited the ICRP to an "Arab Conference on Ionising Radiations and Protection Measures Against Their Hazards." While unhappy that it was "dominantly political in makeup," the ICRP decided to send its newly appointed British Chair, Edward Eric Pochin, but limited his participation to the non-political subjects of health and medical aspects, excluding cooperation among Arab states, national legislation, and French bomb tests in Algeria.[142] At a meeting of ICRP and ICRU officers in 1963, "It was agreed there was a need for broader geographical membership of both commissions."[143] Still reluctant to take on anyone for "political" reasons, the Commissions decided to reach out to the national delegations to the ICR to seek additional experts professionally qualified for their work.

[140] Binks to Professor Sievert, ICRP/55/8(c), November 7, 1955, Taylor, 8-275.

[141] Sievert to Pochin, Stockholm, May 4, 1960, Taylor, 9-301.

[142] "The Arab Conference on Ionising Radiations and Protection Against Their Hazards," ICRP/62/3, Appendix 1, page 2, Taylor, 9-336–7.

[143] "Meeting of ICRP and ICRU Officers," May 8–9, 1963, ICRP/63/MC21, Taylor, 9-939–6.

Participation broadened, but slowly. According to one of its leading lights, radiation protection in the Soviet Union had suffered after World War II from lack of equipment, resources, and training as well as secrecy, restrictions on human rights, and a focus on the military's need for chemicals that would protect exposed people from radiation effects.[144] The LNT hypothesis was taboo as a basis for decision-making, as it allowed risk to workers, contrary to (nominal) Communist doctrine.[145] The first Atoms for Peace Conference in 1955 opened the door to communication with Soviet experts.[146] Physician-radiologist M. N. Pobedinsky became the first Soviet member of an ICRP Committee in 1956. Sievert in a brief retirement letter in 1963 hoped the ICRP would maintain an even number of physical and biological experts among its members and find a Soviet physicist to join.[147] That was not to be. The first Soviet elected to the Main Commission was physician Avgust Andreevich Letavet in 1965. The first ICRP meeting in the Soviet Union appears to have taken place in 1972.[148] Lindell said then he was pleased with the level of Soviet technical competence.[149] Seeking to demonstrate their value added, the Soviets in 1973 prepared for an ICRP task group a 65-page report.[150] It had taken the better part of three decades to expand the epistemic community to encompass the Soviets, who were by then anxious to contribute.

The first Latin American, and for a long time the only one in the ICRP, was Buenos Aires-trained physician and U.S.-experienced physicist

[144] These problems are specified in Scientific Research into Protection of the Public against Radiation: Real Achievements and Lost Opportunities. In: Chapter 2 in Chernobyl: Myth and Reality, translated from the Russian. Moscow: Megalopolis; 1995:28–35.

[145] The Soviet taboo on the LNT hypothesis and on the risk/benefit analysis required to define "acceptable risk" is discussed in ibid., 269–75.

[146] See, for example, Morgan to Krotkov, November 1955, note 3, 8-260–61.

[147] Sievert to the Members of the Main Commission, November 27, 1963, ICRP Archives, Archive Files 46–54, Archive file 47, Archives 47 part 1.pdf, 261.

[148] See "ICRP Committee 3 in Dubna and Moscow" for Lindell's account, with the usual drinking tales, Lindell, note 9, 114–16.

[149] Lindell to Sowby, April 20, 1972, ICRP Archives, Archive Files 43, SOWBY July 1972.pdf, 49.

[150] Yu. I. Moskalev to W. J. Barr, "About the Biological Action of Transuranium Elements which Enter the Animal Body through the Respiratory Tract." Archive Files 1–11, Archive File 11, 65–66 B.pdf, 1–65.

Dan Beninson, elected to the Main Commission in 1963.[151] In that year there was still only one non-European, non-North or South American on an ICRP committee (Egyptian physician and IAEA official Hussein Daw, listed in 1965 as from the United Arab Republic). Asians and other Africans came much later. In 1966 no members of the ICRP task groups, which had far wider participation than the Commission itself, were non-European and non-American.[152] Geographic diversity remained an issue in the following decade, even if the one-time American hegemony had long since declined. In 1973, the four British members of the Main Commission voted out one of two Americans, K. Z. Morgan, causing a brouhaha that ended with his returning as a non-voting Emeritus member.[153] At Whiteshell, Canada in 1976, English speakers still retained a majority on the ICRP main commission, though it was an Anglophone majority that discomforted the Americans:

> The Commission that met in Whiteshell included four Englishmen, two Canadians and one American, so there was a heavy overrepresentation of native English speakers. Since Englishmen and Canadians enjoyed close cooperation, it meant that they had six votes of a total of thirteen. These six votes were also a thorn in the side of the Americans who had just one member in the Commission compared with the four who had been there in Sievert's time and had aroused equivalent criticism then.[154]

Co-optation was bound to generate clubby behavior and insularity.

The leadership of the Commission was not shy about outreach to countries it would like to see represented, but in doing so it targeted the best qualified radiation protection professionals as candidates. Lindell and Sowby reached out to the Chinese in 1972, but apparently without

151 Touzet R. Dan J. Beninson (1931–2003): Obituary. Journal of Radiological Protection. 2003;23:453–5. https://iopscience.iop.org/article/10.1088/0952-4746/23/4/M01/pdf, accessed July 13, 2023.

152 "Membership of ICRP Task Groups; November 1966," Taylor, note 2, 9-490–92.

153 "ICRP in Brighton," Lindell, note 9, 133–43. Lindell thought that incident led to Morgan's subsequent "critical attitude" toward the ICRP, Lindell to Morgan, January 8, 1981, ICRP Archives, Archive files 81, D-Forda Handlingar 81.pdf, 65. Some of the 1973 brouhaha is apparent in letters from Lindell to Sowby and from K. Z. Morgan to Sowby, ICRP Archives, Archive File 42, SOWBY 1970–73.pdf, 54–57.

154 "ICRP in Whiteshell," Lindell, note 9, 184–5.

results.[155] Lindell and Beninson, as Chair of the ICRP and Scientific Secretary of UNSCEAR, met their first Mainland Chinese colleague at a radiation protection meeting in 1978.[156] Lindell welcomed correspondence with Wei Lüxin of the Ministry of Health in 1979, noting especially a common interest in areas with high natural background radioactivity.[157] About the same time, ICRP Scientific Secretary David Sowby took the initiative to meet George Wu, a Mauritius-born Chinese radiation therapist trained in Britain who had returned voluntarily to China after World War II. He was appointed to an ICRP committee in 1979 and hosted some ICRP members on a trip to Hong Kong, Guangzhou, Beijing, and Shanghai in 1981. They found their Chinese colleagues well-prepared:

> We were impressed with our Chinese colleagues' knowledge of ICRP and of what happened in the western world. They had the latest documents and they had had them translated. We were asked many intelligent questions which showed that the asker had looked into the problems thoroughly. They not only understood what was recommended but also why.[158]

Chinese dosimetry expert Li Deping, who had tasked a graduate student with preparing a literature survey that included the work of the ICRP, NCRP, and ICRU in the early 1960s, became the first Chinese member of the ICRP Main Commission in 1985.[159] By the time of the 70th anniversary of the Commission in 1997, the Chinese Society of Radiation Protection was planning a special issue of its official journal Radiation Protection, edited by Li, "concentrating in ICRP's functions and contributions to worldwide radiation protection, present activities of the Main

155 Sowby to Chang and Lindell to Chang, ICRP Archives, Archive File 42, SOWBY 1970–73.pdf, 152–4.

156 "UNEP's scandal meeting in Geneva," Lindell, note 9, 224–7, at 225.

157 Lindell to Wei, August 18, 1979, ICRP Archives, Archive Files 81, Archive Files 81 part 1.pdf, 90. Wei's High Background Radiation Research Group, China soon thereafter published, Health Survey in High Background Radiation Areas in China. Science. 1980 Aug 22;209:877–80.

158 "ICRP in China and Japan," Lindell, note 9, 262–5, at 265. P. Ziqiang refers to the literature survey in his 1996 G. William Morgan lecture, Radiation risk—a Chinese perspective. Health Phys. 1997 Aug;73:295 https://pubmed.ncbi.nlm.nih.gov/9228164/, accessed May 30, 2023.

159 Lindell, note 9, "The ICRP MC in Paris in March—Member Emeritus," pp. 310–11.

Commission and its Committees, and its new concepts."[160] Chinese radiation protection experts had joined the global epistemic community.

Lindell in an address to ICRP main commission and committee members in 1981 noted with pride how its recommendations had continued to gain traction worldwide:

> It is encouraging to see a great uniformity in the fundamental attitude between countries with widely differing economic, social, political and administrative structures. We must realise that this fundamental attitude is usually said to be based on ICRP's recommendations. It places a considerable burden of responsibility on the Commission to develop and formulate well-founded, prudent advice. The circumstances – and hopefully also to some extent dependable work – have put the Commission in a position where much greater importance and weight are attached to each statement than we would give to it ourselves.[161]

By 1981, the IAEA, ILO, OECD/NEA and WHO had all recently revised their Basic Safety Standards based on ICRP's latest 1977 recommendations. This meant, Lindell averred, "that the international significance of the Commission had increased considerably."[162] The authoritative character of the ICRP's recommendations spread geographically even as the Commission itself remained far from representative of the world as a whole.

This was due in part to the phenomenon sociologists known as the "strength of weak ties." A multiplicity of weak ties can transmit messages faster and more widely than a relatively few strong ones, as Granovetter demonstrates.[163] In 1990, a Chinese official of the Southwest Nuclear Power Institute wrote to the ICRP for a copy of its latest recommendations, saying:

[160] Pan Ziqiang to Lindell, November 30, 1997, ICRP Archives, Archive Files 1–11, Archive File 4, 07-25-1994.pdf, 13.

[161] Lindell, note 9, "ICRP in Eastbourne," 272–4.

[162] "Symposium in Madrid regarding ICRP's recommendations," Lindell, note 9, 268.

[163] Granovetter MS. The Strength of Weak Ties. American Journal of Sociology [Internet]. 1973;78(6):1360–80. Available from: https://www.jstor.org/stable/2776392, accessed April 10, 2023.

> Upon drafting the radiological protection criteria of nuclear power plants, we have been mainly referring to No.26 publication [the 1977 recommendations]. But in view of the responsibility of a radiological protection personnel and environmental protector, we are anxious to see the most advanced research results and apply them to engineering design.[164]

While the Commission itself was a tight-knit epistemic group, its members maintained weaker ties both with the many other scientists involved in its subcommittees and task forces as well as with individual scientists and engineers worldwide. Those weaker ties were largely responsible for the wide diffusion of its recommendations.

Authority without representation may appear unexpected at first sight, but this was an epistemic group, where professional reputation counted for more than nationality. In the eyes of experts worldwide, the Commission, its subcommittees, and task forces drew on the best available scholars working on radiation protection issues. It was a first mover in the field of radiation protection and had no competition. The ICRP felt pressured at times to expand in the direction of the Soviet bloc, the People's Republic of China, or what was then known as the Third World. But when and if it gave in to those pressures it did so gradually, considering the expert quality of those selected as well as the longstanding need for balance among different disciplines. It also maintained the influence of leading West Europeans and Americans by keeping their numbers more or less constant, naming some former members as emeriti entitled to attend meetings (but not to have their travel paid by the Commission or to vote), and expanding the total number of Main Commission members to accommodate nominees from other parts of the world. Even in 2023, there are no developing country members of the Main Commission, though China and South Korea are now included. Representation in its committees and task forces is significantly broader, but still premised principally on professional reputation, as judged by the existing members. Co-optation continues.

164 ICRP Archives, Box #@-9 Box #G060, "ICRP New Rec Corres.pdf," 95–6. Comparable requests, from both nuclear industry people and radiation protection people, came from South Korea, Japan, India, Australia, Brazil, Venezuela, Saudi Arabia, and Algeria.

Different Strokes for Different Folks

The ICRP's relationship to national radiation protection institutions was not uniform. Throughout the 1960s, 70s, and 80s, there was considerable variation in the capacities and expectations of different countries with respect to the detail and depth of ICRP norms. With expansion of the nuclear power industry came vastly increased public visibility and concern. The countries with substantial technical capacities of their own preferred to see the international norms focused on basic radiation protection parameters, in particular permissible doses and norms derived from them. They wanted more detailed technical standards required to meet these norms in specific industries and in their own distinct national circumstances set either by their own national analogs of the ICRP or by other international standards bodies with more industry expertise.

The Germans, for example, in 1969 protested against a proposed revision of some ICRP recommendations, claiming they were too detailed, lacked adequate technical grounding, and trespassed on the turf of the International Electrotechnical Commission.[165] Physicians and dentists in Germany in particular objected. Bo Lindell was then the Swedish Vice Chair of the ICRP and chair of the committee making the recommendations the Germans complained about. He responded to them:

> Few countries would consider using other MPDs [maximum permissible doses] than those recommended by ICRP; however, this is not because it is ICRP that has made the recommendations but because the recommendation made by ICRP has met general acceptance.[166]

He received vigorous support from ICRP members, though Taylor confessed privately to concerns about some of the Commission's medical

[165] The protest was a collective one to David Sowby, ICRP Scientific Secretary, from the Deutsche Roentgengesellschaft, the Gesellschaft für medizinische Radiologie, die Strahlenbiologie und Nuklearmedizin Fachnormenausschuss Radiologie im Deutschen Normenausschuss, in Arbeitsgemeinschaft mit der Deutschen Roentgengesellschaft Fachverband 18 im Zentralverband der elektrotechnischen Industrie, "Draft ICRP/69/C3-1 Protection against external radiation," note 3, 10-347. The original letter and annex are in ICRP Archives, Box 26, Archive files 34, "C3 fr Nov 65 to Oct 69.pdf," 133–35.

[166] Lindell to Fachnormenausschuss Radiologie, August 7, 1969, Taylor, note 2, 10-349.

recommendations.[167] In 1965, the Swedes, who had adopted their first radiation protection legislation more than twenty years earlier, had established under Lindell a Radiation Protection Institute within the Ministry of Health and ordered their first two commercial power plants in 1968. Lindell in 1968 initiated "translating" the main existing ICRP recommendations paragraph by paragraph into Scandinavian conditions, for use not only in Sweden but also in Denmark, Finland, and Norway. In 1970, the British shifted responsibility for radiation protection from the Medical Research Council to a National Radiation Protection Board that eventually acquired several hundred personnel. The Americans had in the NCRP a strong national counterpart of the ICRP, albeit a congressionally chartered but nongovernmental one. Like the Germans and the Swedes, the Americans thought national bodies should prevail when it came to more detailed standards. The Johns Hopkins physician Russell Morgan wrote to Lindell in 1968:

> I am convinced that it is the recommendations promulgated by a national body of a given country which will be respected in that country. For this reason, I believe that an international body except under unusual circumstances should not concern itself with the formulation of detailed standards but should leave such matters to national groups.[168]

He wanted to see relations between the ICRP and national radiation protection bodies strengthened, so as to prevent any competition and increase coherence. The need was apparent. The American NCRP often differed on issues, big as well as small, from the ICRP.

Lindell responded to Morgan describing how the ICRP operated through informal channels to constitute what we today should recognize as a well-connected epistemic community. With reference to a committee concerned with application of ICRP recommendations, mainly in medicine, Lindell wrote:

[167] Letters from the U.S., U.K., Canada, Japan are in ICRP Archives, Box 26, Archive files 34, "C3 fr Nov 65 to Oct 69.pdf," 115–25 and 128–30. Taylor's confession is in Taylor to David Sowby, ibid., August 19, 1969, 126–7. Mostly supportive letters to Lindell are also in ICRP Archives, Box 824, C 3 Task Group Rev to Publications 3 & 4 1966–70.pdf, 6–43.

[168] Russell Morgan to Bo Lindell, ICRP Archives, G041, C 3 Task Group on High Radiation 1965–69.pdf, August 7, 1968, 152–4.

> ...the Commission must find the best contacts with the national groups that promulgate standards. It cannot be done in a formal way, since these groups differ from country to country and any formal relationship that would embrace all groups would be too involved to function. It then also follows that ICRP cannot maintain any formal relationship with any one single group. What, then, does the Commission do to maintain the necessary contacts? First, by selecting members to the Commission, its Committees and the various task groups. In most countries there is a central authority responsible for radiation protection. You will find that about 50% of the members are very closely related to such authorities while the other 50% represent more independent scientific interests. Countries such as Canada, Denmark, France, Italy, Japan, Norway, Sweden, USSR and UK have these close contacts or arrangements whereby ICRP members at home maintain very close contacts with the groups that promulgate local standards...
>
> In addition, close relationships are maintained with international organisations such as IAEA, WHO, ILO, ISO, IEC who also promulgate standards.

The Americans, Lindell averred, presented particular problems, because so many different institutions were involved in radiation protection:

> USA constitutes a special problem since you have several groups that are interested in developing radiation protection standards, e. g. NCRP, FRC, PHS. ICRP has tried to follow the work of these groups by relying upon individual Commission and committee members who are also members of the US groups. Such members are L. S. Taylor, K. Z. Morgan, F. P. Cowan, H. 0. Wyckoff, E. Dale Trout, F. Western, R. F. Brown, J. H. Heslep, J. P. Kelley and C. B. Meinhold, to mention some of the persons who, in the Commission, committees or task groups, may influence the present wording of external dose recommendations.[169]

The key to building and sustaining this epistemic community was the selection, by each of the committees and the Main Commission, of their own members. Co-optation favored epistemic leaders at the national level: people with ample publications and sterling professional reputations,

[169] Bo Lindell to Russel H. Morgan, October 30, 1968, ICRP Archives, Box G041, C 3 Task Group on High Radiation 1965–69.pdf, 149–51.

influence in their national institutions, and strong professional networks, including international contacts. Notably, those selected did not exclude people connected to medical and industrial uses of ionizing radiation, who could be expected to bring significant knowledge of how norms would affect practical applications.

Many countries however lacked the technical capacities and confidence of the mainstays of the ICRP—the Americans, British, Swedes, and Germans—who had decades of experience both with national regulations and international norm-setting. Nuclear technology was spreading widely. The organizing congress of the International Radiation Protection Association, an initiative of the American physicist K. Z. Morgan, was held in Rome in 1966 and attracted 845 people from 22 countries, most of them European but also including Argentina, the Philippines, and Mexico. By 1968, the Association had 6000 members from 60 countries.[170] By 1972, the Soviets had their own "NCRP." By 1974, the ICRP had more than 100 of the world's leading radiation experts in its Main Commission, subcommittees, and "task groups." The NCRP had begun to fear that the ICRP, because of its strong connections to UNSCEAR, had the upper hand on evaluating biological effects.[171] In 1983, the ICRP's Annals had a distribution of almost 1400. In 1984 at its Stockholm meeting there were seventy individuals from 17 countries present, including the Main Commission and subcommittee members as well as observers.

Not only science, the environment, and medicine but also trade and technology were in play. In arguing in 1975 for an extension of David Sowby's secondment from the Canadian government as ICRP Scientific Secretary, its Canadian Chairman C. G. Stewart stated bluntly the cost savings and commercial advantages of the ICRP recommendations:

> It has been of great importance to Canada that there has been in existence a set of internationally agreed criteria and standards for radiation protection; at the very least their presence and adoption in considerable part in

[170] Karl Z. Morgan, "The Proper Working Level of Radon and Its Daughter Products in the Uranium Mines of the United States," to be presented at the Hearing on Radiation Standards for Mines, Washington, D.C., November 20, 1968, ICRP Archives, Royal Comm -Health & Safety of Workers in Mines Part 2.pdf, 51–55.

[171] Proposal that the NCRP Initiate a New Activity Concerned with Reassessment of the Maximum Permissible Dose Equivalent Levels," NCRP/BD/72/66, December 6, 1972, Taylor 10-218-9.

> Canadian legislation has obviated the need for Canada to attempt independently the development of its own standards, at considerable expense, and with considerable expenditure of effort. These Recommendations have in no small measure contributed to safety criteria applied in Canadian reactor design and operation that have in the main been found acceptable abroad, as evidenced by Canada's success in marketing nuclear reactors overseas.[172]

At the time, Canada was commercializing the CANDU, a pressurized heavy-water (deuterium) reactor fueled with natural uranium. It would not have been possible to sell the CANDU without being able to demonstrate that their operation would not breach ICRP maximum permissible doses.

Many countries used the ICRP recommendations to fill gaps in their own capabilities. They expected more detailed guidance, not less. A British member of the ICRP reported in 1969 after attending the IAEA Regional Seminar for Asia and the Far East on Radiation Protection Monitoring:

> From the point of view of developing countries, the present trend of ICRP recommendations has some disconcerting features. They accept unquestionably the maximum permissible doses and dose limits but also expect authoritative or perhaps authoritarian guidance on problems of application.[173]

Providing guidance of this sort helped to sustain the ICRP's authority in many countries that could not afford to develop their own more detailed standards. The President of the Polish Radiological Society prepared for the 50th anniversary of the ICRP in 1978 a calligraphed statement:

> Deep knowledge, impartiality and wisdom of the Commission's recommendations lead to great improvements of the conditions of the radiologist's work also in our country. Our national regulations are and have been currently based on the ideas and philosophy developed by the ICRP.[174]

[172] ICRP Archives, specific reference lost.

[173] J. H. Dunster, "ICRP - 1969," note 3, 10-334–5.

[174] Jerzy Zajngner to Sievert, ICRP Archives, Archive Files 56, Stockholm Meeting 1978.pdf, 80.

Many of the ICRP's publications are focused on specific circumstances or applications, not on the basic radiation protection norms that are its main purpose from the perspective of the West Europeans and North Americans who invented and controlled it. Especially since 1990, the last time the ICRP changed its most basic permissible dose limits, the Commission has labored more to diffuse its recommendations and adapt them to particular applications.

The Commission still continued, however, to prefer to think of itself as providing guidance, not requirements. Lindell's first point (of 23!) in a talk given in 1981 was this: "The ICRP recommendations cannot supersede national regulations."[175] The Commission itself had made this point in its 1977 recommendations:

> The Commission wishes to reiterate that its policy is to consider the fundamental principles upon which appropriate radiation protection measures can be based. Because of the differing conditions that apply in various countries, detailed guidance on the application of its recommendations, either in regulations or in codes of practice, should be elaborated by the various international and national bodies that are familiar with what is best for their needs.[176]

The recommendations were not intended to constrain other international and national authorities, but rather to act as a basis for their own decisions. This leeway was reassuring both to those with technical capacities and to those who lacked them. The former might resist the recommendations but, in the end, could and sometimes did depart from them, as the Americans did. The latter could still use them. As ICRP Secretary in 1959, Lindell had opposed making compliance obligatory in an ILO convention. He explained later: "I quite simply thought it was not possible to assume that ICRP would always issue wise recommendations in the future, although that was what I did hope."[177]

[175] Lindell, note 9, "ICRP in Eastbourne," 270–74 at 273.

[176] "Recommendations of the ICRP," ICRP Publication 26 (Pergamon, 1977). This point was reiterated in the new "Constitution of the International Commission on Radiological Protection," ICRP Archives, Misc Box 4, "ICRU," 77–82.

[177] Hercules, 275.

The international recommendations could nevertheless steer national authorities in the right direction. Lindell wrote to Russell Morgan in 1969:

> There are recommendations that could be made - even should be made - but that may not be made at the national level because the local "pressure group" is not strong enough. There are other recommendations that should not be made but are nevertheless made because the local pressure groups are inappropriately strong.[178]

The ICRP and its many committees and task groups amplified the voices of government officials who specialized in radiation protection as well as people with other relevant specialties, like physics, radiation biology, genetics, and oncology. The far more numerous practicing physician radiologists and the nuclear power industry were weightier at the national level. Redressing this imbalance was one of the ICRP's de facto roles. As the Deputy Director of the UK National Radiological Protection Board put it in 1977, ICRP members

> ...represent no-one but themselves and are chosen for their eminence in the relevant field of science. The authority of the Commission's recommendations depends entirely on the regard in which its members are held by their peers and, given a high regard, by the consequential persuasion of governments to adopt the recommendations. Such is their reputation that some governments boast that they allow no practice which will cause radiation doses to be given in excess if ICRP's dose equivalent limits *irrespective of the cost* of achieving this. The British government have adopted this attitude in respect of the discharge of radioactive waste.[179]

That was not the attitude of all agencies of the U.S. Government. The Nuclear Regulatory Commission (NRC) created in 1975 followed the ICRP deliberations carefully and contributed funding to the Commission but relied on the NCRP for advice on when and how to implement recommendations. The NCRP did not follow the ICRP's 1977 recommendations until 1987. The NRC then followed with new standards in

[178] Bo Lindell to Russell Morgan, 30 October 1968, Box G041, C 3 Task Group on High Radiation 1965–69.pdf, 149–51.

[179] L. D. G. Richings, "Risks Dose Equivalent Limits and ICRP," ICRP Archives, Archive Files 100, MC.pdf, 95–106, at 96–97.

1991 based on the ICRP's 1977 recommendation, after which it declined to implement the ICRP's 1990 recommendations. As a result, the NRC in 2014 described its own "regulatory framework" as

> ...a mixture of radiological standards, concepts and quantities, ranging from the 1959 recommendations in ICRP Publication 1 (1959) to the modeling and numeric values of the 1990 recommendations in ICRP Publication 60 (1991).[180]

The NRC was still aiming in 2014 "to align more closely with the ICRP Publication 103 (2007) dose assessment methodology and terminology."[181] One of the issues concerned the permissible dose for radiation workers, which the Americans still have not lowered to 20 mSv, due in part to concern about inhibiting medical applications and in part to different procedures for measuring doses in American clinics. The international norms are the ideal to which American national regulations aspire rather than an obligation they feel bound by. Hegemony is long gone but exceptionalism persists.

Delays in conforming to the international norms were common in some other countries as well. Adaptation of national regulations to the international norms necessarily took time. Optionality was still a feature of the international radiation protection norms, not a glitch. The international norms were as soft as law can get.[182] Their extra-legal, voluntary character proved a strength: whatever was decided, everyone had the opportunity to adjust the norms as needed to particular national circumstances and timetables. It also meant that there was little reason to bolt if national circumstances required something different from what the ICRP recommended. There would always be an opportunity to revisit the recommendations and try to convince the Commission to revise them. The authority of the ICRP was resilient in part because it had the best expertise available and in part because compliance was voluntary.

[180] "A Proposed Rule by the Nuclear Regulatory Commission on 07/25/2014," Federal Register, 10 CFR Part 20 [NRC–2009–0279], RIN 3150–AJ29, https://www.govinfo.gov/content/pkg/FR-2014-07-25/pdf/2014-17252.pdf, accessed August 25, 2023.

[181] Ibid.

[182] Weiss EB. Conclusions: Understanding Compliance with Soft Law, Chapter 9. In: Commitment and Compliance: The Role of Non-Binding Norms in the International Legal System. Oxford: Oxford University Press; 2000.

By the 1980s, national radiation authorities were demonstrating their satisfaction with the ICRP through financial contributions that covered about half of its still modest budget of around $160,000 per year.[183] The rest came from intergovernmental organizations like WHO, IAEA, and the Commission of the European Community as well as the nongovernmental International Society for Radiology, the International Radiation Protection Association, and the Pergamon Press. The United States and Europe still dominated the governmental financial contributions, as they did the norm-setting. But there was little sign of dissatisfaction in other countries, which stood to benefit from the ICRP's deliberations and norm-setting. That general pattern has continued, albeit with increasing membership and contributions from Asia. In addition to publication sales, 2016–20 funding for the four-person secretariat as well as meetings and publications was provided by voluntary contributions, three-quarters were governmental and three-quarters still came from the United States and Europe.[184] Total incoming resources in 2022 amount to about $1 million.[185] ICRP is still a bargain.

The Public Gets Its Say

The scientists involved with radiation dosimetry and protection after World War II were anxious to keep norm-setting within their own professional circles and to insulate it from the broader society. The ICRP in 1959 had adopted a policy "that pre-publication information should be restricted as much as possible with the details left at the discretion of the Chairman."[186] Meetings were held behind closed doors, with little or no input from the lay world beyond them. At least since the 1950s, low-key and often technical statements were issued after meetings of the

[183] "ICRP Budget 1982–1984," attached to "Proposed Agenda for Washington Meeting," ICRP/83/MC-08, July 29, 1983, ICRP Archives, Archive File 94, MC 1960–1983B.pdf, 102–7.

[184] ICRP Funding [Internet]. www.icrp.org. Available from: https://www.icrp.org/page.asp?id=172#:~:text=As%20an%20independent%20registered%20charity, accessed October 16, 2023.

[185] ICRP Annual Report 2022 [Internet]. Available from: https://www.icrp.org/admin/AnnualReport2022_Digital-FINAL.pdf, accessed October 16, 2023.

[186] Bo Lindell to Lauriston Taylor, December 18, 1959, ICRP Archives, Box W-18, Archive file 26, 3–5.

Main Commission, but this one-way communication did not allow for public input. As late as 1987, the Commission saw a "need to maintain confidentiality to prevent premature leakage of evolving concepts."[187] The anti-bomb movements of the 1950s and early 1960s as well as the 1970s attack on their recommendations made the NCRP and ICRP wary of the broader society, which was roiled with civil rights protests in the United States and anti-Vietnam War protests in both the United States and Europe. The NCRP in particular did not want to let those issues, in which its members "might have strong beliefs but little scientific or professional qualifications," impinge on radiation protection.[188]

By contrast, the impact of ionizing radiation on society was clearly a sphere in which the NCRP participants had vital scientific and professional qualifications. The LNT hypothesis, reaffirmed repeatedly, meant that the norms implied a balance between risk and benefit, even if those risks and benefits resisted quantification. Norm-setting was no longer a question of "tolerance" in the biological sense but rather one of tolerance from the perspective of the broader society. What risks would the public bear in order to gain the benefits of ionizing radiation? This issue was resolved for medical irradiation by leaving it up to the doctor and patient. While continuing to urge improved radiation protection practice in clinics, the NCRP, its counterparts in other countries, and the ICRP no longer counted doses from medical irradiation when setting maximum permissible doses, even though medical irradiation contributed more than other sources to the exposure of the general population.

The NCRP Board began to discuss in the early 1970s what it termed the "social responsiveness" of NCRP activities, including "popular level" publications, explanatory events and resources, modification of its operating rules, more open scientific forums, and assessing the public impact of its draft recommendations.[189] This effort made little progress. As a radiologist asked to lead the ad hoc committee on social responsiveness put it:

[187] Minutes of the ICRP Meeting, Washington USA 1987," ICRP/87/MC16, dated March 18, 1987, ICRP Archives, Box W-18, Archive files 32, ICRP Como 1987.pdf, 41–56, at p. 14.

[188] [Eugene] Saenger, "Social Responsiveness of NCRP Activities," July 3, 1973, Taylor, note 2, 10-240–42.

[189] "Topics That Might Be Included in a Study of Social Responsiveness of NCRP Activities," ibid., 10-217.

> The NCRP is essentially, and almost solely, a scientific organization whose major contribution to society is in the form of rigorously edited communications wherein available scientific data is reviewed to reach conclusions justified by the data.[190]

The epistemic community found it difficult to respond to public concerns that came from beyond the realm of data and resisted opening its process to those without professional qualifications. In 1973, the NCRP Board, which had rejected risk calculations based on the LNT hypothesis as the basis for norms, agreed "that there was no need to offer explanations of how the NCRP reached agreement on the current levels for maximum permissible doses and dose limits."[191] ICRP meetings through the mid-1980s were still conducted behind closed doors, albeit with an increasing number of observers from interested and professionally qualified intergovernmental, professional, and regional organizations as well as the ICRU.[192] Environmental and labor organizations concerned with ICRP decisions had no established route into the process, though they tried to communicate both privately and in public. Lindell as Chair made a serious effort to correspond with ICRP critics.[193] Taylor in 1980 reviewed the many "nonscientific" influences on radiation protection standards, which he classified as philosophical, the media, morality, laws and regulations, and economics. He averred that he felt "strongly that we must turn to the much larger group of citizens generally" for wisdom in combining nonscientific approaches with scientific ones. But he complained, as he

[190] Saenger E. Social Responsiveness of NCRP Activities. July 3, 1973, ibid., 10-240–42.

[191] 31st Meeting of the Board of Directors, "Radiation Protection Philosophy," ibid., 10-249–50.

[192] Sowby to Members of the Commission, "Observers at the 1980 ICRP Meeting," March 6, 1980, ICRP/80/MC-04, ICRP Archives, Archive Files 55–65, Archive File 65, Cirk 1979–1980.pdf, 59.

[193] For samples, see Alvarez R. [U.S.] Environmental Policy Institute, Radiation Exposure Limits. Bull At Sci. 1980 Nov;58–9. and "La Confédération Générale du Travail Force Ouvrière et les Recommandations de la C.I.P.R. 26," ICRP Archives, Box W-26, Archive Files 91, "Sowby.pdf," 73–83.

had many times over previous decades, that the public was not sufficiently well-informed to play its role, due largely to misinformation in the media.[194]

The intense public interest in the ICRP's Como meeting in 1987, held in the aftermath of the Three Mile Island and Chernobyl incidents, marked a significant break with past practices. During the session, a meeting was held with observers, "who stressed the need for early consultation with them on the practical problems in implementing the recommendations."[195] Consulting much more widely than in the past, the Commission "task group" that prepared the 1990 recommendations received more than 1000 comments on its drafts.[196] These included a 52-page submission from UK Friends of the Earth that Roger Clarke, Director of the UK National Radiation Protection Board, had solicited.[197] Lindell commented at the time:

> It is quite obvious from most of the comments that the Commission made a very wise move when it let draft number 9 [of what became the Commission's 1990 recommendations] be available for an informal outside consultation procedure. This has created valuable good will, and comments are, in general, friendly or even respectful.[198]

194 Taylor LS. Some Non-Scientific Influences on Radiation Protection Standards and Practice: the 1980 Sievert Lecture. Health Physics [Internet]. 1980 Dec 1;39(6):851. Available from: https://journals.lww.com/health-physics/Citation/1980/12000/SOME_NONSCIENTIFIC_INFLUENCES_ON_RADIATION.1.aspx, accessed May 30, 2023.

195 Hylton Smith to Main Commission members, "Record and Minutes of the ICRP Meetings in Como 1987," ICRP/87/MC-28, 1987-10-09, ICRP Archives, Box #5, Constitution, Rules, Procedures A.pdf.

196 Dozens of these totaling close to 600 pages can be viewed in the ICRP Archives, "Comments on draft 90-G01.pdf," file A805. These include comments from government institutions, intergovernmental organizations, environmental organizations, and individual scientists. The first batch are summarized in "Responses received and summarised by the Scientific Secretary (1/6/90) (for Mr Dunster)", ibid., at 237–47. Additional comments are in ICRP Archives, Box 1163, Misc dossie.pdf.

197 ICRP Archives, "Letters from Friends of the Earth.pdf," file 805.

198 "Comments on ICRP/90/G-1 submitted through Bo Lindell," 1990-06-16 ICRP/90/MC-, ICRP Archives, Box W-26, Archive Files 92, "92-10-08.pdf," 13–23. Tamplin was among those submitting comments in 1990, see Tamplin and Bjorn O. Gillberg, Miljocentrum's "Comments on Draft ICRP 190/G-01 Recommendations of the Commission –1990," May 11, 1990, ICRP Archives, Box W-26, 92-10-08.pdf, 34–9. The draft recommendations were sent in early 1990 to the International Society of Radiology, the

As Lindell noted later, this opening to broader input was partly due to the spirit of the times, in which Glasnost was blooming, and partly due to generational change.[199] ICRP was not the only institution opening up by the 1990s and might be considered more tardy than anticipatory in this dimension of what amounts to isomorphic mimicry.

The generational change later culminated when Clarke was appointed the ICRP Chair in 1993. He proposed a reform and simplification of the ICRP's recommendations as well as a "unique extensive consultation process where firstly the conceptual basis and later the detailed recommendations text were analysed and discussed publicly on several occasions."[200] Clarke's reform proposal involved the concept of "controllable dose" that would have permitted low doses to individuals to be ignored, a notion Lindell and Beninson had long opposed.[201] It ultimately failed to gain traction with the Commission.[202] Lindell, who felt the younger Clarke did not show appropriate deference to the

Soviet-led Council of Mutual Economic Assistance (COMECON), the International Radiation Protection Association, the International Confederation of Free Trade Unions, the Commission of the European Communities, the International Labor Office, the Organization for Economic Cooperation and Development, the (U.S.) Health Physics Society as well as national radiation protection authorities and the Main Commission and committee members both for their own comments and for circulation to professional colleagues. This wider distribution than in the past generated dozens of responses, ICRP Archives, Box G041, Nuclear Safety circa 1990.pdf, 36-211 and 219-311 and G042, 03-26-1990.pdf. Some Canadian comments are to be found scattered in Box 042, Recommendations Draft 1990 A.pdf.

199 "Generational change for radiation protection" Lindell, note 9, 409–11.

200 "The conclusion of a century," Lindell, note 9, 454–5.

201 Clarke R. Control of low-level Radiation Exposure: Time for a Change? Journal of Radiological Protection. 1999;19:107–25. https://iopscience.iop.org/article/10.1088/0952-4746/19/2/301/pdf, accessed July 14, 2023. For a taste of the opposition his proposals aroused, see Lecomte JF, Schieber C. Contribution of the French Society for Radiation Protection to the Current Reflections on the Possible Improvements of the Radiological Risk Management System. Journal of Radiological Protection. 2001;21(277). https://doi.org/10.1088/0952-4746/21/3/306, accessed July 14, 2023.

202 By 2003, the ICRP had decided against a "radical revision," see ICRP. The Evolution of the System of Radiological protection: the Justification for New ICRP Recommendations. Journal of Radiological Protection. 2003;23:129–42. https://doi.org/10.1088/0952-4746/23/2/301, accessed July 14, 2023. Nine national member societies of the International Radiation Protection Association had critiqued Clarke's proposals, see IRPA Member Societies' Contributions to the Development of new ICRP Recommendations, July 2000, ICRP Archives, Box #5, Controllable Doses, IRPA Members Societies Contributions-2000.pdf, 6–145.

ICRP *emirati* like himself, nevertheless still credited him generously in another direction: "Important components were openness, information and consultation. This is where Roger made a substantial and important contribution."[203]

This ICRP Glasnost has lasted longer than the Russian version. The 2007 ICRP recommendations resulted from a broad process of international consultation with stakeholders, including government officials, international organizations, and nongovernmental organizations.[204] Initiated in 1997, the process included two public consultations as well as multiple reviews arranged by the International Radiation Protection Association, the Nuclear Energy Agency of the OECD, the European Commission, and United Nations agencies. Draft recommendations for public comment were posted on the ICRP website in June 2004. Within six months, 200 comments had been received. Nothing like this level of transparency had been attempted previously.[205] A second international consultation elicited more than 700 pages of comments.[206] For the previous 1990 recommendations, ICRP had solicited comments only from governmental radiation protection authorities, who had become its main source of funds.[207] Allergy to politics continued but no longer meant allergy to governments.

[203] Lindell, note 9 above, at 409–11, at 411.

[204] "The 2007 Recommendations of the International Commission on Radiological Protection," Annals of the ICRP, Vol. 37 Nos. 2–4, ICRP Publication 103, 2007, p. 4. For samples from this process, see "Development of the Draft 2005 Recommendations of the ICRP: a Collection of Papers," ICRP Supporting Guidance 4 Commissioned/approved by ICRP, April 1998–April 2004, https://journals.sagepub.com/doi/suppl/10.1177/ANIB_34_1/suppl_file/ANI_34_1.pdf, accessed July 13, 2023.

[205] J. W. Stather, L.-E. Holm, J. Valentina "Meeting of ICRP Main Commission and Committees: 11–18 September 2005, Geneva, Switzerland," Archives, 2004–2006 Box 13, File A64, Dossie 00 MC.pdf, 5–8. The results of the consultation are summarized in "Summary of the Results of the Consultation on the Proposed 2005 Recommendations," Note by Chairman, Vice-Chairman, and Scientific Secretary, 00/47/0, ibid., 124–44.

[206] ICRP Chair Lars-Erik Holm to Nuclear Regulatory Commission Chair Dale E. Klein, January 10, 2007, ICRP Archives, 2004–2006 Box-13, File A73, Reg No. 02-276 2006 Recommendations.pdf, 1–2. Klein wanted a third round of public consultation, Klein to Holm, January 3, 2007, ibid., 3. The remainder of this file contains many of the comments.

[207] Some of these are ICRP Archives, Box G043, Minutes of C1 Bethesda.

The twenty-first-century openness elicited some tough critiques. A German critic thought the existing norms unjustifiably exigent:

> ICRP 2005 [a draft that preceded the 2007 recommendations] looks somewhat like "jumping as a lion and landing as a bed-rug". There have even been suggestions to develop some alternative to current basic radiation protection recommendations, taking into account many of the recent results in radiation biology, epidemiology, but also socio-economic factors, cost/benefit considerations, and so on.[208]

However, he regretted, in a backhanded tribute to ICRP's resilient institutionalization, "it would be impossible to compete with the accumulated know-how, infrastructure, high-level support, and still rather high reputation which ICRP enjoys." Greenpeace objected to what it saw as loosening of the norms in emergency situations and argued essentially for tightening the 1990 recommendations or at least keeping them constant, which was what was done.[209] That, too, was a backhanded tribute to ICRP's norms. At least these two critics–from opposite ends of the spectrum–accepted the ICRP's dominance of norm-setting, even if grudgingly. Stakeholder involvement, once resisted as an encroachment on professional prerogatives, had gone from a taboo subject to one explicitly discussed and encouraged. "Optimization" was no longer only a quantitative exercise in weighing costs and benefits but included the views of stakeholders on both sides of the cost/benefit equation.[210] Since 2013, qualified stakeholders have also had the opportunity to gain membership in ICRP and its committees and task forces through an open nomination process.[211]

[208] Klaus Becker, "ICRP 2005—Much Ado About Nothing? Draft of an Open Letter to ICRP," Manuscript for *Strahlenschutzpraxis*, 2004-09-03, Box #5, LC3, "12-16-2004.pdf," 74–8, p. 1.

[209] McSorley J. Commenting on Behalf of the Organization [Internet]. Icrp.org. Greenpeace; 2004. Available from: https://www.icrp.org/consultation_viewitem.asp?guid=%7b07A7B32B-137B-4009-8F24-45A21B36B98B%7d, accessed July 13, 2023.

[210] ICRP, 2006. The Optimisation of Radiological Protection—Broadening the Process. ICRP Publication 101b. Ann. ICRP 36 (3), https://www.icrp.org/publication.asp?id=ICRP%20Publication%20101b, accessed August 25, 2023.

[211] This and other institutional developments are reviewed in Cousins C. The future of ICRP: toward a centenary and beyond. Annals of the ICRP Volume 45, Issue 1_

Another broad consultative process is being undertaken at present in preparation for the issuance of new recommendations within the next several years after 2023. The ICRP Scientific Secretary and members of the Commission have laid out in public their suggestions of where the system for radiation protection may require adjustments to keep it "fit for purpose."[212] They foresee no need for a change in the numerical permissible limits but suggest many other respects in which the system might be improved. The Commission has outlined priority areas of research to support the revision of its recommendations.[213] It has in addition followed the trend among environmental regimes toward more formal rules for outside participation.[214] It now maintains formal relations with several dozen other organizations–governmental, intergovernmental, and nongovernmental–interested in radiation protection as well as "special liaison relations" with other institutions. The ICRP however remains an epistemic group of global experts. It is far more interested in scientific and technical input, including from those who apply radiation, than political advocacy. Its recent meeting with its special liaison organizations, for example, was co-sponsored with the nuclear industry's World Nuclear Association and dealt mainly with technical issues in applying the ICRP recommendations.[215]

Perhaps as remarkable as its openness in recent decades to stakeholder input is the ICRP's explicit attention to ethics. This includes a code of ethics for itself adopted in 2014 that emphasizes commitment to public benefit, independence, transparency, and accountability. It also extends

suppl, June 2016, Pages 5–8, https://doi.org/10.1177/0146645315613480, accessed November 13, 2023.

212 Clement C, Ruehm W, Harrison JD, Applegate KE, Cool D, Larsson CM, et al. Keeping the ICRP recommendations fit for purpose. Journal of Radiological Protection. 41(1390) 2021 Jul 20; https://iopscience.iop.org/article/10.1088/1361-6498/ac1611, accessed June 25, 2023.

213 Laurier D, Rühm W, Paquet F, Applegate K, Cool D, Clement C. Areas of Research to Support the System of Radiological Protection. Radiation and Environmental Biophysics. 2021 Oct 17;60(4):519–30. https://doi.org/10.1007/s00411-021-00947-1, accessed June 25, 2023.

214 This trend is documented in Breitmeier H. Chapter 10: Non-State Actors and Participation in Regime Politics. The Legitimacy of International Regimes. Routledge; 2016.

215 World Nuclear Association. Bristol, September 27–28. ICRP Workshop Programme, https://na.eventscloud.com/website/57139/programme/, accessed November 11, 2023.

to ethical considerations in both its suggested areas for possible revision and for research.[216] Apart from citing the three principles discussed in earlier chapters of "justification, optimization, and individual dose limitation," ethical considerations in the past were discussed only behind closed doors at the ICRP. They did not enter into its recommendations explicitly, even if they were implicit in consideration of risks and benefits. Stakeholder communication and involvement from beyond the Commission and its subsidiary bodies date as an intentional ICRP practice only from the 1990s, even if social pressures are evident in much of its history. Both ethics and stakeholders are now a focus of ICRP public disquisition.[217] The Commission identifies the main values underlying its work as:

> Beneficence/non-maleficence: promoting or doing good, and avoiding doing harm. This is reflected, for example, in the primary aim of the system of radiological protection: ... an appropriate level of protection ... without unduly limiting ... desirable human actions.
>
> Prudence: making informed and carefully considered choices without full knowledge of the scope and consequences of an action. Prudence is reflected, for example, in the consideration of uncertainty of radiation risks for both humans and the environment.
>
> Justice: fairness in the distribution of advantages and disadvantages. Justice is a key value underlying, for example, individual dose restrictions that aim to prevent any individual from receiving an unfair burden of risk.
>
> Dignity: the unconditional respect that every person deserves, irrespective of personal attributes or circumstances. Personal autonomy is a corollary of human dignity. This underlies, for example, the importance placed on stakeholder participation and the empowerment of individuals to make their own informed decisions.

[216] ICRP. Code of Ethics. Approved by the Main Commission on 2014 April 10. https://www.icrp.org/admin/ICRP%20Code%20of%20Ethics.pdf, accessed November 12, 2023.

[217] ICRP, 2018. Ethical foundations of the system of radiological protection. ICRP Publication 138.

Ann. ICRP 47(1), https://www.icrp.org/publication.asp?id=ICRP%20Publication%20138, accessed June 25, 2023.

It also cites three "procedural values": accountability, transparency, and inclusiveness (stakeholder participation). This is a gigantic evolution from the closed-door efforts of a self-anointed epistemic group to set norms intended to protect enterprises using radiation from societal pressures that might otherwise have limited benefits to medicine, national security, and energy supplies over the past almost 100 years.

This positive evolution of the relationship of the ICRP with the broader society is however a recent development. Its role as norm setter for radiation protection worldwide predated its opening to the public. Nor did this global role derive from geographical diversity, legal authority, or institutional weight. It evolved organically from a knowledge-based epistemic community concerned with protecting both the uses of radiation and those affected by it. In the words of the ICRP itself:

> The primary aim of radiological protection is to provide an appropriate standard of protection for man without unduly limiting the beneficial practices giving rise to radiation exposure.[218]

In the next chapter, we will look at lessons from the history of radiation protection that might be applied in setting international norms for other knowledge-rich enterprises where a balance between risks and benefits is needed.

[218] Note 131 above, para. 15.

CHAPTER 9

What Radiation Protection Suggests About Other Issues, 1990–Present

Two organizations have been very important in radiation protection work. One of these, UNSCEAR, ought to be an exemplary model for what can be accomplished within the framework of the UN. The other, ICRP, is so unconventional that it unfortunately appears to be impossible to copy it within the other fields.[1]

–Bo Lindell

Lindell knew the two organizations well. He had chaired them both and participated for many years in their activities, in addition to his scientific contributions to their work. He and his Argentine friend Dan Beninson led the tightening of the International Commission on Radiological Protection norms in the 1980s, as discussed in Chapter 8. Humility should guide any effort to draw conclusions from the international regime for radiation protection to other risks associated with contemporary technology. There are many irreproducible aspects of the history that created a long-lasting, resilient regime for ionizing radiation. It evolved organically, not as the result of planning or even intention.

[1] Lindell B. The Toil of Sisyphus, Part IV (1967–1999+). Bo Lindell and Nordic Society for Radiation Protection. 2020;53.

D. Serwer, *Strengthening International Regimes*, Palgrave Studies in International Relations, https://doi.org/10.1007/978-3-031-53724-0_9

It would be easy to fault the scientists and physicians involved at each stage for not having anticipated the next tightening of the norms. X-rays and radium moved unusually quickly from the laboratory into the medical clinic, where they caused readily recognizable harm but initially little professional reaction despite the impact on the medical practitioners themselves. Only lawsuits and press coverage motivated national professional organizations to respond, in order to protect the medical applications. Thereafter, two world wars created essential components of the international radiation protection regime. During World War I, German physicists invented accurate means of measuring and delivering radiation doses deep inside the human body. That cutting-edge technique, however unacceptable some of its applications were from the perspective of the twenty-first century, made international comparison of radiation doses a necessity and international norms for radiation protection a possibility realized in the 1930s. During World War II, the Americans adopted in a secret weapons program pre-war norms developed for medical radiology and applied them more broadly to handling not only X-rays and radium but also other types of ionizing radiation as well as a multitude of radioactive isotopes. They did this to protect an urgent program from disruption by resignations, labor unrest, and lawsuits.

Post-World War II, Americans associated with the pre-war national and international radiation protection institutions revived their own nongovernmental institution for setting radiation protection norms as well as the relevant pre-war international organization. But the Americans, concerned not to interfere with atomic bomb testing, hesitated to set norms for the general public that took genetic effects into account. Their foot dragging opened the door to competitive institutions that paid attention to American and British geneticists concerned about long-term radiation effects. Pressure from the geneticists and those institutions caused the 1950s tightening of the national and international norms. Effluent from nuclear power reactors then raised questions about carcinogenic effects associated with relatively low levels of exposure to ionizing radiation. As public concern about nuclear power loomed in the aftermath of the Three Mile Island and Chernobyl incidents, radiation protection specialists, one Argentine and the other Swedish, led the international regime into again tightening its norms.

None of these details is likely to be repeated for any other technology.

Nor would we want it to be. The sporadic tightening of norms for ionizing radiation entailed the deaths of at least hundreds (more likely thousands) of people over decades, not to mention those whose diseases were not recognized as due to radiation. Lives were shortened, cancers developed, and harmful mutations were inherited for decades before the norms were tightened to levels that today are deemed acceptable. The closed-door approach of the ICRP at the beginning of the twentieth century was possible in a world with only 176 international nongovernmental organizations, but not at the beginning of the twenty-first century, by which time there were 40,000.[2] Equipped with formidable digital and communication capacities, they can no longer be locked out of deliberations at either the national or international levels.[3] Even today's permissible limits may someday be viewed as inadequate, or too strict, despite their persistence for more than 30 years while open to public scrutiny and criticism. Science, technology, medicine, society, and values can all change with time. We do not know the future of radiation protection norms, even if many of those serving on the ICRP and in national radiation protection institutions today might anticipate little change in the decades to come. Their predecessors thought likewise and were wrong.

If You Want the Benefits, Limit the Risks

What we do know is that the norms set by an epistemic community of global experts have helped valuable technologies to be used without causing the kind of harm that might have led to prohibition or limitation of their continued use. The pre-World War I national radiation norms protected both medicine and society, enabling X-rays to be used for diagnostic and therapeutic purposes while protecting physicians and patients from obvious harm. After World War I, international norms based on the tolerance dose enabled not only X-rays but also radium to be used extensively in medicine, even if failure to apply the norms beyond medicine harmed radium dial painters and uranium miners. During World War II and for a year thereafter, Manhattan Project workers fabricated the deadliest weapons known while observing norms thought at the time to suffice, with only a few acute incidents and no known impact on

[2] Clark I. International Legitimacy and World Society. Oxford; New York: Oxford University Press; 2007:189.

[3] Hall N. Transnational Advocacy in the Digital Era: Think Global, Act Local. Oxford, 2022; online edn, Oxford Academic; 2022 Jun 23. https://doi-org.proxy1.library.jhu.edu/10.1093/oso/9780198858744.003.0009, accessed September 29, 2023.

the health of tens of thousands of employees. The norms contributed to political decisions in the early 1960s that sharply reduced nuclear weapons testing in the atmosphere. Thereafter, they protected not only medicine but also the many industrial applications of radioisotopes and an entirely new industry using nuclear reactors to produce electricity. While in some countries that industry has been closed or is phasing down, those decisions were based more on the risk of accidents than the routine environmental effluents the international norms sought principally to regulate.

The main norm-setting mechanism in the case of radiation protection is an "epistemic" (knowledge-based) group of global experts seeking to enable the use of technology in medicine, industry, electricity production, and weaponry. This group, both at the national and international levels, was interdisciplinary and included people with interests in using radiation as well as those studying its physical and biological effects. They sought not to block the use of technology, but rather to enable its use by limiting its negative impacts on human health and eventually also the environment. Rolf Sievert put it this way in 1958 while chairing the ICRP for the second time:

> I will begin by defining the establishment of maximum permissible radiation levels as a non-scientific task which must primarily be based on scientific knowledge and judgement. It must be carried out independently of the demands of persons or organizations who are responsible for the increase of ionizing radiation in the world, but nevertheless in close contact with them.

He elaborated:

> The only way to arrive at useful and well balanced maximum permissible levels seems then to be to bring people together representing extensive knowledge and experience on the one hand of the relevant biological effects, and on the other, on the working conditions and protections possibilities. Such a group is capable of discussing the fundamental protection problems from the various aspects relevant for establishment of sound principles in the assessment of maximum permissible levels.[4]

[4] Rolf Sievert. "The Work of the International Commission on Radiological Protection," submitted to the Conference on the Peaceful Uses of Atomic Energy by the World Health

This mixture of interests in our contemporary world is often frowned upon. Regulators, it is believed, need to be separated from the industry regulated. Many standard-setting processes in today's world are adversarial, not cooperative. Those for and against a particular standard argue for their respective perspectives in administrative, judicial, or political proceedings. That logic and process are compelling when the regulators are governmental. But if your objective is science-based value judgments that allow the use of risk-laden technology, there is good reason for people concerned about a particular technology to know and appreciate the people who want to use it. There is also good reason for the people using a particular technology to know and appreciate those who are concerned about it. Effective advocacy in both directions requires epistemic depth, mutual understanding, and competent expert groups focused on providing norms that protect the public as well as the technology.

Public, Specialist, and Competitive Pressures Are Key

That said, the history of radiation protection is not limited to closed expert groups or supposed professional self-regulation. It is replete with public concern as a driver of norm-tightening, as we have seen in previous chapters. The professionals often tried to insulate themselves and consistently denied its efficacy, but when public concern found resonance among professionals its impact was palpable. That resonance was often associated with moments in which new data became available or norm-setters thought they might face competition from other professional bodies. Specialists inside the world of radiation protection were particularly effective in advocating for tighter norms. The post-World War I physicists in medical radiology and the post-World War II geneticists in radiobiology had an outsized influence on the course of radiation protection, as did professional radiation protection experts from the 1970s on. Endowed with more prestige than general practitioners, specialists collaborated nationally and internationally to tighten norms they thought

Organization, ICRP Archives Box W-18, Archive File 23, Correspondence 1958.pdf, 300–8, at p. 5.

necessary to protect human health and believed the affected industries could meet.

Knowledge-based norm-setting in radiation protection however did not start with norms. It started with reproducible measurement of doses and scientific investigation of effects. Radiation protection norms pre-World War I were inadequate because little was understood about how to accurately assess exposure or the biological effects of X-rays and radium, the nature of which was disputed in the early years. Clinical medicine that claimed to be scientific in fact had little basis in contemporary science. The measurement of X-rays and radium was a matter of significant dispute into the 1930s. Understanding of the biological effects of ionizing radiation greatly expanded during and after World War II. Without scientific dosimetry and knowledge of the genetic and carcinogenic effects of ionizing radiation, norm-setting was at best limited to avoiding, with a margin of safety, the more easily observable harm to skin, blood-forming organs, and lens of the eye. The norms were more often too loose than too strict, judging with the benefit of hindsight from the subsequent tightening.

The right lesson from radiation protection is that any norm-setting process for a new technology should have a firm basis in the assessment of effects, including both risks and benefits, which will both need to be considered in many cases. This assessment need not be entirely divorced from industry or government. There is far more likelihood that governments and industries will agree with scientific experts on effects than on norms. Norm-setting will be easier if industry and government contribute their own knowledge and can agree with experts on effects, even if they have different utility functions for the technology in question. The international group establishing norms in the case of ionizing radiation was and still is nongovernmental, but that is not a necessary feature. Norm-setting by governments and intergovernmental organizations is today more the rule. Still, the basic mechanisms at work in radiation protection are worth notice. International norms can be set to establish a basis or limits for competition, with specialists playing a stronger role at the international level than they can at the national level, where they are outnumbered and where economic considerations may be stronger.

Any such effort in the future should anticipate and welcome public criticism, competitive professional consideration, and input from outside the epistemic community, as the radiation protection regime eventually did. Those are essential ingredients in ensuring that the process moves forward. Much as scientists may have good reason to doubt how much the public really understands, the professional institutions dedicated to radiation protection would not have moved as far and fast as they did without pressure from insurance companies, the courts, public hearings, the media, public protests, and other fora for expression of concern. While the national and international institutions concerned with radiation protection tried for many decades to seal themselves off from politics and public scrutiny, and denied their influence, the epistemic groups not only failed but also risked losing their dominance of the norm-setting process, which at several junctures might have been assumed by other professional organizations or government institutions. Opening the institutions to more public scrutiny and input, and to wider geographic diversity in the case of the international institutions, has not hurt their dominance. To the contrary, it has augmented their legitimacy and authority.

If these are the lessons available from the regime for radiation protection, the question is whether they have been applied to other comparable issues, if not why, and whether they offer guidance for future challenges, both technological and non-technological.

Adversarial Approach Fails for Air Pollution and Toxic Chemicals

Air Pollution

WHO, recognizing that air pollution lagged far behind ionizing radiation as a subject of international norm-setting, wanted comparable work done on air pollutants in the 1970s. It convened in March 1977 a "task group" for this purpose explicitly focused on dose–response relationships and on whether the approach used in radiation protection could be applied to pollutants from burning fossil fuels.[5] The scientists agreed that "from the risk assessment point of view, the same approach as for radioactive substances should be applied as regards carcinogenic air contaminants."[6] Discussions in Sweden ensued about the need to emulate the radiation

[5] Air Pollution and Cancer: Risk Assessment Methodology and Epidemiological evidence. Report of a Task Group. Environmental Health Perspectives. 1978 Feb;22:1–12. https://ehp.niehs.nih.gov/doi/10.1289/ehp.22-1637148, accessed May 26, 2023. Lindell recounts this meeting in note 1, 201.

[6] Note 1, Meeting of Scientists at Karolinska Institutet, March 8–11:201.

protection regime, including its linear, no-threshold (LNT) hypothesis, for toxic chemicals.[7] That would have allowed a more direct comparison of the health and environmental risks of nuclear and fossil fuel electricity production. At about the same time, Brookhaven National Laboratory's Leonard Hamilton was purveying the same idea, with explicit reference to modeling the effort on ICRP and UNSCEAR. Hamilton was certain that an objective assessment would show nuclear power, still nascent, far less harmful to human health than fossil fuels.[8]

Whatever its merits, this idea did not gain traction. No professional epistemic institution comparable to the ICRU and ICRP formed around the dosimetry and effects of air pollutants. The fossil fuel industry, which was producing in one way or the other many of the pollutants of concern, knew about the health effects but chose for decades to defend itself by repressing information about them.[9] This effort to conceal what it knew has led to an inundation of lawsuits against the fossil fuels industry in the United States.[10] Without a dedicated epistemic group to weigh risks and benefits, industry and the public engaged in a more adversarial, but arguably slower and ultimately costly, standard-setting process than would otherwise have been the case. It was not until 1987 that WHO started setting "Air Quality Guidelines," analogous to the maximum permissible limits for exposure to ionizing radiation, based on the deliberations

[7] Ibid., Discussion Lars Friberg – Bo Lindell in Läkartidningen:206–8.

[8] Ibid., Snihs and Boge to COGEMA?:209–11. Caveat emptor: I had drafted for Hamilton, who was my boss at Brookhaven in 1976–1977, the proposal. For a contemporary sample comparison of impacts of different energy sources, see Comar CL, Sagan LA. "Health Effects of Energy Production and Conversion," Hollander, JM and Simmons, MK. Annual Review of Energy; 1976;1.

[9] Milman O. Oil Firms Knew Decades Ago Fossil Fuels Posed Grave Health risks, Files Reveal [Internet]. The Guardian. 2021. Available from: https://www.theguardian.com/environment/2021/mar/18/oil-industry-fossil-fuels-air-pollution-documents, accessed June 1, 2023. Or Eaton C, Matthew CM. WSJ News Exclusive | Inside Exxon's Strategy to Downplay Climate Change [Internet]. WSJ. 2023. Available from: https://www.wsj.com/business/energy-oil/exxon-climate-change-documents-e2e9e6af, accessed September 14, 2023.

[10] Climate Accountability Lawsuits: Cases Underway to Make Climate Polluters Pay [Internet]. https://climateintegrity.org/. Center for Climate Integrity; Available from: https://climateintegrity.org/cases, accessed September 17, 2023.

of expert groups it convenes.[11] The guidelines cover particulate matter, ozone, nitrogen oxide, sulfur dioxide, and carbon monoxide. According to WHO itself, 99% of the world's population in 2019 was living in places where the WHO air quality guidelines levels were not met.[12]

One important aspect of controlling air pollution has been more effective. Many governments since the 1970s have used taxes, prohibitions, and public information campaigns against smoking, with more effect in developed countries and with women.[13] In the United States, adult cigarette smoking has declined by 68%.[14] There is no public health benefit to cigarette smoking, despite the satisfaction and dependence that it creates for smokers. There is therefore no need to balance risks and benefits. Public policy can and often does aim to eliminate smoking, consistent with individuals' right to choose (though that has also come into question given the addictive character of nicotine and the alleged effects of second-hand smoking).[15]

Toxic Chemicals

As with air pollutants, by the time of the first United Nations Conference on the Human Environment, held in Stockholm in June 1972, it was clear that radiation protection had progressed far more rapidly than protection against toxic chemicals, where internationally divergent

[11] World Health Organization. What Are the WHO Air Quality Guidelines? [Internet]. 2021. https://www.who.int. Available from: https://www.who.int/news-room/feature-stories/detail/what-are-the-who-air-quality-guidelines, accessed June 4, 2023.

[12] WHO. Ambient (outdoor) Air Quality and Health [Internet]. World Health Organization: WHO. 2022. https://www.who.int/. Available from: https://www.who.int/news-room/fact-sheets/detail/ambient-(outdoor)-air-quality-and-health, accessed June 4, 2023.

[13] Dai X, Gakidou E, Lopez AD. Evolution of the Global Smoking Epidemic Over the Past Half Century: Strengthening the Evidence Base for Policy Action. Tobacco Control [Internet]. 2022 Mar 1;31(2):129–37. Available from: https://tobaccocontrol.bmj.com/content/31/2/129, accessed June 1, 2023.

[14] American Lung Association. Overall Tobacco Trends | American Lung Association [Internet]. American Lung Association. 2021. www.lung.org. Available from: https://www.lung.org/research/trends-in-lung-disease/tobacco-trends-brief/overall-tobacco-trends, accessed June 1, 2023.

[15] Cole HM, Fiore MC. The War Against Tobacco: 50 Years and Counting. JAMA. 2014 Jan 8;311(2):131–2. https://doi.org/10.1001/jama.2013.280767. PMID: 24399546; PMCID: PMC4465196.

standards were the rule rather than the exception.[16] At the UN Conference, the main proposal to remedy this situation was the establishment of an international Registry of Data on Chemicals in the Environment.[17] A wide divergence of views initially hampered its creation. Some countries, mainly in the more developed world, wanted an intensive focus on a relatively few chemicals posing the greatest risks. Other countries, mainly in the developing world, wanted a far more extensive catalog of all the many chemicals about which their scientists knew little. The United Nations Environment Programme, which was established following the Stockholm Conference, created the International Register of Potentially Toxic Chemicals in 1976 more on the "extensive" model than the "intensive." It was a database, but with provisions for preparing more detailed profiles on a relatively few chemicals. At the time, perhaps 60,000 chemicals were in common use, with 1000 more added annually. In parallel with this effort, a veteran Chair of UNSCEAR, Dutch geneticist Frits Sobels, spawned an International Commission for Protection against Environmental Mutagens and Carcinogens (ICPEMC) modeled on ICRP.[18]

Neither ICPEMC nor IRPTC would survive into the twenty-first century. The ICPEMC soldiered on at least until the early 1990s but struggled for resources. Its last trace on today's internet, a report modeled on the ICRP's approach to radiation, appeared in 1992.[19] By 1997,

[16] Truhaut R. "Les limites tolérables pour les substances toxiques dans l'industrie," Extrait des Archives des Maladies Professionnelles. T. 26, 1965, no 1–2 (pp. 41–56), ICRP Archives, Box 039, C2 Internal Exposure 1965–1968 C.pdf, 189–204. He compares U.S. and Soviet maximum permissible concentrations.

[17] Caveat emptor: I was in the secretariat of the Conference and was responsible for pursuing the IRPTC idea during 1974–1975. Its history and then current state is told in Huismans JW. The International Register of Potentially Toxic Chemicals (IRPTC): Its Present State of Development and Future Plans. No. 5/6, Toxics and Their Control: A Special Issue (1978) Ambio [Internet]. 1978;7(5/6):275–7. Available from: https://www.jstor.org/stable/4312399, accessed June 2, 2023.

[18] Jansen JD. The International Commission for Protection against Environmental Mutagens and Carcinogens (ICPEMC): The First Seven Years. Regulatory Toxicology and Pharmacology. 1984 Jun;4(2):138–44. https://www.sciencedirect.com/science/article/pii/0273230084900369?via%3Dihub, accessed July 24, 2023 Early ICPEMC activities are reported in "ICPEMC News No. 2," stamped July 2, 1979, ICRP Archives, Archive Files 81, Archive Files 81 part 1.pdf, 178–84.

[19] Brusick DJ, Gopalan HNB, Heseltine E, Huismans JW, Lohmay, PHM. Assessing the Risk of Genetic Damage [Internet]. Gabarone: Hodder and Stoughton. 1992. Available

IRPTC contained data on 8000 chemicals.[20] The database existed until the late 1990s, but its value added declined with the internet's capacity to make the latest data available on (almost) everything from (almost) anywhere.[21] It eventually got reorganized into "UNEP Chemicals." UNEP tried in the 1990s to convince UNSCEAR to shift its focus to a few, top-priority toxic chemicals but failed. The radiation protection experts thought it would be a bridge too far for their own professional capacities and did not want to give up UNSCEAR's focus on ionizing radiation.[22]

The 1992 Earth Summit (the UN Conference on Development and Environment) in Rio de Janeiro called for an Intergovernmental Forum on Chemical Safety, which led to the creation of the UNEP-sponsored Strategic Approach to International Chemicals Management (SAICM) in 2006.[23] SAICM aims to achieve "the sound management of chemicals throughout their life cycle…so that chemicals are produced and used in ways that minimize significant adverse impacts on the environment and

from: https://wedocs.unep.org/bitstream/handle/20.500.11822/29186/ATGD.pdf?sequence=1&isAllowed=y, accessed December 22, 2023.

[20] U.S. EPA. Chemicals in the Environment: International Chemicals Management [Internet]. EPA. 749-R-97-001a (Spring/Summer 1997); [cited 2023 Jun 2]. Available from: https://nepis.epa.gov/Exe/ZyNET.exe/20001KYX.TXT?ZyActionD=ZyDocument&Client=EPA&Index=1995+Thru+1999&Docs=&Query=&Time=&EndTime=&SearchMethod=1&TocRestrict=n&Toc=&TocEntry=&QField=&QFieldYear=&QFieldMonth=&QFieldDay=&IntQFieldOp=0&ExtQFieldOp=0&XmlQuery=&File=D%3A%5Czyfiles%5CIndex%20Data%5C95thru99%5CTxt%5C00000008%5C20001KYX.txt&User=ANONYMOUS&Password=anonymous&SortMethod=h%7C-&MaximumDocuments=1&FuzzyDegree=0&ImageQuality=r75g8/r75g8/x150y150g16/i425&Display=hpfr&DefSeekPage=x&SearchBack=ZyActionL&Back=ZyActionS&BackDesc=Results%20page&MaximumPages=1&ZyEntry=1&SeekPage=x&ZyPURL, accessed December 23, 2023.

[21] Caroli S, Menditto A, Chiodo F. The International Register of Potentially Toxic Chemicals. Environmental Science and Pollution Research. 1996 Jun 1;3(2):104–7, accessed June 2, 2023.

[22] Note 1, "UNSCEAR's 34th Session in Vienna," p. 313; and "Tolba's Proposal for UNSCEAR," p. 414. Only 8 of UNSCEAR's 21 representatives favored broadening its focus.

[23] Intergovernmental Forum on Chemical Safety—IFCS [Internet]. IISD Earth Negotiations Bulletin. Available from: https://enb.iisd.org/negotiations/intergovernmental-forum-chemical-safety-ifcs#:~:text=The%20Intergovernmental%20Forum%20on%20Chemical, accessed December 23, 2023.

human health," in accordance with the Sustainable Development Goals.[24] SAICM has generated a convention on persistent organic pollutants (Stockholm Convention), which joined two earlier UNEP-supported conventions that set standards in the 1990s for the export and import of chemicals and waste.[25] The 2013 Japan-sponsored Minamata Convention aims to end mercury mining, phase out existing mines and uses of mercury, and control releases to air and water. Leaded petrol disappeared worldwide in 2021 without an international convention, when Algeria ended its use more than a century after its invention in the U.S.[26] None of these international steps has sought to protect the use of the chemicals in question in addition to protecting against their risks. The cooperating states have judged that the risks to human health and the environment of these specific chemicals are greater than the conceivable benefits, though the Stockholm Convention has a specific exemption for DDT disease vector control (mainly against malaria) and one other group of chemicals. They all aim at phasing down and out their use. In this sense they deal with low-hanging fruit, either because the chemicals are no longer necessary or because adequate alternatives are available.

Norm-setting on chemicals and air pollution has progressed since the 1970s, but all is still not right in setting norms for the many toxic chemicals that offer benefits as well as risks. Individual scientists do research on specific chemicals and groups of chemicals, but interdisciplinary epistemic groups with shared normative and causal beliefs as well as shared notions of validity and engagement in a common policy enterprise have not emerged. The chemical industry, which has substantial scientific expertise, has chosen to try to protect itself from regulation not through such collaboration but rather through well-funded chemical associations

[24] Overview: Strategic Approach to International Chemicals Management [Internet]. www.saicm.org. Available from: https://www.saicm.org/About/Overview/tabid/5522/language/en-US/Default.aspx, accessed June 2, 2023.

[25] Basel/Rotterdam/Stockholm Conventions [Internet]. Available from: http://www.brsmeas.org/, accessed June 2, 2023. The 1989 Basel Convention governs transboundary movements of hazardous wastes and their disposal. The 1998 Rotterdam Convention governs prior informed consent for trade in certain hazardous chemicals and pesticides. Its list of "candidate" chemicals is long and the process of approving them for listing is slow due the requirement for unanimous consent.

[26] Inside the 20-year Campaign to Rid the World of Leaded Fuel [Internet]. UNEP. 2021. Available from: https://www.unep.org/news-and-stories/story/inside-20-year-campaign-rid-world-leaded-fuel, accessed June 2, 2023.

and broad claims of confidentiality concerning proprietary business data. Critics have responded with pressure for prohibitions. This has created an adversarial space for norm-setting, rather than the more cooperative one that emerged for ionizing radiation. Progress has depended not on epistemic communities but rather on advocacy by coalitions of states, intergovernmental organizations, and nongovernmental organizations. These advocates share interests and beliefs that have expanded restraints on toxic chemicals as well as diffusing the regime and making it more effective, but they have also left many priority toxic chemicals unregulated internationally.[27]

The adversarial approach is ill-suited to balancing risks and benefits. It can result in binary and sometimes exaggerated risk assessments. The WHO International Agency for Research on Cancer, established in 1965, has adopted a "hazard" approach to classifying chemicals as carcinogens, ignoring dose–response relationships and the associated quantification of risks. Geoffrey Kabat has documented unscientific hyping of health risks of organochlorine compounds and combustion products, electromagnetic fields, radiofrequency radiation (from cell phones and other sources), residential radon, passive smoking, bisphenol-A (BPA), the pesticide DDT, and glyphosate (the main ingredient of the weedkiller Roundup).[28] In his view, many millions of dollars have been spent on poorly designed and executed studies that ignored the fundamental dictum of toxicology: "the dose makes the poison." In several of these cases, the doses are so low compared to what would be required to demonstrate an effect, or so low compared to natural exposures, that it is no surprise the studies failed.

[27] Selin H. Global Governance of Hazardous Chemicals: Challenges of Multilevel Management. Cambridge, Mass.: MIT Press; 2010, especially Chapter 8.

[28] Kabat GC. Hyping Health Risks: Environmental Hazards in Daily Life and the Science of Epidemiology. New York: Columbia University Press; 2008; and Kabat GC. Getting Risk Right: Understanding the Science of Elusive Health Risks. New York: Columbia University Press; 2017. On glyphosate, see Kabat GC, Price WJ, Tarone RE. On Recent Meta-Analyses of Exposure to Glyphosate and Risk of non-Hodgkin's Lymphoma in Humans. Cancer Causes & Control. 2021 Jan 15;32(4):409–14. https://doi.org/10.1007/s10552-020-01387-w; https://link.springer.com/article/10.1007/s10552-020-01387-w, accessed June 10, 2023. For Kabat's layman's version, Kabat G. Who's Afraid of Roundup? Issues in Science and Technology [Internet]. 2019;36(1):64–73. Available from: https://issues.org/whos-afraid-of-roundup/, accessed November 9, 2023 and the responses Reassessing Roundup. Issues in Science and Technology [Internet]. 2020;36(2). Available from: https://issues.org/reassessing-roundup-carcinogen-kabat-forum/, accessed November 9, 2023.

In others, known confounding factors make it impossible to discern cause and effect, or data has been cherry-picked. In still others, measurement of doses is highly uncertain. It is difficult to believe these issues would not have been highlighted more quickly and much effort conserved if there had been competent, dedicated epistemic groups nationally and internationally to examine the scientific evidence. The more usual practice, peer review conducted by professional journals, is unreliable when it comes to weeding out dubious science.[29]

Several dozen scientists representing multiple disciplines have identified what they regard as key outstanding issues in the regulation of chemicals in the United States, mainly by the Environmental Protection Agency (EPA).[30] While their views on specific chemicals differ from Kabat's, they are also critical of the system as a whole. They describe a wide divergence between the legally fragmented U.S. approach, which often relies on the government to identify chemical hazards, and the more unified European approach, which assigns that responsibility to industry, before marketing. The results in the United States are underwhelming: an asbestos ban proposed in 1989 is still not in effect, whereas the European Union banned all use of asbestos in 2005 (and some member states had banned it previously). The recommendations of the interdisciplinary American group include shifting the financial burden of data generation to industry (though they also warn about possible conflicts of interest), recognizing that lack of data is not evidence of a lack of hazard, exposure, or risk, identifying populations at greater risk, and applying a no-threshold assumption to non-cancer risks (EPA already applies it to carcinogens). It is also important to recognize that conflict of interest can apply to government-sponsored research, which needs to be examined with the same sharp eyes as industry-sponsored research.

While the Americans cite a European Environment Agency paper that bemoans the delay in the development of radiation norms by the ICRP, they do not comment on how that eventually successful institutional

[29] Velterop J. Peer Review—Issues, Limitations, and Future Development. ScienceOpen Research. 2015 Sep 29;0(0):1–5. https://www.scienceopen.com/hosted-document?doi=10.14293/S2199-1006.1.SOR-EDU.AYXIPS.v1, accessed June 11, 2023.

[30] Woodruff TJ, Rayasam SDG, Axelrad DA, Koman PD, Chartres N, Bennett DH, et al. A Science-Based Agenda for Health-Protective Chemical Assessments and Decisions: Overview and Consensus Statement. Environmental Health. 2023 Jan 12;21(S1). https://doi.org/10.1186/s12940-022-00930-3, accessed June 5, 2023.

precedent might be applied to chemicals.[31] It would not be easy. Radiation is complicated because there are many different isotopes that produce radiation of different types over a wide energy range, but there is a single mechanism, ionization, that is believed to cause their "stochastic" biological effects. Chemicals come in daunting numbers and can cause biological effects in many different ways. Over 350,000 chemicals and chemical mixtures have been registered for production and use in 19 countries.[32] It is not possible to picture epistemic groups dedicated to more than a tiny fraction of these, or to a few priority groups of them. The United States EPA is required to prioritize 20 chemicals at a time for risk evaluation, which assesses whether they present an unreasonable risk to public health or the environment under current conditions of use. Provided the conflict of interest issue can be neutralized, it makes more sense for the industry to pay for the initial assessment, as it has an incentive to bring new chemicals to market and to justify the use of those already marketed. The companies producing chemicals also know, or should know, a good deal about their biological effects, or absence of them, as their workers are likely to have been exposed. But if American industry were to be tasked in the future with this responsibility, it would be judicious to do it via arms-length epistemic groups, as the AEC did with the NCRP, prepared to spend not weeks or months but years getting to the level of quantitative sophistication concerning doses and effects that the ICRP and UNSCEAR have achieved for ionizing radiation. Doing this cooperatively with Europeans, Chinese, and other more research-focused countries could spread the burden.

The adversarial approach stands in the way. Jessica Templeton concluded more than a decade ago that for persistent organic pollutants:

[31] The paper they cite is Harremoës P, et al. Late Lessons from Early Warnings: The Precautionary Principle 1896–2000—European Environment Agency. Environmental Issue Report No. 22 [Internet]. www.eea.europa.eu. Available from: https://www.eea.europa.eu/publications/environmental_issue_report_2001_22#:~:text=Late%20lessons%20from%20early%20warnings%20is%20about%20the%20gathering%20of, accessed June 5, 2023.

[32] Wang Z, Walker GW, Muir DCG, Nagatani-Yoshida K. Toward a Global Understanding of Chemical Pollution: A First Comprehensive Analysis of National and Regional Chemical Inventories. Environmental Science and Technology. 2020;54(5):2575–84.

1. the formation of epistemic communities of technical experts is precluded by political pressure on scientists to represent government/organizational interests, and
2. scientists strategically frame issues in ways that support the social, economic or political interests of the governments or organizations with which they are affiliated, thus contributing to the politicization of science-based decision-making.[33]

It is one thing to phase down and out the use of chemicals whose risks clearly exceed their benefits. It is another to manage exposure to chemicals so that the benefits exceed the risks. UNEP's Environment Assembly has authorized discussions in an open-ended working group intended to create "a science-policy panel to contribute to sound management of chemicals and waste and prevention of pollution."[34] The focus of the discussions thus far has been on scanning the horizon for emerging hazards, scientific assessments, information provision and dissemination, information sharing, and capacity building.[35] This effort to bring the scientific and policy communities together could eventually help to catalyze the creation of international epistemic communities focused on priority chemicals requiring normative balance between risks and benefits. But that would entail a change in industry and advocacy attitudes toward acceptance of such balancing and willingness to contribute to a more cooperative, less adversarial approach to norm-setting for chemicals.

[33] Templeton J. Framing Elite Policy Discourse: Science and the Stockholm Convention on Persistent Organic Pollutants [Internet]. PhD Thesis, London School of Economics and Political Science. 2011. Available from: http://etheses.lse.ac.uk/361/, accessed June 25, 2023.

[34] Summary Report 30 January–3 February 2023. OEWG1-2: Science-Policy Panel to Contribute Further to the Sound Management of Chemicals and Waste and to Prevent Pollution. [Internet]. IISD Earth Negotiations Bulletin. Available from: https://enb.iisd.org/oewg1-2-science-policy-panel-contribute-further-sound-management-chemicals-waste-prevent-pollution-summary, accessed June 13, 2023.

[35] I am indebted to Templeton, now at the International Institute for Sustainable Development, for drawing my attention to this UNEP activity and its possible future evolution, in addition to answering many questions on international chemicals issues.

Better Results with Global Atmospheric Challenges

Global atmospheric challenges like ozone depleting and climate change chemicals pose "collective action" problems. These involve a conflict between the interests of individual actors who use the chemicals and the collective interest in preventing ozone depletion or climate change that would harm life on earth. The benefits of chemical emissions and the resulting harm often accrue to different countries, making these issues particularly knotty. Nevertheless, protecting the ozone layer is today about as close to solved as an international environmental issue gets to be, due in part to an epistemic community that played vital roles. Climate change is still a pressing problem, but in some respects it has proven less resistant to international norms than toxic chemicals.

Ozone-Depleting Chemicals

Like the efforts to phase out and end the production of selected chemicals toxic to human health, the 1987 Montreal Protocol to a 1985 Vienna Convention aimed at phasing out the production and use of chemicals that deplete the atmosphere's ozone layer as well as contribute to climate change.[36] This was an important and innovative first step that has proven, with its several amendments, remarkably resilient and effective.[37] It has been 99% successful, in part because viable alternatives became available, as anticipated in the Protocol.[38] Attention to ozone-depleting chemicals (especially chlorofluorocarbons, or CFCs, and other halogenated compounds, or halons) originated in 1974 in a paper based on known chemical and physical phenomena and sponsored by the U.S.

[36] Institutions | Ozone Secretariat [Internet]. 2020. https://unep.org/. Available from: https://ozone.unep.org/institutions, accessed June 11, 2023.

[37] Koehler J, Hajost SA. The Montreal Protocol: A Dynamic Agreement for Protecting the Ozone Layer. Ambio [Internet]. 1990;19(2):82–6. Available from: http://www.jstor.org/stable/4313664, accessed June 11, 2023.

[38] World Meteorological Organization. Executive Summary: Scientific Assessment of Depletion [Internet]. Ozone Research and Monitoring—GAW Report No. 278. 2022. Available from: https://ozone.unep.org/system/files/documents/Scientific-Assessment-of-Ozone-Depletion-2022-Executive-Summary.pdf, accessed June 4, 2023.

Atomic Energy Commission.[39] The ozone layer of the stratosphere (at 20–25 km altitude) is essential to human and other life on earth because it blocks harmful ultraviolet radiation. Its disruption can also affect military communications.[40] The potential impact of chlorofluorocarbons was substantial but so too were their benefits, as they were widely used in industrial and consumer products.

Parts of the American scientific community reacted quickly, as did industry, which initially defended the production and use of CFCs. UNEP mounted an International Conference on the Ozone Layer and launched a World Plan of Action on the Ozone Layer in 1977 that called for a treaty on protecting it and also created a continuing Coordinating Committee on the Ozone Layer. The issue attracted political and public attention by the mid-1980s, partly due to the discovery of a "hole" in the ozone layer over Antarctica. The decisive role of a transnational "ecological" epistemic community in arousing public opinion and shaping the U.S. government and industry positions as well as preparing the ground for compromise that enabled international action is well-documented:

> ...the ecological epistemic community played a primary role in gathering information, forming a consensus regarding the available scientific evidence, disseminating information to government and corporate decision makers, and helping them formulate policies regarding CFC consumption and production.[41]

Specialists who did computer modeling of the atmosphere were particularly influential participants in this epistemic community, as their work

[39] Molina MJ, Rowland FS. Stratospheric Sink for Chlorofluoromethanes: Chlorine Atom-Catalysed Destruction of Ozone. Nature. 1974 Jun;249(5460):810–2. https://doi.org/10.1038/249810a0, accessed June 11, 2023.

[40] The risks to military communications are not usually mentioned in this connection, but I negotiated an agreement for, and as the Science Counselor for the U.S. Embassy in Brasilia was present at, a U.S. Air Force launch in Natal of a sounding rocket designed for studying implications of ozone layer depletion for military communications in 1984.

[41] Haas PM. Introduction: Epistemic Communities and International Policy Coordination. International Organization. 1992;46(1):1–35. https://www.cambridge.org/core/journals/international-organization/article/abs/banning-chlorofluorocarbons-epistemic-community-efforts-to-protect-stratospheric-ozone/6325DC982B4573C378334D80F8835B72, accessed June 11, 2023.

limited the range of alternatives considered.[42] Some CFC-producing companies, including the leading one in the United States (Dupont), decided to search for alternatives and eventually supported a phaseout. The ingredients of success included, according to the chief American negotiator, Richard Benedick:

1. scientific collaboration;
2. the public information and opinion;
3. a respected international institution (UNEP);
4. U.S. leadership;
5. participation of both industry and citizens' groups;
6. an effective process of subdividing the problem and brainstorming before formal negotiations;
7. a flexible and dynamic agreement.[43]

Laura Thoms adds the "common but differentiated responsibility for developing nations."[44] The ecological epistemic group rendered the risks of ozone depletion clear and present, specialists within that group used their expertise to eliminate minimalist options as ineffective, and public concern aroused politicians to begin acting in the United States and elsewhere even before the Montreal Protocol negotiations had begun. These are factors familiar from the history of protection against ionizing radiation.

Climate Change Gases

The issue of chemicals that cause global warming is a tougher one. Climate change is a "malign" collective action problem because it involves many chemicals and their interaction with the atmosphere, its impacts are long-term, and it has broad implications for the burning of fossil fuels and

[42] UNEP. Ad Hoc Scientific Meeting to Compare Model Generated Assessments of Ozone Layer Change for Various Strategies for CFC Control. Wurzburg, Federal Republic of Germany; 1987 Apr 9–10. https://ozone.unep.org/system/files/documents/adhoc-vg-167-infl-add1-compare_model_assmnts.87-02-23.pdf, accessed August 31, 2023.

[43] Benedick RE. Ozone Diplomacy New Directions in Safeguarding the Planet. Cambridge: Harvard University Press; 1991.

[44] Thoms L. International Regimes on Ozone and Climate Change. Columbia Journal of Transnational Law. 2003;41(3):95–860.

other greenhouse gas-producing activities. The benefits of those activities are enormous, as oil, gas, and coal are still vital to the world's current economy. At best, it will take decades to phase them out, in the process shifting benefits and costs dramatically. As a result, the United States was not prepared to play the leadership role on climate change that it had played on ozone depletion, which concerned fewer chemicals of less economic importance. Unlike radiation protection, climate change norms are decided in multilateral fora with virtually universal state participation subject to elaborate procedural rules and treaty-based legal obligations.[45] Legal authority makes agreement harder, not easier.

In addition, many countries see an economic interest in continuing to produce greenhouse gases, although doing so may produce harm not only to other countries but eventually also to themselves. China is a glaring example: global warming threatens it with large-scale coastal flooding, but it is still planning a giant expansion of its coal-burning electrical generation (alongside extensive use of renewables).[46] This collective action problem was avoided in the Montreal Protocol, because U.S., European, and developing country negotiators compromised on the transition to an eventual complete halt to production and consumption, which proved feasible within a reasonable time frame because alternatives to CFCs became available. But the failure of collective action vitiated the 1997 Kyoto Protocol to the 1992 United Nations Framework Convention on Climate Change, as alternatives seemed still far off and states could not agree on how the enormous costs of reducing greenhouse gases would be divided. Developing countries wanted industrialized countries to shoulder the burden, as they have produced the bulk of greenhouse gases in the past. Industrialized countries wanted China and other rapidly developing countries who will produce more greenhouse gasses in the future to shoulder more of the burden. The United States never ratified the Kyoto Protocol and Canada withdrew from it. Despite 192 ratifications, it has remained a dead letter.

[45] Schiele S. Evolution of International Environmental Regimes the Case of Climate Change. Cambridge Studies in International and Comparative Law. Cambridge University Press; 2014.

[46] China's New Great Wall [Internet]. The Economist. Available from: https://www.economist.com/china/2023/06/05/chinas-new-great-walland; and Who Is Keeping Coal Alive? [Internet]. The Economist. 2023 Jun 10. Available from: https://www.economist.com/finance-and-economics/2023/06/04/who-is-keeping-coal-alive, accessed June 13, 2023.

The 2015 Paris climate agreement has been modestly more successful. It allowed states to set their own "nationally determined contributions" and enunciated for the first-time overall goals: to keep global warming "well below 2 °C above pre-industrial levels" while "pursuing efforts to limit the temperature increase to 1.5 °C."[47] These norms are conceptually analogous to the performance-focused permissible doses used in radiation protection. They aim to protect a specified "target" (in this case the world's average atmospheric temperature) from the effects of human activity. The nationally determined contributions set to date will not meet the 1.5 °C norm, and there is well-founded doubt they will be tightened sufficiently in time to do so, but the existence and acceptance of the overall norm have nevertheless become a widely shared objective and measure of success or failure.

The climate change norms emerged from the Intergovernmental Panel on Climate Change (IPCC), created in 1988 by the World Meteorological Society and UNEP. All UN member states can be members of the IPCC, but its periodic assessments (every 5–7 years) are written by experts based on thousands of scientific contributions from sources worldwide. The IPCC plays a role roughly comparable to the combined roles UNSCEAR and ICRP played for ionizing radiation. It assesses the effects of climate change and recommends a performance goal. Its experts essentially constitute an epistemic group of remarkable size, range, and diversity who have managed to enunciate norms (1.5/2 °C) that are grudgingly accepted worldwide as desirable, even if so far ineffectively.[48] The fact that the lower number will be missed does not, however, diminish its role in marking a milestone that connotes failure. That is an important normative function. The projected failure to meet the norm was one of the factors that forced the Dubai Climate Change Conference in December 2023 to acknowledge the necessity of "transitioning away" from fossil fuels.[49]

[47] Paris Agreement. United Nations. 2015. https://unfccc.int/sites/default/files/english_paris_agreement.pdf, accessed June 10, 2023.

[48] The IPCC experts are not the only epistemic group effective on climate change issues. The Green Diplomacy Network constitutes another, see Cross MKD. Partners at Paris? Climate Negotiations and Transatlantic Relations. Journal of European Integration. 2018 Jul 11;40(5):571–86. https://doi.org/10.1080/07036337.2018.1487962, accessed December 13, 2023.

[49] Outcome of the First Global Stocktake [Internet]. Available from: https://unfccc.int/sites/default/files/resource/cma2023_L17_adv.pdf, accessed December 22, 2023.

Potential for Other Hi-Tech Hazards

Nonionizing Radiation

An obvious analogue to ionizing radiation is nonionizing radiation, that is rays that have insufficient energy to expel an electron from a gas like air. These include microwave transmissions, emissions from magnetic resonance imaging (MRI), electromagnetic fields surrounding powerlines, emissions from cell phones, lasers, sunlamps, radio transmitters, radar stations, microwave ovens, and ultrasonic cleaners. The ICRP considered but declined repeatedly to take on responsibility for nonionizing radiation, following a pattern set earlier by the American NCRP. People whose professional identity became associated with ionization as the cause of biological effects sometimes found it hard to imagine dealing with phenomena that by definition did not cause ionization but were still alleged to have biological effects whose physical basis was often obscure.[50]

Informed that the ICRP did not want to take on the task, the WHO, which wanted an institution comparable to the ICRP to set norms for nonionizing radiation, turned to the International Radiation Protection Association (IRPA). Like Bo Lindell's Swedish Radiation Protection Institute, IRPA had decided to include nonionizing radiation in its remit, if only to reduce public anxiety. It convened a "task group" in 1972 that became the International Non-Ionizing Committee (INIRC) in 1977 with a French member of the ICRP Main Commission, Henri Jammet, as Chair. This Committee was spun off in 1992 as the still existing International Commission on Non-Ionizing Radiation Protection (ICNIRP).[51]

ICNIRP's norms have not gained the same universal adherence as the ICRP's. The United States and Europe still differ in how they formulate norms for nonionizing radiation, though not by much.[52] That was also

[50] There was a lengthy discussion at the ICRP of adding nonionizing radiation to its agenda, and a decision not to do so, in 1971, Minutes of the Commission Meeting in London: April 1971, ICRP/71/MC-17, ICRP Archives, Box W-10, "Minutes 1953–1972.pdf," 22–40, at p. 5-9.

[51] ICNIRP | Aim, Status & History [Internet]. www.icnirp.org. Available from: https://www.icnirp.org/en/about-icnirp/aim-status-history/index.htmland, "Creation of the INIRC," accessed December 23, 2023.

[52] Note 28, Getting Risk Right:63.

the case for the ICRP up until about 1965. Local content is not necessarily inconsistent with the eventual establishment of broad authority. Notably, the ICNIRP assesses that "Acute and long-term effects of RF [radiofrequency] EMF [electromagnetic field] exposure from the use of mobile phones have been studied extensively without showing any conclusive evidence of adverse health effects."[53] Admittedly it is difficult to imagine any health effect, even the alleged brain cancer, that would keep the world's population from using cell phones, but reassurance from an epistemic group is welcome.

Pharmaceuticals, Medical Devices, and Vaccines

Compared to toxic chemicals, the situation is strikingly different for pharmaceuticals, medical devices, and vaccines. The importance of safety and effectiveness as well as the need to bring medically beneficial innovations quickly into use are widely shared. No one in the industry, the scientific community, or government regulatory authorities will want to forget the thalidomide disaster, though even thalidomide has approved beneficial uses today.[54] The World Health Organization runs an International Pharmacopoeia, which aims "to provide specifications and test methods for priority medicines of major public health importance."[55] It also sets norms for production, quality control, prequalification, regulatory standards, development, distribution, inspections, and quality assurance.[56] It

[53] ICNIRP | Mobile Phones: Radiofrequency—RF EMF [Internet]. www.icnirp.org. Available from: https://www.icnirp.org/en/applications/mobile-phones/index.html, accessed June 26, 2023.

[54] Rehman W, Arfons LM, Lazarus HM. The Rise, Fall and Subsequent Triumph of Thalidomide: Lessons Learned in Drug Development. Therapeutic Advances in Hematology [Internet]. 2011 Aug 4;2(5):291–308, PMID: 23556097; PMCID: PMC3573415, accessed June 8, 2023. Available from: https://www.ncbi.nlm.nih.gov/pmc/articles/PMC3573415/.

[55] WHO. The International Pharmacopoeia. [Internet]. Available from: https://www.who.int/teams/health-product-policy-and-standards/standards-and-specifications/norms-and-standards-for-pharmaceuticals/international-pharmacopoeia, accessed December 22, 2023.

[56] WHO. Guidelines: Norms and Standards for Pharmaceuticals. [Internet]. Available from: https://www.who.int/teams/health-product-and-policy-standards/standards-and-specifications/norms-and-standards-for-pharmaceuticals/guidelines, accessed December 22, 2023.

relies on expert groups and national regulatory authorities, but the registration of specific pharmaceuticals is not an international responsibility.

Pharmaceutical research and development is concentrated in the United States and Europe. U.S. regulation is centralized in the Food and Drug Administration (FDA), while the European Union approves pharmaceuticals and medical devices "through a network of centralized and decentralized agencies throughout its member states."[57] According to Gail Van Norman, the FDA review process for pharmaceuticals in 2016 was generally a bit quicker than the centralized European one administered by the European Medicines Agency (EMA), but most European applications are submitted at the member state level in more than one of the 27 member states, rather than to the EMA. Companies applying to register pharmaceuticals and medical devices are responsible for development costs, but many clinical trials are sponsored by government agencies, all the data from which is available to the public in principle in the United States but not in Europe if it is unpublished. Requirements for medical devices in Europe are less stringent than in the United States, where some (but not all) approvals are slower than in Europe. But in both Europe and the United States some devices can get to market with minimal clinical scrutiny of safety or effectiveness, and post-market surveillance is often inadequate.

Regulatory authorities, including those in the United States and Europe, have been trying to harmonize their processes through the nongovernmental International Council for Harmonisation of Technical Requirements for Pharmaceuticals for Human Use, which "brings together regulatory authorities and pharmaceutical industry representatives to discuss scientific and technical aspects of drug registration." Established in 1990, it had issued by 2023 fifty-nine guidelines on salient issues in the categories of quality, safety, efficacy, and "interdisciplinary" intended to promote harmonization of registration processes, without however recommending specific registrations. The implementation of the guidelines in some countries is spotty, but strong in the United States and

[57] Van Norman GA. Drugs and Devices. JACC: Basic to Translational Science [Internet]. 2016 Aug;1(5):399–412. Available from: https://www.sciencedirect.com/science/article/pii/S2452302X16300638, accessed June 6, 2023.

EU.[58] Pharmaceutical regulators also participate in an intergovernmental program that aims at regulatory convergence, a cooperative scheme among pharmaceutical inspectors with 52 participating authorities, and an "an executive-level" forum of medicines regulatory authorities.[59] The United States and EU since 2019 have relied on each other's inspections for human medicines, and since 2023 for veterinary medicines, produced in their own territories. They thereby avoid duplicative work while cooperating in inspections in other countries.[60]

The U.S. market for pharmaceuticals is about 49% of the world market, while Europe's is about 24%.[61] Not surprisingly, most of the rest of the world therefore follows the United States and European leads when it comes to regulation of many pharmaceuticals and medical devices. Even if they have their own approval processes, they must meet U.S. or EU standards if they have production facilities and want to export to these dominant markets, and many countries lack the expertise required to do the elaborate clinical trials and technological development required for pharmaceuticals and some medical devices on their own. There might be economies of scale if international epistemic groups formed to recommend norms for safety and effectiveness of at least some pharmaceuticals or medical devices, but there are also high barriers to such normative collaboration, including national pride, commercial interests, diverse population genetics, and differing regulatory systems.

If the Americans and Europeans have not been able to combine forces to coordinate on specific registrations, it is difficult to imagine either group doing it with others (though the EMA does include non-EU but still European Iceland, Norway, and Liechtenstein). Both the FDA

[58] Harmonisation for Better Health [Internet]. Available from: https://www.ich.org/; and ICH Guideline Implementation [Internet]. Available from: https://www.ich.org/page/ich-guideline-implementation, accessed June 6, 2023.

[59] International Regulatory Harmonization. US FDA [Internet]. 2020 Mar 26. Available from: https://www.fda.gov/drugs/cder-international-program/international-regulatory-harmonization, accessed June 6, 2023.

[60] Hrabovszki G. EU and US Reach a Milestone in Mutual Recognition of Inspections Medicines Manufacturers—European Medicines Agency [Internet]. European Medicines Agency. 2019. Available from: https://www.ema.europa.eu/en/news/eu-us-reach-milestone-mutual-recognition-inspections-medicines-manufacturers, accessed June 6, 2023.

[61] EFPIA. The Pharmaceutical Industry in Figures [Internet]. European Federation of Pharmaceutical Industries and Associations. 2022. Available from: https://www.efpia.eu/media/637143/the-pharmaceutical-industry-in-figures-2022.pdf, accessed June 27, 2023.

and EMA cooperate with other countries, however, and it is possible to imagine nongovernmental initiatives like the ICRP for a few higher priority pharmaceuticals or technologies, especially cardiovascular devices that often pose thorny issues. No doubt the executive-level meetings among regulatory authorities do already include some informal discussion of specific items. The rapidly growing number of pharmaceuticals and medical devices being brought to market will make some sort of international cooperation on norms highly desirable, though it may continue to take the form of many countries copycatting EU and U.S. decisions.

WHO does recommend specific vaccines, nominally for international travel purposes. But it had a hard time keeping up with the COVID-19 pandemic, as everyone did. National governments took the lead in that emergency situation, which meant that recommendations and requirements varied widely worldwide. The Chinese resisted acknowledging the virus and letting its origins be investigated. The Americans initially refused to take action against it and announced that the United States would withdraw from WHO. These stances put WHO in a difficult situation, as it depends on both China and the United States not only for budget but also for political support and technical expertise. As an intergovernmental organization, not an epistemic community, WHO is vulnerable to political conflict, especially when its Director General shies away from vigorous independence. The timeline of WHO's response to the pandemic is impressive, but its efforts lacked impact.[62] Governments "retreated to national policies," weakening WHO and the role of its extensive expert network.[63] While no doubt some of its expert committees gave good advice, none had the traction with national authorities or the global public that a longstanding, independent, epistemic group can acquire.

[62] WHO. Timeline: WHO's COVID-19 Response. [Internet]: Available from: https://www.who.int/emergencies/diseases/novel-coronavirus-2019/interactive-timeline, accessed December 22, 2023.

[63] Buranyi S. The WHO V Coronavirus: Why It Can't Handle the Pandemic. [Internet]. Available from: https://www.theguardian.com/news/2020/apr/10/world-health-organization-who-v-coronavirus-why-it-cant-handle-pandemic, accessed December 22, 2023.

Artificial Intelligence

The internet and social media were initially greeted with the innocent enthusiasm that X-rays and radium once enjoyed. Their evolution in recent decades has given the world good reason to react with caution and even alarm to artificial intelligence (AI), which simulates human intelligence using "software that mimics human cognition or perception."[64] AI nevertheless promises colossal economic benefits. It could spur productivity and growth while disrupting existing economies.[65] Goldman Sachs guesstimates that generative AI (software that can produce text, video, audio, and data, like ChatGPT) can lift global productivity growth by as much as 1.5% annually over 10 years, driving a $7 trillion increase in global GDP.[66] Like other revolutionary technologies, AI will shift employment and affect competition in many different spheres. Services (including supply chain management, logistics, marketing, and sales) stand to gain in productivity more than other sectors.

Such specific predictions are less important than the broad understanding that AI can make an enormous difference over the next several decades in many economic sectors as well as in the military and intelligence worlds. It needs to be subjected to reasonable norms if its benefits are to be maximized and its risks minimized. Some of the risks are already apparent. Self-driving cars cause accidents, machine-aided hiring can systematize prejudice, generative software can produce fiction as well as fact, and AI-guided weapons can make choices that are not ethically defensible. The Pentagon's Replicator initiative aims to produce large numbers of "attritable" land, sea, and air drones operating autonomously

[64] Ruta FL. Do the Benefits of Artificial Intelligence Outweigh the Risks? We Need to Develop AI That Aligns with Human Values [Internet]. The Economist. 2018. Available from: https://www.economist.com/open-future/2018/09/10/do-the-benefits-of-artificial-intelligence-outweigh-the-risks, accessed June 7, 2023.

[65] Economic Impacts of Artificial Intelligence (AI) [Internet]. European Parliament Briefing. Available from: https://www.europarl.europa.eu/RegData/etudes/BRIE/2019/637967/EPRS_BRI(2019)637967_EN.pdf, accessed June 7, 2023.

[66] Goldman Sachs. Generative AI Could Raise Global GDP by 7% [Internet]. Goldman Sachs. Goldman Sachs; 2023. Available from: https://www.goldmansachs.com/intelligence/pages/generative-ai-could-raise-global-gdp-by-7-percent.html, accessed June 7, 2023. PwC's earlier publication is broadly consistent with Goldman Sachs, PwC. The Macroeconomic Impact of Artificial Intelligence [Internet]. 2017. Available from: https://www.pwc.co.uk/economic-services/assets/macroeconomic-impact-of-ai-technical-report-feb-18.pdf, accessed June 7, 2023.

but ostensibly subject to human judgment when force is used.[67] Yet even in these obviously troubling instances, one can question whether AI is better or worse than its human-controlled analogs. At the least, it seems reasonable to argue that AI decisions should have no worse outcomes on average than human-informed decisions. Such an expectation would constitute a performance norm roughly analogous to the expectation in radiation protection that the general population not be exposed to artificial levels of ionizing radiation greater than the natural background. With both radiation and AI, we do not start from ground zero but from already existing risks, at least in some AI applications. It is also possible we will want stricter norms for AI than current human performance, as has been the case for ionizing radiation in relation to natural background in some parts of the world.

There are many national or international institutions that might set norms to govern the adoption and use of AI. Among them are the Association for the Advancement of Artificial Intelligence (AAAI is an international scientific society), the industry-based AI Association, the European Association for Artificial Intelligence, the American non-profit Center for AI Safety, and the Global Partnership on Artificial Intelligence (GPAI), in addition to many other profit and non-profit think tanks, scientific laboratories, and networks. To their credit, "Responsible AI" is the watchword of many. In 2019, AAAI adopted a Code of Professional Ethics and Conduct focused mainly on the behavior of professionals involved in AI research, development, and applications.[68] GPAI is an OECD-generated "multistakeholder" activity of 29 governments as well as experts from science, industry, civil society, international

[67] Dress B. Why the Pentagon's "Killer Robots" Are Spurring Major Concerns [Internet]. The Hill. 2023. Available from: https://thehill.com/policy/defense/4225909-why-the-pentagons-killer-robots-are-spurring-major-concerns/?email=fda599a7134fd2ace7187ec8a1ff88353214111d&emaila=f09a46c0cf6dd50778c9b1b231196449&emailb=80b8321492a8ab396ee67ece2081dcacc65d403744c5c136fa446ca628fddb0c&utm_source=Sailthru&utm_medium=email&utm_campaign=09.28.23%20RNS%20%E2%80%93%20News%20Alert%20-%20killerrobots, accessed September 28, 2023. For more details, see O'Connor M. Replicator: A Bold New Path for DoD—Center for Security and Emerging Technology % [Internet]. Center for Security and Emerging Technology. 2023 Sep 18. Available from: https://cset.georgetown.edu/article/replicator-a-bold-new-path-for-dod/, accessed September 28, 2023.

[68] Code of Professional Ethics and Conduct AAAI Ethics and Diversity [Internet]. AAAI. Available from: https://aaai.org/about-aaai/ethics-and-diversity/, accessed June 7, 2023.

organizations, and governments. It seeks to "guide the responsible development and use of artificial intelligence consistent with human rights, fundamental freedoms, and shared democratic values."[69] Its Responsible AI Working Group focuses on environment, gender, social media, and pandemics. These are eminently worthy priorities but do not deal with the full spectrum of AI risks and benefits.[70]

In May 2023, the Hiroshima G7 Summit tasked its governments to work with GPAI and the OECD to create a working group on generative AI by the end of the year. Its discussions could include a far broader risk assessment and governance agenda.[71] This will not however suffice. An OECD-focused initiative cannot claim global legitimacy today, especially as it is devoted to shared democratic values. China did join 27 other countries and the European Union in the November 2023 Bletchley Declaration of the AI Safety Summit, which projects a broad agenda for identifying and responding to AI risks.[72] But an explicitly democratically oriented scheme would be unlikely to attract either the Russians or Chinese, who are already major factors in AI use. A broader, global "technoprudential" approach "to identify and mitigate risks to global stability without choking off AI innovation and the benefits that flow from it" will be needed.[73] Ian Bremmer and Mustafa Suleyman have proposed some "governance principles" for AI intended to meet that

[69] OECD. Recommendation of the Council on Artificial Intelligence. OECD Legal Instruments [Internet]. 2019. https://www.oecd.org/. Available from: https://legalinstruments.oecd.org/en/instruments/OECD-LEGAL-0449, accessed June 7, 2023.

[70] Responsible AI—GPAI [Internet]. https://gpai.ai/. Available from: https://gpai.ai/projects/responsible-ai/, accessed December 23, 2023.

[71] G7 Hiroshima Leaders' Communiqué [Internet]. 2023 May 20, para 38. Available from: https://www.g7hiroshima.go.jp/documents/pdf/Leaders_Communique_01_en.pdf, accessed August 29, 2023.

[72] The Bletchley Declaration by Countries Attending the AI Safety Summit [Internet]. GOV.UK. 2023 Nov 1–2. Available from: https://www.gov.uk/government/publications/ai-safety-summit-2023-the-bletchley-declaration/the-bletchley-declaration-by-countries-attending-the-ai-safety-summit-1-2-november-2023, accessed November 1, 2023.

[73] Bremmer I, Suleyman M. The AI Power Paradox: Can States Learn to Govern Artificial Intelligence–Before It's Too Late. Foreign Affairs [Internet]. 2023 Oct;102(5). Available from: https://www.foreignaffairs.com/world/artificial-intelligence-power-paradox, accessed August 29, 2023.

need.[74] The extraordinarily rapid progress in AI and its highly technical character will necessitate participation by the people and companies producing it. An adversarial norm-setting process for AI will be unable to ensure its benefits while minimizing its risks in a timely way.

Governments are not waiting for international norms. The U.S. Congress mounted a bipartisan National Security Commission on Artificial Intelligence in 2019 and has held multiple hearings on AI-related issues since. The Commission report issued in 2021 focused on the opportunities and risks of artificial intelligence for military purposes, including both defense and warfighting, as well as on winning the global technological competition. Thirty-two countries have endorsed a U.S.-proposed Political Declaration on Responsible Military Use of Artificial Intelligence and Autonomy, which the United States plans to use as a basis for a proposal at the United Nations.[75] President Biden has succeeded in getting some still vague voluntary commitments focused on safety, security, and trust from major AI companies.[76] The White House has offered a more specific "Blueprint for an AI Bill of Rights" focused on safety and effectiveness, algorithmic discrimination protections, data privacy, notice and explanation, and access to human alternatives, consideration, and fallback.[77] The United States National Institute of Standards and Technology (NIST) has developed, under a Congressional mandate,

[74] Bremmer I, Suleyman M. Building Blocks for AI Governance by Bremmer and Suleyman [Internet]. IMF. 2023. Available from: https://www.imf.org/en/Publications/fandd/issues/2023/12/POV-building-blocks-for-AI-governance-Bremmer-Suleyman, accessed December 11, 2023.

[75] Political Declaration on Responsible Military Use of Artificial Intelligence and Autonomy [Internet]. United States Department of State. 2023. Available from: https://www.state.gov/political-declaration-on-responsible-military-use-of-artificial-intelligence-and-autonomy-2/, accessed November 12, 2023.

[76] FACT SHEET: Biden-Harris Administration Secures Voluntary Commitments from Leading Artificial Intelligence Companies to Manage the Risks Posed by AI [Internet]. The White House. 2023. Available from: https://www.whitehouse.gov/briefing-room/statements-releases/2023/07/21/fact-sheet-biden-harris-administration-secures-voluntary-commitments-from-leading-artificial-intelligence-companies-to-manage-the-risks-posed-by-ai/#:~:text=As%20part%20of%20this%20commitment, accessed July 30, 2023.

[77] The White House. Blueprint for an AI Bill of Rights [Internet]. The White House. 2022. Available from: https://www.whitehouse.gov/ostp/ai-bill-of-rights/, accessed June 7, 2023.

"a voluntary risk management framework for trustworthy artificial intelligence systems."[78] That framework has an institutional base focused on implementation in a NIST United States AI Safety Institute. The U.S. government has also published draft policy guidance on its own use of AI and is mobilizing private funding to support responsible AI as well as beginning the process of setting standards intended to make AI safe and secure.[79] There is even concern that American regulation may be moving too far, too fast.[80]

UNESCO has already published a recommendation on the ethics of artificial intelligence that focuses on the intersection between the technology and existing internationally shared ideals, but more detailed AI norms will not be easy to agree internationally.[81] Concerns vary markedly around the world. Europe and China, like the U.S., are also considering legislation and administrative action to control risks, but with different goals and outcomes. President Xi Jinping has warned of risks to Chinese

[78] Artificial Intelligence Risk Management Framework (AI RMF 1.0) [Internet]. NIST. NIST AI 100-1; Available from: https://nvlpubs.nist.gov/nistpubs/ai/nist.ai.100-1.pdf, accessed June 16, 2023.

[79] FACT SHEET: Vice President Harris Announces New U.S. Initiatives to Advance the Safe and Responsible Use of Artificial Intelligence [Internet]. The White House. 2023. Available from: https://www.whitehouse.gov/briefing-room/statements-releases/2023/11/01/fact-sheet-vice-president-harris-announces-new-u-s-initiatives-to-advance-the-safe-and-responsible-use-of-artificial-intelligence/, accessed November 1, 2023; and FACT SHEET: President Biden Issues Executive Order on Safe, Secure, and Trustworthy Artificial Intelligence [Internet]. The White House. 2023. Available from: https://www.whitehouse.gov/briefing-room/statements-releases/2023/10/30/fact-sheet-president-biden-issues-executive-order-on-safe-secure-and-trustworthy-artificial-intelligence/, accessed November 10, 2023.

[80] Wu T. Opinion | In Regulating A.I., We May Be Doing Too Much. And Too Little. The New York Times [Internet]. 2023 Nov 7; Available from: https://www.nytimes.com/2023/11/07/opinion/biden-ai-regulation.html.

[81] Recommendation on the Ethics of Artificial Intelligence [Internet]. 2021 Nov 23. https://unesco.org/. Available from: https://unesdoc.unesco.org/ark:/48223/pf0000381137, accessed November 10, 2023.

national security from AI.[82] Beijing is focused on maintaining government control and censorship. Some fear China's autocratic "disaster amnesia" and growth-fueling "techno-optimism" as well as its enthusiasm for surpassing the United States in AI will lead to catastrophe.[83] The European Parliament has agreed to an AI Act that rates the risks of some AI applications as "unacceptable" (and therefore banned) and "high-risk" (and therefore regulated (as well as "limited" and "minimal/none").[84] It lacks only European Council approval, which is expected by June 2024. The European Parliament lists "untargeted scraping of facial images from the internet or CCTV footage to create facial recognition databases" as "high risk," but it is already in common use in China and the United States This kind of divergence could potentially create serious international misunderstandings and friction. North Americans and Europeans are already less convinced than people from other parts of the world that "Products and services using artificial intelligence have more benefits than drawbacks."[85] More Asians and Latin Americans believe they have a good understanding of AI and trust AI companies as much as other companies.

[82] China Warns of Artificial Intelligence risks, Calls for beefed-up National Security Measures [Internet]. AP News. 2023. Available from: https://apnews.com/article/china-artificial-intelligence-national-security-00a38e550ef6b4ac12cd1fd418363d2b#:~:text=Government%20shutdown-,China%20warns%20of%20artificial%20intelligence%20risks%2C%20calls,beefed%2Dup%20national%20security%20measures&text=BEIJING%20(AP)%20%E2%80%94%20China's%20ruling,for%20heightened%20national%20security%20measures, accessed June 16, 2023.

[83] Drexel B, Kelley H. China Is Flirting With AI Catastrophe [Internet]. Foreign Affairs. 2023 May 30. Available from: https://www.foreignaffairs.com/china/china-flirting-ai-catastrophe?check_logged_in=1, accessed June 7, 2023.

[84] The Artificial Intelligence Act [Internet]. The Artificial Intelligence Act. European Union. 2021. Available from: https://artificialintelligenceact.eu/, accessed June 16, 2023; and Hoffman M. The EU AI Act: A Primer [Internet]. Center for Security and Emerging Technology. 2023 Sep 23. Available from: https://cset.georgetown.edu/article/the-eu-ai-act-a-primer/#:~:text=The%20AI%20Act%20is%20a,systems%20across%20EU%20member%20states, accessed November 1, 2023. The final version is described in Artificial Intelligence Act: Deal on Comprehensive Rules for Trustworthy AI | News | European Parliament [Internet]. 2023. www.europarl.europa.eu. Available from: https://www.europarl.europa.eu/news/en/press-room/20231206IPR15699/artificial-intelligence-act-deal-on-comprehensive-rules-for-trustworthy-ai, accessed December 11, 2023.

[85] Expectations About Artificial Intelligence [Internet]. IPSOS. Available from: https://www.ipsos.com/sites/default/files/ct/news/documents/2022-01/Global-opinions-and-expectations-about-AI-2022.pdf, accessed June 7, 2023.

It is not going to be easy in this diverging global environment to establish a few broadly accepted norms, even for Europe and the United States.

Failure to do so will have consequences. The handwriting is on the wall. If greater efforts are not forthcoming to limit AI risks, the benefits of AI could be delayed or even vitiated. One of Google's key AI researchers has resigned in part to speak out about the risks.[86] More than 31,000 people, including Tesla magnate and Twitter owner Elon Musk, by June 2023 had signed an open letter asking to "Pause Giant AI Experiments" so the risks could be evaluated.[87] The letter also urges the U.S. government to step in to impose a moratorium if the industry does not accept the pause. Another group of leading AI researchers has signed a strikingly stark statement: "Mitigating the risk of extinction from AI should be a global priority alongside other societal-scale risks such as pandemics and nuclear war."[88] The AI industry is not yet prepared for the controls on hardware and software that will be required.[89] To ensure that these do not unnecessarily inhibit innovation and its benefits, the AI companies and researchers need to take more vigorous action to suggest norms and avoid a backlash. Its leading experts should be among those most anxious to do so, working with critics as well as government agencies, especially in the United States and Europe. This seems an ideal situation for the emergence of an epistemic group concerned with protecting both the technology and the public: an international commission on safe and secure artificial intelligence.

Genome Editing

Editing of the human genome is a close competitor to AI in offering enormous potential benefits and substantial attendant risks both to individuals

[86] Kleinman Z, Vallance C. AI "godfather" Geoffrey Hinton Warns of Dangers as He Quits Google. BBC News [Internet]. 2023 May 2. Available from: https://www.bbc.com/news/world-us-canada-65452940, accessed June 7, 2023.

[87] Future of Life Institute. Pause Giant AI Experiments: An Open Letter [Internet]. Future of Life Institute. Future of Life Institute; 2023. Available from: https://futureoflife.org/open-letter/pause-giant-ai-experiments/, accessed June 7, 2023.

[88] Statement on AI Risk | Center for AI Security [Internet]. www.safe.ai. Available from: https://www.safe.ai/statement-on-ai-risk#open-letter, accessed June 26, 2023.

[89] Scharre P. AI's Gatekeepers Aren't Prepared for What's Coming [Internet]. Foreign Policy. 2023 Jun 19. Available from: https://foreignpolicy.com/2023/06/19/ai-regulation-development-us-china-competition-technology/, accessed June 26, 2023.

and populations. The increasingly precise genome mapping of individuals and populations, combined with the current ease of editing DNA with a decade-old tool known as CRISPR (as well as other biochemical tools), has opened up the promise of interventions to maintain and improve health as well as counter disease. Somatic (non-reproductive) human genome editing is expected to cure diseases that have so far proven intractable, though the cost is still high.[90] Sickle cell disease is the first, but others are on the way: congenital blindness, heart disease, diabetes, cancer, and HIV.[91] Many clinical trials were ongoing by 2023. Existing national regulations for safety and effectiveness have proven adequate so far in dealing with somatic human genome editing in many countries, though questions of cost and equitable access still loom over the technology's future. Editing of the human germline genome for non-reproductive purposes is useful to research and likewise poses issues that existing laws and regulations are handling.

By contrast, heritable "germline" human genome editing for reproductive purposes raises serious ethical questions about whether to eliminate supposed "disabilities" or improve "desirable" characteristics. Consent of the individual in question is not possible. Even people with disabilities may object to fixing them in embryos.[92] American adults are evenly divided on whether they would want such an intervention for the benefit of their own offspring, with more religious people more doubtful.[93] A

[90] Muigai AWT. Expanding Global Access to Genetic Therapies. Nature Biotechnology [Internet]. 2022 Jan 1;40(1):20–1. Available from: https://www.nature.com/articles/s41587-021-01191-0, accessed June 8, 2023.

[91] Stein R. Sickle Cell Patient's Success with Gene Editing Raises Hopes and Questions [Internet]. NPR. 2023. Available from: https://www.npr.org/sections/health-shots/2023/03/16/1163104822/crispr-gene-editing-sickle-cell-success-cost-ethics#:~:text=Press-,CRISPR%20gene%2Dediting%20success%20for%20sickle%20cell%20raises%20new%20questions,once%20thought%20incurable%20have%20disappeared, accessed June 8, 2023.

[92] Sufian S Garland-Thomson R. The Dark Side of CRISPR [Internet]. Scientific American. 2021 Feb 16. Available from: https://www.scientificamerican.com/article/the-dark-side-of-crispr/#:~:text=Genome%20editing%20is%20a%20powerful,categorize%20as%20diseased%20or%20genetically, accessed June 8, 2023.

[93] Nadeem R. Americans Are Closely Divided Over Editing a Baby's Genes to Reduce Serious Health Risk [Internet]. Pew Research Center: Internet, Science & Tech. 2022 Mar 17. Available from: https://www.pewresearch.org/internet/2022/03/17/americans-are-closely-divided-over-editing-a-babys-genes-to-reduce-serious-health-risk/, accessed June 8, 2023.

meta review of work published in English worldwide on ethical issues from philosophical, theological, public, and research perspectives suggests that germline editing for therapeutic and medical purposes is more widely, but not universally, accepted within and across these perspectives than for enhancement purposes.[94] Premature experiments and overweening ambition to "design" the genome could cause irreparable harm to individuals and even to populations. Eugenics in a test tube is a dubious enterprise.

The ethical issues have not gone unnoticed. Many countries already have explicit government policies on human genome editing.[95] Seventy-five of nine-six countries surveyed in 2019/20 prohibited heritable human genome editing (though 5 of the 75 allow some exceptions). The Director General of WHO issued a statement in July 2019 saying "it would be irresponsible at this time for anyone to proceed with clinical applications of human germline genome editing."[96] WHO has convened an Expert Advisory Committee on Developing Global Standards for Governance and Oversight of Human Genome Editing. It has urged continued restraint. The third International Summit on Genome Editing (convened by the UK Royal Society, UK Academy of Medical Sciences, US National Academies of Sciences and Medicine, and The World Academy of Sciences) in March 2023 likewise reiterated the call for a moratorium on heritable human genome editing, which it deemed "unacceptable at this time."[97]

[94] Joseph AM, Karas M, Ramadan Y, Joubran E, Jacobs RJ. Ethical Perspectives of Therapeutic Human Genome Editing From Multiple and Diverse Viewpoints: A Scoping Review. Cureus. 2022 Nov 27;14(11):e31927. https://doi.org/10.7759/cureus.31927. PMID: 36582559; PMCID: PMC9793437, accessed June 10, 2023.

[95] Baylis F, Darnovsky M, Hasson K, Krahn TM. Human Germ Line and Heritable Genome Editing: The Global Policy Landscape. CRISPR J. 2020 Oct;3(5):365–77. https://doi.org/10.1089/crispr.2020.0082. Erratum in: CRISPR J. 2021 Apr;4(2):301–2. PMID: 33095042. https://www.liebertpub.com/doi/10.1089/crispr.2020.0082, accessed June 8, 2023.

[96] Statement on Governance and Oversight of Human Genome Editing, WHO [Internet]. 2019. www.who.int. Available from: https://www.who.int/news/item/26-07-2019-statement-on-governance-and-oversight-of-human-genome-editing, accessed December 23, 2023.

[97] Statement from the Organising Committee of the Third International Summit on Human Genome Editing [Internet]. Available from: https://royalsociety.org/-/media/events/2023/03/human-genome-editing-summit/statement-from-the-organising-committee-of-the-third-international-summit-on-human-genome-editing.pdf, accessed June 8, 2023.

Not everyone will want to remain restrained. Already in 2018, an American-trained Chinese biophysicist experimented with genetic editing of twin human embryos, for which he garnered a three-year prison sentence for "illegal medical practices" in China.[98] The outcome for the twins is not known. The biophysicist is still banned from working on reproduction, but he has completed his prison sentence and says he is returning to his own laboratory to do somatic genome editing. Scientific colleagues in China have objected vehemently in a consensus statement denouncing his work as unethical and calling on the authorities to block his renewed efforts in genome editing.[99] Other scientists in the United States and Russia are working on editing human embryo genomes, in preparation for requesting permission to implant them.[100] In the past, governments abused eugenics, but in the future it seems likely consumer demand will drive the diffusion of eugenic technologies.[101] It is not going to be possible to continue the moratorium on germline genome editing forever. Clearer and weightier guidance to scientists, medical doctors, and the public is needed.

WHO has so far failed to provide such guidance. The initial questions are all too clear. Some are the traditional ones about safety and effectiveness of medical treatments and devices. Others have been termed "non-physical" and concern the ethical appropriateness of "shaping" the

[98] Ruwitch J. His Baby Gene Editing Shocked Ethicists. Now He's in the Lab Again [Internet]. 2023. Available from: https://www.npr.org/2023/06/08/1178695152/china-scientist-he-jiankui-crispr-baby-gene-editing#:~:text=Press-,He%20Jiankui%2C%20Chinese%20scientist%20scorned%20for%20gene%2Dedited%20babies%2C,cure%20for%20Duchenne%20muscular%20dystrophy, accessed June 9, 2023.

[99] Zhai X. Chinese Academic Community Speaks out on He Jiankui Again: Consensus Statement on the Challenges and Responses of Science and Technology Ethics Governance. Health Care Science. 2023 Apr;2(2):79–81. https://doi.org/10.1002/hcs2.41, accessed June 9, 2023.

[100] Ma H, Marti-Gutierrez N, Park SW, Wu J, Lee Y, Suzuki K, et al. Correction of a Pathogenic Gene Mutation in Human Embryos. Nature [Internet]. 2017 Aug 2;548(7668):413–9. Available from: http://i2.cdn.turner.com/cnn/2017/images/08/02/nature23305_proof4.pdf, accessed June 9, 2023; and Cohen J. Embattled Russian Scientist Sharpens Plans to Create Gene-Edited Babies. Science. 2019. https://www.science.org/content/article/embattled-russian-scientist-sharpens-plans-create-gene-edited-babies, accessed June 9, 2023.

[101] Kevles DJ. The History of Eugenics. Issues in Science and Technology [Internet]. 2016;32(3):45–50. Available from: http://www.jstor.org/stable/24727059.

human genome, as opposed to "accepting" its natural order, and the broader consequences for human society:

> Might such technologies push us toward thinking of human beings in increasingly mechanistic terms? Might they push us toward ever-narrower conceptions of acceptable ways to be human? Might they undermine healthy relationships between parents and children? Might they exacerbate the obscene gap between the haves and have-nots?[102]

Some general ethical principles may apply, as they did in radiation protection: any unnecessary risk of harm should be avoided, benefits from specific interventions should outweigh costs, agreed norms should be respected. Individual scholars have elaborated on these and other issues like informed consent and protection of vulnerable groups, but how to apply them has not been codified in international norms, beyond the moratorium on heritable genome editing. Limitation to "therapeutic" or "medical" purposes without further guidance could prove meaningless, as some practitioners might regard height, strength, or skin color as medically necessary. Nor is it clear whether new principles might be required. If the issue is how to balance "shaping" the human genome with "acceptance" of the genome that exists, there is today precious little guidance on how to do it, either at the individual or the societal level. In this day and age, public consultation and participation should be anticipated for any such effort to balance social preferences.

The paucity of norms is surprising. Many of the issues surrounding CRISPR were previewed in the 1970s and 1980s, when artificial "recombinant" DNA from different species held the limelight. But now the technology for changing the human genome in heritable ways is progressing rapidly and inexorably. The normative vacuum leaves room for its more enthusiastic advocates to breach the moratorium and even the laws and policies in countries restricting the use of CRISPR on human embryos intended for reproduction. It is more than time that countries leading this technological race begin to consult each other on normative issues, not necessarily in the formal international sphere so much as in the professional one. Leading researchers should be talking with each other and

[102] Parens E, Johnston J. Introduction to Human Flourishing in an Age of Gene Editing. Oxford University Press eBooks. 2019 Aug 22;1–12. https://doi-org.proxy1.library.jhu.edu/10.1093/oso/9780190940362.003.0001, accessed June 9, 2023.

with their colleagues in other countries, as well as hearing from the public about societal needs. It may be excessively idealistic, but the world needs in this moment of heightened geopolitical tension a challenge that it can confront in a thoughtful way that emphasizes our common humanity. A nongovernmental International Commission on Gene Editing aiming to develop and elaborate norms would be a worthy way of trying to bridge the gaps among Russia, China, and the United States, with the participation of other countries as well. It is no more unrealistic to propose this in 2023 than it was for the ICRP to invite Soviet membership during the height of the Cold War and Chinese membership in the 1990s.

Arms Control

Bilateral arms control applied to long-range, "strategic," nuclear weapons capabilities of the United States and U.S.S.R./Russia has been pursued for more than fifty years. The first twenty were a successful uphill climb against long odds. An American epistemic community played an important role in the early part of this history. It gained traction in the United States even as it diffused its ideas to a Soviet group, helping to create the necessary conditions that generated the 1972 Anti-Ballistic Missile Treaty and the SALT I (Strategic Arms Limitation Talks) interim agreement.[103] President Jimmy Carter and General Secretary Leonid Brezhnev signed an expanded SALT II agreement in 1979 that was never ratified, but both the United States and the U.S.S.R agreed to abide by its provisions until 1985. A new Strategic Arms Reduction Treaty (START I) limiting nuclear warheads and intercontinental ballistic missiles (ICBMs) and bombers was signed in 1991 and START II (banning multiple independently targetable reentry vehicles on ICBMs) was signed in 1993. Both the United States and Russia sharply decreased their nuclear weapons inventories after 1990.

While the numbers of American and Russian warheads have remained low compared to previous decades, since 2000 arms control between the United States and Russia has been on a bumpy ride downhill. When the United States withdrew from the ABM Treaty in 2002, Russia withdrew from START II, which had never come into effect. Instead, Russia

[103] Adler E. The Emergence of Cooperation: National Epistemic Communities and the International Evolution of the Idea of Nuclear Arms Control. International Organization [Internet]. 1992;46(1):101–45. Available from: https://www.jstor.org/stable/2706953, accessed June 17, 2023.

and the United States then negotiated the Strategic Offensive Reductions Treaty (SORT), which was superseded by New START in 2011. The Intermediate-Range Nuclear Forces (INF) Treaty collapsed when the U.S., asserting Russia was cheating on its provisions, withdrew in 2019. Citing NATO wartime support for Ukraine, Russia suspended its participation in New START in February 2023 but has not withdrawn from the treaty and says it will abide by its numerical limits on deployed strategic warheads. Notifications and inspections required by the treaty have however been suspended on both sides. New START expires in February 2026, but talks on a replacement have been suspended since the Russian invasion of Ukraine in February 2022. The United States has also signaled willingness to adhere to the New START numerical limits as well as to return to a dialogue on strategic nuclear arms control.[104]

Restarting negotiations on nuclear weapons is now more a political question than an epistemic one. The advantages of strategic arms control are well known. It provides a more stable and predictable environment than a nuclear arms race. But so too are the challenges. Rebecca Lissner has elucidated both.[105] As she sees it, strategic arms control is now a triangular affair involving China as well as Russia and the United States. Russia can still claim nominal strategic nuclear parity with the U.S., but it is a much-reduced conventional military, economic, and ideological challenger compared to the Soviet Union. Moscow nevertheless is trying to regain superpower status and will be loath to sacrifice strategic capabilities in the future, no matter the outcome of the Ukraine war. The Chinese military challenge has been less nuclear than conventional, but Beijing is rapidly expanding its strategic nuclear force from its relatively low base. By 2035 Beijing could equal the American and Russian strategic nuclear forces if it continues to arm itself at the current pace. In addition, new technologies like cyber-dependent command and control, AI, anti-satellite weapons, and hypersonic glide missiles present both benefits and risks. Polarized domestic politics in the United States make formal

[104] Madhani A. White House Wants to Engage Russia on Nuclear Arms Control in Post-Treaty World [Internet]. PBS NewsHour. 2023. Available from: https://www.pbs.org/newshour/politics/white-house-wants-to-engage-russia-on-nuclear-arms-control-in-post-treaty-world, accessed June 18, 2023.

[105] Lissner R. The Future of Strategic Arms Control [Internet]. Council on Foreign Relations. 2021 Apr. Available from: https://www.cfr.org/report/future-strategic-arms-control, accessed June 17, 2023.

approval of any new arms control treaties difficult, undermining American credibility in future negotiations. The most recent U.S. Nuclear Posture Review was a disappointment to those favoring arms control and risk reduction, even if it does not suggest increases in the U.S. nuclear arsenal.[106] Neither Moscow nor Beijing seems readier than Washington to pursue nuclear arms control under current tense circumstances.

The high point of recent nuclear arms control was a 2022 joint statement in which the five nuclear weapons states recognized under the Non-Proliferation Treaty (aka the Perm 5 in the UN Security Council) affirmed "that a nuclear war cannot be won and must never be fought" (reiterating a Reagan-Gorbachev dictum) and that nuclear weapons "should serve defensive purposes, deter aggression, and prevent war."[107] Moving beyond such worthy generalities to detailed treaty obligations appears unlikely under the current highly charged geopolitical circumstances. There are however less formal measures that could be considered. Lissner suggests a piecemeal approach could include trilateral (U.S.-Russia-China), bilateral (U.S.-Russia, U.S.-China), multilateral (P5), and unilateral steps. The objective would be to enhance strategic stability by preventing crises and discouraging a nuclear arms race. It is hard to picture how such steps could be successful without epistemic input, but there are few signs at present of anything like a transnational epistemic community that includes Americans, Russians, and Chinese working for nuclear arms control. Nor is there a popular outcry for nuclear arms control or a strong domestic lobby in its favor. Arms control is suffering a moment of political and epistemic neglect. We may well be headed for an extended period of uncertainty, rearmament, and heightened risks.

[106] Kristensen H, Korda M. The 2022 Nuclear Posture Review: Arms Control Subdued by Military Rivalry [Internet]. Federation of American Scientists. 2022 Oct 27. Available from: https://fas.org/publication/2022-nuclear-posture-review/, accessed June 18, 2023; and Kimball DG. Biden's Disappointing Nuclear Posture Review | Arms Control Association [Internet]. 2022 Dec. www.armscontrol.org. Available from: https://www.armscontrol.org/act/2022-12/focus/bidens-disappointing-nuclear-posture-review, accessed June 18, 2023.

[107] Joint Statement of the Leaders of the Five Nuclear-Weapon States on Preventing Nuclear War and Avoiding Arms Races [Internet]. The White House. 2022 Jan 3. Available from: https://www.whitehouse.gov/briefing-room/statements-releases/2022/01/03/p5-statement-on-preventing-nuclear-war-and-avoiding-arms-races/, accessed June 18, 2023.

One aspect of arms control that might still benefit from a transnational epistemic community involving Americans, Russians, Chinese, and Europeans is nuclear nonproliferation. Their countries' joint efforts in negotiating the 2015 Iran nuclear deal were a triumph, even if largely vitiated by the American withdrawal in 2018.[108] An epistemic group of their experts could still play a critical role in signaling risks associated with supply of nuclear technology to potential proliferators while also enabling importers to benefit from nuclear energy and radioisotope production. Such a group would aim to give the existing Nuclear Suppliers Group and the International Atomic Energy Agency early warning of any problematic transfers insufficiently regulated by existing agreements. It would keep track of known factors that influence nuclear decisions and the indicators that can signal potential proliferation in the hope of constructing a "firewall" against it.[109]

Other Issues

It would not be difficult to continue enumerating contemporary technological issues amenable to epistemic group treatment. For example, neurotechnologies, which entail risks as well as benefits, seem ripe for norms, rooted in human rights law.[110] But neurotechnologies have not as yet benefitted from the careful analysis of risks and benefits that an epistemic group might provide. Failure to do that analysis and establish widely accepted norms for cryptocurrencies and for 5G communications has wrought international confusion, unscrupulous competition, and colossal financial losses.

[108] The Joint Comprehensive Plan of Action [Internet]. Vienna. 2015. Available from: https://www.documentcloud.org/documents/2165399-full-text-of-the-iran-nuclear-deal, accessed December 13, 2023.

[109] Dalton T et al. Toward a Nuclear Firewall: Bridging the NPT's Three Pillars. Carnegie Endowment for International Peace. 2017. https://carnegieendowment.org/files/CP_301_Dalton_et_al_Firewall_Final_Web.pdf, accessed December 13, 2023; and Kamil A, Noor Z, Serwer D. Assessing Proliferation Risks in the Middle East. Survival. 2023 Mar 4;65(2):141–64. https://doi.org/10.1080/00396338.2023.2193105, accessed December 13, 2023.

[110] Bublitz JC. What an International Declaration on Neurotechnologies and Human Rights Could Look like: Ideas, Suggestions, Desiderata. AJOB Neuroscience. 2023 Nov 3;1–17. https://doi.org/10.1080/21507740.2023.2270512, accessed November 10, 2023.

Dealing with Knowledge-Rich Non-Technological Issues

It is clear that epistemic groups can sometimes add substantial value to normative enterprises dealing with risk/benefit issues that have high scientific and technological content. Norms also emerge on issues that have low scientific and technological quotients. Some have been shown to emerge from "world society," that is the community of individuals, as opposed to "international society," the community of states.[111] These norms convey, or deny, legitimacy in a particular set of historical circumstances. Epistemic communities are distinguishable from the broader category of world society, as they are constituted by professionals with policy-relevant expertise in a particular area. They are arguably a subset of world society and, as we have seen, can have strong impacts on the norms chosen by states (i.e., international society) in areas that require technical know-how, especially where the inherently uncertain balancing of risks and benefits is required. But can they do so also in areas of state behavior less insulated by the requirement for scientific and technological expertise? Mai'a K. Davis Cross argues that they can and do.[112] She suggests military officers and diplomats in Europe, and religious leaders in particular national contexts.

Interstate war is one such possible state behavior. After more than two decades of fits and starts, the United Nations reached agreement on a definition of aggression in the General Assembly in 1974.[113] The UN Security Council has apparently not used the definition. Both the International Court of Justice and the International Criminal Court have.[114]

[111] Clark I. International Legitimacy and World Society. Oxford Academic; online edn: Oxford University Press; 2007 May 1. https://doi.org/10.1093/acprof:oso/9780199297009.001.0001, accessed June 19, 2023.

[112] Cross MKD. Rethinking Epistemic Communities Twenty Years Later. Review of International Studies. 2012 Apr 11;39(1):137–60. https://doi.org/10.1017/S0260210512000034.

[113] UNGA 3314 (XXIX). Definition of Aggression [Internet]. 1974 Dec 14. https://documents-dds-ny.un.org/. Available from: https://documents-dds-ny.un.org/doc/RESOLUTION/GEN/NR0/739/16/PDF/NR073916.pdf?OpenElement. accessed June 26, 2023.

[114] See also Wilmshurst E. Definition of Aggression General Assembly Resolution 3314 (XXIX) [Internet]. 1974. https://legal.un.org/. Available from: https://legal.un.org/avl/ha/da/da.html, accessed June 26, 2023.

Their focus on determining whether a particular act constitutes aggression has, however, been sporadic and necessarily post-facto. "Aggression" when it occurs has been left to the eye of the beholder. Saddam Hussein regarded Kuwait as the 19th province of Iraq and therefore his for the taking. George H.W. Bush regarded that act as aggression and swore to reverse it. Serbia regarded the 1999 NATO war against it as aggression, but Bill Clinton saw it as justified humanitarian intervention to protect civilians in Kosovo. George W. Bush defined the invasions of Afghanistan in 2001 and Iraq in 2003 as self-defense in the wake of 9/11, but the Taliban and Saddam Hussein saw those invasions as aggression.

The question of what constitutes aggression has been complicated by the 2005 General Assembly World Summit Outcome Document on the Responsibility to Protect (R2P).[115] This obligates states to protect their own populations "from genocide, war crimes, ethnic cleansing and crimes against humanity," including incitement thereof It also declares states prepared:

> to take collective action, in a timely and decisive manner, through the Security Council, in accordance with the Charter, including Chapter VII, on a case-by-case basis and in cooperation with relevant regional organizations as appropriate, should peaceful means be inadequate and national authorities manifestly fail to protect their populations from genocide, war crimes, ethnic cleansing and crimes against humanity.

R2P has been invoked more than 80 times by the Security Council, more than 50 times by the UN Human Rights Council, and in 13 General Assembly resolutions. While not mentioned in the UNSC resolution authorizing intervention against Muammar Qaddafi in Libya in 2011, it had been mentioned in the preamble to a prior resolution and is often regarded as having justified that intervention.[116]

[115] What Is R2P? [Internet]. Global Centre for the Responsibility to Protect. Available from: https://www.globalr2p.org/what-is-r2p/#:~:text=R2P%20has%20been%20invoked%20in,of%20genocide%2C%20prevention%20of%20armed, accessed June 26, 2023.

[116] Resolution 1973 (2011) Adopted by the Security Council at its 6498th meeting, on 17 March 2011, S/RES/1973 (2011). https://documents-dds-ny.un.org/doc/UNDOC/GEN/N11/268/39/PDF/N1126839.pdf?OpenElement, accessed June 26, 2023. The prior resolution is Resolution 1970 (2011) Adopted by the Security Council at its 6491st meeting, on 26 February 2011, S/RES/

The R2P doctrine has good epistemic credentials, with deep roots in an academic book on conflict in Africa.[117] The theme was amplified in 2001 in the report of a Canada-convened Commission on Intervention and State Sovereignty.[118] The UN Secretary General issues annual reports on R2P that catalog failures to protect civilian populations as well as remedies. There are also nongovernmental organizations that advocate for and against R2P, or against a particular alleged aggression by one state against another, but there is no continuing, professional epistemic community trying to establish the norms that should govern whether any particular act constitutes aggression or not. The Courts and the UN pay only sporadic attention. In principle, the International Court of Justice or the International Criminal Court might eventually decide whether a particular act constitutes aggression in a specific case, but it will be years if not decades after the fact.

It is plain enough that R2P cannot be used to justify armed intervention without UN Security Council approval, but it is more often than not blocked from blowing the whistle because its permanent five members hold vetoes. The recent egregious case of the Russian invasion of Ukraine is a case in point. The West says the February 2022 invasion was aggression. Vladimir Putin claims it was humanitarian intervention akin to NATO's intervention in Kosovo, likewise not authorized by the UNSC. What is needed is an authoritative, professional, knowledge-based group that will monitor such claims and call them out when they are invalid. An epistemic group of global experts focused on interstate war could be a useful restraining influence on the temptation to invade neighbors, as well as provide grounds for post-war legal actions.

This is but one example, but modern life is data- and knowledge-rich so there will be others. Currency manipulation is a notoriously difficult phenomenon to demonstrate that entails both benefits (to the country

1970 (2011). https://documents-dds-ny.un.org/doc/UNDOC/GEN/N11/245/58/PDF/N1124558.pdf?OpenElement, accessed June 26, 2023.

[117] Deng FM, Kimaro S, Lyons T, Rothchild ID, Zartman W. Sovereignty as Responsibility: Conflict Management in Africa. Washington D.C: The Brookings Institution: Conflict Management in Africa; 1996.

[118] The Responsibility to Protect: 10th Anniversary of the Report of the International Commission on Intervention and State Sovereignty, 2001 [Internet]. Global Centre for the Responsibility to Protect. 2001. Available from: https://www.globalr2p.org/resources/the-responsibility-to-protect-report-of-the-international-commission-on-intervention-and-state-sovereignty-2001/, accessed June 26, 2023.

doing it) and risks (to others). Intergovernmental agreement, bilaterally or through an organization such as the International Monetary Fund, on currency manipulation is difficult to achieve. Might an epistemic group of economists, central and private bankers, government officials, labor unions, and multinational companies enlighten us on when it is occurring and when it is not? The World Trade Organization considers complaints against national authorities who levy tariffs on subsidized products, but would it not be quicker and better to have available an epistemic group ready to act more quickly than the years of deliberation required at the WTO? The rules-based world order is today too dependent on post-facto, adversarial, and necessarily delayed administrative and legal proceedings to act expeditiously and satisfy legitimate requirements for quick, preventive action. Epistemic communities, like the one that eventually emerged for ionizing radiation, could fill at least part of the gap.

The point can be stretched further, at risk of breaking it. There exist today quantitative indices that purport to define and measure democracy, rule of law, governance, peace, and other parameters that provide benefits but are all too often at risk from state fragility, insurrection, terrorism, organized crime, and economic failure. The nongovernmental groups publishing these indices set performance norms in order to produce quantitative estimates of the parameters they purport to measure. They could go further and constitute epistemic groups of global experts to recommend ways of countering these risks. That would extend an analytical exercise into the normative realm. Such epistemic groups could also engage directly with those wanting to improve their performance to help them design means of doing so.

Conclusions

Where epistemic communities emerge to analyze the risks of beneficial technologies–in radiation protection, ozone-depleting chemicals, and climate change, twentieth-century strategic arms control–we have documented some success in setting international performance norms. Where they have failed to emerge–for toxic chemicals, air pollution, and recent strategic arms control–international norms have either not emerged or have been ineffective. The jury is still out for nonionizing radiation, pharmaceuticals, medical devices, nuclear nonproliferation, and pandemic response, artificial intelligence, and genome editing. It is possible that either existing epistemic groups or emerging ones will set international norms that balance the risks and benefits of these technologies in ways that will prevent the former and still enable realization of the latter.

Even then, success will depend on convincing decisionmakers, which is of course not guaranteed and likely much harder today than it was in the 1920s and 1930s when the international radiation protection regime originated.[119] Multiplication of priorities does not favor concentrating the resources needed for a committed, independent, dominant, and effective epistemic group. Nor does the prevalence of public or commercial forces that impinge on policymakers in directions opposed to the certification of an expert group and its recommendations. Policymaker "learning" can be shifted away from an epistemic mode, sometimes using an epistemic group's own expertise.[120] If the radiation protection norms are a useful guide, effectiveness will also depend on specialist pressure within an epistemic group and the risk of encroachment by competitive institutions.

When it comes to knowledge-rich but non-technological issues like aggression, currency manipulation, and trade subsidies, international and world society have generally engaged through adversarial processes that are slow, uncertain, ill-adapted to balancing risks and benefits, and often backward looking. Use of epistemic groups in these areas to set forward-looking performance norms would be challenging but potentially rewarding. It might also encourage healthy state restraint in engaging in activities that create risks for other countries even if they deliver benefits for their own. Epistemic groups of global experts might also help to improve state performance with regard to parameters like democracy, rule of law, governance, and peace. Strengthening international regimes is vital to bringing order to our conflictual world.

[119] See, for examples of failure: Löblová O. When Epistemic Communities Fail: Exploring the Mechanism of Policy Influence. Policy Studies Journal. 2017 Aug 26;46(1):160–89. https://doi.org/10.1111/psj.12213.

[120] Dunlop CA. The Irony of Epistemic Learning: Epistemic Communities, Policy Learning and the Case of Europe's Hormones Saga. Policy and Society. 2017 Apr 3;36(2):215–32. https://doi.org/10.1080/14494035.2017.1322260, accessed December 12, 2023.

Index

D. Serwer, *Strengthening International Regimes*, Palgrave Studies in International Relations,
https://doi.org/10.1007/978-3-031-53724-0

C

Z

GPSR Compliance

The European Union's (EU) General Product Safety Regulation (GPSR) is a set of rules that requires consumer products to be safe and our obligations to ensure this.

If you have any concerns about our products, you can contact us on ProductSafety@springernature.com

In case Publisher is established outside the EU, the EU authorized representative is:

Springer Nature Customer Service Center GmbH
Europaplatz 3
69115 Heidelberg, Germany

FSC
www.fsc.org
MIX
Papier | Fördert gute Waldnutzung
FSC® C083411

Kolibri 360 GmbH
Ferdinand-Jühlke-Straße 7
99095 Erfurt, Deutschland
produktsicherheit@kolibri360.de